Veteran Psychiatry in the US

Elspeth Cameron Ritchie • Maria D. Llorente
Editors

Veteran Psychiatry in the US

Optimizing Clinical Outcomes

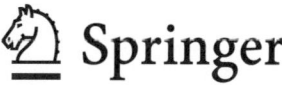

Editors
Elspeth Cameron Ritchie
Mental Health Community
Based Outpatient
Georgetown University
Mental Health Community
Based Outpatient
Silver Spring, MD
USA

Maria D. Llorente
Georgetown University School of Medicine
Washington DC VA Medical Center
Department of Psychiatry
Washington, DC
USA

ISBN 978-3-030-05383-3   ISBN 978-3-030-05384-0   (eBook)
https://doi.org/10.1007/978-3-030-05384-0

Library of Congress Control Number: 2019934812

© Springer Nature Switzerland AG 2019
This work is subject to copyright. All rights are reserved by the Publisher, whether the whole or part of the material is concerned, specifically the rights of translation, reprinting, reuse of illustrations, recitation, broadcasting, reproduction on microfilms or in any other physical way, and transmission or information storage and retrieval, electronic adaptation, computer software, or by similar or dissimilar methodology now known or hereafter developed.
The use of general descriptive names, registered names, trademarks, service marks, etc. in this publication does not imply, even in the absence of a specific statement, that such names are exempt from the relevant protective laws and regulations and therefore free for general use.
The publisher, the authors, and the editors are safe to assume that the advice and information in this book are believed to be true and accurate at the date of publication. Neither the publisher nor the authors or the editors give a warranty, express or implied, with respect to the material contained herein or for any errors or omissions that may have been made. The publisher remains neutral with regard to jurisdictional claims in published maps and institutional affiliations.

This Springer imprint is published by the registered company Springer Nature Switzerland AG
The registered company address is: Gewerbestrasse 11, 6330 Cham, Switzerland

This volume is dedicated to US service members, veterans, and their families with acknowledgment to many new contributions to science and practice in the areas of PTSD, TBI, and other psychological responses to the stress of deployment and combat. Knowledge gained through clinical trials in diverse areas, including schizophrenia, bipolar disorder, depression, sexual trauma, substance abuse, and population health, is shared here in hopes of enriching the awareness and education of present and future generations of medical students, residents, psychiatrists, primary care physicians, psychologists, and other clinical disciplines.

Preface

Introduction

War and politics are always intertwined, and both impact the health care of the active duty service member. The health of veterans may be still more sensitive to this interconnection because politicians often rally to their cause in order to further their own careers.

The current President fires up his base by stressing veterans' health issues, although it is unclear whether his efforts are helpful or harmful. His VA Secretaries and Senior Executives seem to come and go as if through a revolving door.

At the time of the writing of this preface, a former Navy aviator, prisoner of war, and Senator, John McCain, has just been laid to rest in the cemetery at the Naval Academy. Most agree that this veteran epitomized the principles of service to country and leadership in government, but it's difficult for one person, even a remarkable one, to prevail when national perspectives and aims are so much in conflict.

Unquestionably, military service and the health of those who serve are a top priority of the nations' leaders whether in war or peace. This volume seeks to go beyond the politics to lay out what is known and not known about the best way to care for veterans facing the psychological challenges of war.

Background

There is a rich literature on the psychological issues affecting the active duty military. The Textbooks of Military Medicine from the Borden Institute summarize lessons learned from numerous aspects of combat surgery, medicine, and psychiatry. For psychiatry, there are two volumes which focus on lessons from the first two World Wars and from the military psychiatry in peacetime [1, 2]. Two more recent psychiatric texts concentrate on lessons learned from the Vietnam War, the Gulf War, and the wars on Afghanistan and Iraq [3, 4].

On the veteran side, the Vietnam War spawned a rich literature focusing on PTSD. Military sexual trauma has also been an area of considerable research and publication.

More recently, the Long War, i.e., the wars in Iraq and Afghanistan since 9/11, has led to numerous publications on behavioral health issues in active duty service members. Groundbreaking research on behavioral health issues in the recent theaters of war has mounted rapidly [5–8]. Much of it has been published in high-profile civilian journals, such as the NEJM and JAMA, rather than the traditional venues of military medicine.

On the other hand, and surprisingly, despite all the research published on psychiatric health and illness in veterans, this will be the first volume that presents a comprehensive array of topics on psychiatric issues for veterans between one set of book covers.

Discussion of the Volume

There is often confusion about what is a veteran, compared to the active duty military. Further, it is safe to assume that many readers will not even be sure what terms such as "veterans" and "combat veterans" really mean. These are further defined herein. Some chapters focus only on veterans, while others include service members and the transitions between military and civilian life.

Another question is "what is the VA?" Many think the Military Health System (MHS) and the Veterans Health Administration (VHA) system are the same, but they are actually distinct health-care systems. In turn, the VHA is part of the broader Veterans Administration (VA). So this volume opens with some definitions and context about these health-care systems [9].

The importance of the VHA is highlighted in the chapter by Dr. Kudler, who worked in it for almost 40 years and ended his career leading the mental health system. Another chapter by Dr. Cheryl Lowman outlines some of the best practices present in the VA.

Veterans generally accumulate trauma during their military and/or wartime service, which may lead to diagnoses of PTSD, military sexual trauma (MST), or traumatic brain injury (TBI). Much has been published in the psychiatric and psychological literature on these topics, as mentioned above. There are clearly defined clinical practice guidelines and evidence-based practices for each. However, while important, these topics alone do not define the broad range of combat and deployment stress and the veteran experiences.

Of relevance, the veterans usually enter the military in their late teens or early 20s. Their past lives include, in some cases, histories of depression, bipolar illness, psychotic illnesses, substance use, and physical and/or sexual trauma. Potential recruits may or may not disclose these conditions. Although there are some screening protocols in place, there is no easy way to detect this prior history. Thus treatment of veterans must include common psychiatric illnesses that occur in the civilian world as well.

Professionals and the public at large are increasingly aware of the significance of past history of head trauma and its possible consequences for military members at war. PTSD and TBI often co-occur as a result of combat, as a result to exposure to bombs and other weapons. Of course other injuries do as well, leading to short- or long-term pain and disability.

Suicide and opioid safety are critically important issues for civilians and the military alike. Both may reflect a combination of issues stemming from premilitary experience, service in war, and readjustment to civilian life. The chapters in this volume cover these topics in more detail.

Other veteran topics have received less attention in civilian clinical journals. These include psychosis, bipolar illness, depression, and homelessness among recent veterans. This volume contains chapters on these issues. It also expands the literature on smaller subsets of veterans including female, gay, lesbian, and transgendered veterans.

Conclusion

Wars, even this long one, are relatively brief, compared with the long tail of their impact on the health of combat veterans. We anticipate that the psychological sequelae of the wars since 9/11 will last for decades.

This volume seeks to deepen the understanding of the health-care systems designed for service members and veterans as well as the specific psychiatric disorders and problem behaviors which they are prone to.

It builds upon the work of numerous distinguished psychiatrists whose work has focused on American military and VA health systems. They include Thomas Salmon, Albert Glass, Kenneth Artiss, Frank Jones, Harry Holloway, Norman (Mike) Camp, Paul Errera, Art Blank, Robert Ursano, Charles Engel, and Charles Hoge. Many of these authors have been instrumental in the publications mentioned above. The authors in this current volume have also either been major contributors or hopefully will be in their future professional careers.

Finally, this volume also seeks to honor the blood, sweat, and sacrifice of America's sons and daughters: our nation's military and veterans.

Silver Spring, MD, USA	Elspeth Cameron Ritchie
Washington, DC, USA	Maria D. Llorente

References

1. Jones FD, Sparacino LR, Wilcox VL, Rothberg JM, Stokes JW, editors. War psychiatry, textbook of military medicine, Borden Pavilion. Washington, DC: Office of The Surgeon General, US Department of the Army and Borden Institute; 1995.
2. Jones FD, Sparacino LR, Wilcox VL, Rothberg JM, editors. Military psychiatry preparing in peace for war, textbook of military medicine, Borden Pavilion. Washington, DC: Office of The Surgeon General, US Department of the Army and Borden Institute; 1993.
3. Ritchie EC. Senior Editor, Combat and operational behavioral health, textbook of military medicine, Borden Pavilion. Washington, DC: Office of The Surgeon General, US Department of the Army and Borden Institute; 2011.
4. Ritchie EC, Senior Editor. Forensic and ethical issues in military behavioral health. Textbook of military medicine, Borden Pavilion. Washington, DC: Office of The Surgeon General, US Department of the Army and Borden Institute; 2014.
5. Hoge CW, Castro CA, Messer SC, McGurk D, Cotting DI, Koffman RL. Combat Duty in Iraq and Afghanistan, mental health problems, and barriers to care, N Engl J Med 2004;351:13–22.
6. Ursano RJ, Kessler KC, Naifeh JA, et al. Associations of time-related deployment variables with risk of suicide attempt among soldiers: results from the Army Study to Assess Risk and Resilience in Servicemembers (Army STARRS). JAMA Psychiatry 2018;75(6):596–604.
7. Nock MK, Stein MB, Heerings SG et al. Prevalence and correlates of suicidal behavior among soldiers: results from the Army Study to Assess Risk and Resilience in Service members (Army STARRS). JAMA Psychiatry. 2014;71(5):514–22.
8. Galloway MS, Millikan A, Bell M, Ritchie EC. Epidemiological consultation teams. In: Ritchie EC, editor. Forensic and ethical issues in military behavioral health. Textbook of military medicine, Borden Institute; 2014.
9. Ritchie EC. The DoD and VA health care system overview. In: Cozza S, Goldenberg M, editors. Clinical manual for the care of military service members, veterans and their families, APPI; 2014.

Contents

Part I Overview of the VA and Military

1. **Introduction**... 3
   Elspeth Cameron Ritchie, Harold Stephen Kudler,
   and Robert L. Koffman

2. **Outline of Military Culture and Military and VA Health Systems** ... 9
   Elspeth Cameron Ritchie

3. **Psychiatry in the United States Department of Veterans Affairs:
   A History and a Future**.. 17
   Harold Stephen Kudler

4. **Optimizing Clinical Outcomes in VA Mental Health Care**........... 29
   Cheryl A. Lowman

Part II Clinical Issues—General

5. **Military and Veteran Suicide Prevention**........................ 51
   David A. Jobes, Leslie A. Haddock, and Michael R. Olivares

6. **Treatment for Trauma-Related Disorders:
   The "Three Buckets" Model**..................................... 73
   Elspeth Cameron Ritchie, Rachel M. Sullivan, and Kyle J. Gray

7. **Treatment-Resistant Depression Among US Military Veterans**...... 93
   R. Gregory Lande

8. **Psychotic Disorders and Best Models of Care**................... 113
   Philip M. Yam, Dinesh Mittal, and Ayman H. Fanous

9. **Alcohol and Alcohol Use Disorder**.............................. 135
   Thomas W. Meeks, Nicole M. Bekman, Nicole M. Lanouette,
   Kathryn A. Yung, and Ryan P. Vienna

10. **Alcohol Pharmacotherapy**...................................... 157
    Jasmine Carpenter and Shannon Tulk

11	**Opiate Use in the Military Context** .... 169 Mike Colston	
12	**Use of Stimulants for ADHD and TBI in Veterans**................ 177 Donna L. Ticknor and Antoinette M. Valenti	
13	**Use of Complementary and Integrative Health for Chronic Pain Management** .... 191 Marina A. Khusid, Elissa L. Stern, and Kathleen Reed	
14	**Traumatic Brain Injury** .... 211 Blessen C. Eapen and Bruno Subbarao	
15	**Homeless Veterans and Mental Health** .... 233 Kaitlin Slaven and Maria D. Llorente	
16	**Contextual Frameworks for Addressing Risk and Fostering Resilience Among Sexual and Gender Minority Veterans** .... 241 Rebecca Gitlin and Michael R. Kauth	
17	**Older Veterans**... 265 John T. Little, Bryan A. Llorente, and Maria D. Llorente	
18	**Women Veterans** .... 281 Kasey M. Llorente, Keelan K. O'Connell, Margaret Valverde, and Elspeth Cameron Ritchie	
19	**Military Environmental Exposures and Mental Health** .... 299 Matthew J. Reinhard, Michelle Kennedy Prisco, Nicholas G. Lezama, and Elspeth Cameron Ritchie	
20	**Neuropsychiatric Quinism: Chronic Encephalopathy Caused by Poisoning by Mefloquine and Related Quinoline Drugs** .... 315 Remington L. Nevin	
21	**Listening to Trauma, and Caring for the Caregiver: A Psychodynamic Reflection in the Age of Burnout** .... 333 Joseph E. Wise	

Index..343

Contributors

Nicole M. Bekman, PhD Naval Medical Center San Diego, Substance Abuse Rehabilitation Program, San Diego, CA, USA

Jasmine Carpenter, PharmD, BCPS, BCPP Veterans Affairs Medical Center, Washington DC, Pharmacy Service/Mental Health Service, Washington, DC, USA

Mike Colston, MD Fort Belvoir Community Hospital, Mental Health Department, Fort Belvoir, VA, USA

Blessen C. Eapen, MD Chief, Physical Medicine and Rehabilitation, VA Greater Los Angeles Health Care System, Associate Professor, David Geffen School of Medicine at UCLA, Los Angeles, CA, USA

Ayman H. Fanous, MD SUNY Downstate Medical Center, Psychiatry and Behavioral Sciences, Brooklyn, NY, USA

Rebecca Gitlin, PhD Los Angeles County Department of Mental Health, Los Angeles, CA, USA

Kyle J. Gray, MD, MA Walter Reed National Military Medical Center, Behavioral Health, Bethesda, MD, USA

Leslie A. Haddock, BS Department of Psychology, The Catholic University of America, Washington, DC, USA

David A. Jobes, PhD Department of Psychology, The Catholic University of America, Washington, DC, USA

Michael R. Kauth, PhD VHA LGBT Health Program, Washington, DC, USA

VA South Central Mental Illness Research, Education, and Clinical Center, Houston, TX, USA

Department of Psychiatry, Baylor College of Medicine, Michael E. DeBakey Veterans Affairs Medical Center, Houston, TX, USA

Marina A. Khusid, MD, ND, MSA Jesse Brown Veterans Affairs Medical Center, University of Illinois at Chicago, Department of Family Medicine, Chicago, IL, USA

Robert L. Koffman, MD, MPH Walter Reed National Military Medical Center, NICoE, Bethesda, MD, USA

Harold Stephen Kudler, MD United States Department of Veterans Affairs Medical Center, Durham, NC, USA

Duke University School of Medicine, Psychiatry and Behavioral Sciences, Durham, NC, USA

R. Gregory Lande, DO Psychiatry Continuity Service, Walter Reed National Military Medical Center, Behavioral Health, Bethesda, MD, USA

Nicole M. Lanouette, MD Uniformed Services University of the Health Sciences, Naval Medical Center San Diego, Substance Abuse Rehabilitation Program, Point Loma, San Diego, CA, USA

Nicholas G. Lezama, MD, MPH War Related Illness and Injury Study Center, Washington DC Veterans Affairs Medical Center, Washington, DC, USA

John T. Little, MD Departments of Psychiatry and Neurology, Georgetown University School of Medicine, Washington, DC, USA

Geriatric Mental Health Services, Department of Veterans Affairs Medical Center, Department of Psychiatry, Washington, DC, USA

Bryan A. Llorente, BA Social Work College of Health Professions and Sciences, University of Central Florida, Orlando, FL, USA

Kasey M. Llorente, BS Creighton University, Omaha, NE, USA

Maria D. Llorente, MD Georgetown University School of Medicine, Washington DC VA Medical Center, Department of Psychiatry, Washington, DC, USA

Cheryl A. Lowman, PhD VA Capitol Health Care Network, VISN 5, Linthicum, MD, USA

Thomas W. Meeks, MD University of California, Davis, Davis, CA, USA

Sacramento VA Medical Center, Department of Psychiatry, Mather, CA, USA

Dinesh Mittal, MD G. V. (Sonny) Montgomery VA Medical Center, Department of Mental Health, Jackson, MS, USA

Remington L. Nevin, MD, MPH, DrPH The Quinism Foundation, White River Junction, VT, USA

Keelan K. O'Connell, MD, BS, LT, MC, USN Walter Reed National Military Medical Center, Department of Behavioral Health, Bethesda, MD, USA

Michael R. Olivares, BA Department of Psychology, The Catholic University of America, Washington, DC, USA

Michelle Kennedy Prisco, MSN War Related Illness and Injury Study Center, Washington DC Veterans Affairs Medical Center, Washington, DC, USA

Kathleen Reed, MS in Nursing Jesse Brown Veterans Affairs Medical Center, Women Veteran Health Center, Chicago, IL, USA

Matthew J. Reinhard, PsyD War Related Illness and Injury Study Center, Washington DC Veterans Affairs Medical Center, Washington, DC, USA

Department of Psychiatry, Georgetown University Medical School, Washington DC Veterans Affairs Medical Center, Washington, DC, USA

Uniformed Services University of the Health Sciences, Silver Spring, MD, USA

Elspeth Cameron Ritchie, MD, MPH Department of Psychiatry, Georgetown University Medical School, Washington DC Veterans Affairs Medical Center, Washington, DC, USA

Department of Psychiatry, MedStar Washington Hospital Center, Washington, DC, USA

George Washington University School of Medicine, Washington, DC, USA

Uniformed Services University of the Health Sciences, Silver Spring, MD, USA

Mental Health Community Based Outpatient, Washington, DC, USA

Kaitlin Slaven, MD George Washington University, Department of Psychiatry, Washington, DC, USA

Elissa L. Stern, MD Jesse Brown Veterans Affairs Medical Center, Northwestern University Feinberg School of Medicine, Department of Medicine, Chicago, IL, USA

Bruno Subbarao, DO Medical Director, Polytrauma/Transition and Care Management Programs, Phoenix Veterans Healthcare System, Physical Medicine and Rehabilitation, Phoenix, AZ, USA

Rachel M. Sullivan, MD Psychiatry Residency Program, Tripler Army Medical Center, Behavioral Health, Honolulu, HI, USA

Donna L. Ticknor, MD Washington DC Veterans Affairs Medical Center, Department of Psychiatry, Camp Springs, MD, USA

Shannon Tulk, Pharm D, BCPS Minneapolis VA Health Care System, Pharmacy Service, Minneapolis, MN, USA

Antoinette M. Valenti, MD Washington DC VA Medical Center, Department of Mental Health, Washington, DC, USA

Margaret Valverde, MD George Washington University Hospital, Psychiatry and Behavioral Sciences, Washington, DC, USA

Ryan P. Vienna, MD Naval Medical Center San Diego, Substance Abuse Rehabilitation Program, San Diego, CA, USA

Joseph E. Wise, MD US Army, Walter Reed National Military Medical Center, Brooklyn, NY, USA

Private Practice, Brooklyn, NY, USA

Philip M. Yam, MD Naval Branch Health Clinic Belle Chasse, Department of Behavioral Health, Belle Chasse, LA, USA

Kathryn A. Yung, MD Uniformed Services University of the Health Sciences, Naval Medical Center San Diego, Substance Abuse Rehabilitation Program, Point Loma, San Diego, CA, USA

Part I

Overview of the VA and Military

Introduction

Elspeth Cameron Ritchie, Harold Stephen Kudler, and Robert L. Koffman

Background

Approximately 2.7 million people have served in the military since September 11, 2001. For these recent veterans, posttraumatic stress disorder (PTSD), traumatic brain injury (TBI), other mental and physical consequences of accidents, combat, other military-related occupational exposure, and re-integration into the civilian world are pressing issues. Veterans of past eras may face the same problems and others as well.

The veteran population has both specific needs and strengths. Their needs revolve around the sequelae of exposure to war. These needs will likely change as the veteran ages. For example, Vietnam veterans, most of whom are currently in their seventies, may continue to experience symptoms of PTSD or the re-emergence of these symptoms when they retire, suffer the death of a spouse, and/or develop serious medical or neurocognitive disorders. (Definitions of service members and veterans are covered in the next chapter.)

E. C. Ritchie
Department of Psychiatry, MedStar Washington Hospital Center, Washington, DC, USA

Georgetown University School of Medicine, Washington, DC, USA

George Washington University School of Medicine, Washington, DC, USA

Uniformed Services University of the Health Sciences, Silver Spring, MD, USA

Mental Health Community Based Outpatient, Washington, DC, USA

H. S. Kudler (✉)
United States Department of Veterans Affairs Medical Center,
Durham, NC, USA

Duke University School of Medicine, Psychiatry and Behavioral Sciences,
Durham, NC, USA
e-mail: hkudler@duke.edu

R. L. Koffman
Walter Reed National Military Medical Center, NICoE, Bethesda, MD, USA

© Springer Nature Switzerland AG 2019
E. C. Ritchie, M. D. Llorente (eds.), *Veteran Psychiatry in the US*,
https://doi.org/10.1007/978-3-030-05384-0_1

More recent veterans have benefited from strong support systems both in deployment and back home, but some still fall through the cracks and experience unemployment, homelessness, and/or substance use disorders.

The strengths of the veteran population include pride in having served the nation and access to educational benefits, mortgages, and other support from the Department of Veterans Affairs (VA) civilian providers. In particular, their veteran status gives them access to VA health care. However, at the time of this writing, only about a third of all American veterans are enrolled in VA care, and a significant portion of these are receiving that care from VA's network of civilian providers, many of whom lack an understanding of a veteran's specific needs, nor are they even familiar with the concepts of veteran and military "culture". Many are not even aware of the full range of resources available to their patients through VA.

This volume addresses the many specific clinical issues facing the veteran population, including PTSD, TBI, depression, and other related topics. The contributors are experts who treat veterans and will describe optimal care and treatment recommendations. To the best of our knowledge, there is no other volume which brings this crucial clinical information about veterans together. There are, however, recent books which cover many of these topics from the perspective of the active service member and/or active duty behavioral health providers; this volume should complement those [1–6]. Later chapters will have many more references depending on their topic.

Our review begins with systems issues. Military and veteran cultural competences are first covered. The next chapter takes a look at the history of the psychological needs of service members and veterans and covers the development of the Veterans Administration. The final chapter in this opening section covers the best practices within.

The next section focuses on clinical issues, such as depression, psychosis, pain, suicide prevention, addiction, and trauma-related disorders, focusing on military- and veteran-specific issues. Complementary and alternative medicine or integrated medicine is discussed in the chapter on pain management but is also interwoven in many other chapters.

These writings cover a large body of general medical knowledge which, at times, may also be generalizable to civilian populations. They attempt to strike a balance, both on clinical issues and research findings. The latter draws from the evidence base, which often comes from civilian subjects, versus studies that were conducted in military and veteran populations. However, the intent is to always focus on veteran-specific issues.

The latter chapters cover the environmental exposures faced by veterans although civilians may face them as well. For example, taking mefloquine is an exposure in the military, the State Department, the Peace Corps, and among all travelers to countries where malaria is endemic.

The last chapter focuses on the burden to providers. This may result in "clinician burnout." Strategies to minimize this consequence are outlined.

Themes

A number of themes permeate this volume. These are summarized below and will be more fully developed in the following chapters:

- The need to bridge the gap separating military and civilian worlds and ease the transition between
- The desire to share information about military and veterans' experience with the provider who has not served in the military
- The importance of looking at veterans through the lens of when and where they served and in which branch of the military
- The veterans experience of "moral injury"
- The shame and stigma of having a psychiatric diagnosis among military service members and the potential impact on future career options
- The importance of the Veterans Health Administration and what benefits it offers
- The critical need to prevent suicide among veterans
- The importance of evidence-based therapies informed by clinical judgment as well as newer strategies including complementary and alternative medicine or concepts of integrative health and wellness
- Comorbidities among the varied physical and mental effects of war, including pain, disability, and traumatic brain injury
- The tensions surrounding disability evaluations as well as assessments and determinations for compensation and pension
- Special populations such as women and LGBTQ members in the military and, subsequently, as veterans

This volume is not a comprehensive discussion of all issues related to veterans. But we hope that it highlights the most relevant ones and stimulates further exploration of others.

Moral Injury

A major theme in the lives of many veterans is the concept of "moral injury." This normally refers to a veteran's feelings of loss, shame, guilt, or betrayal.

The feelings of shame and guilt are often intertwined with the service member or veteran feeling that he/she could or should have done something differently to save another colleague from being killed or injured. In addition, it often harkens back to the killing of others, whether enemy combatants or civilians.

Moral injury may also develop from a feeling of having been betrayed by the command chain or by the government. Sometimes that is related to combat experiences. Often it is linked to the benefits system, either from the military or VA disability process.

Many veterans believe that they have symptoms related to toxic exposures and may feel betrayed when the government denies the connection. These themes are also developed in the chapters on toxic exposures.

Stigma vs Fitness for Duty

All agree that stigma about mental health disorders should be lessened. That is easier said than done.

Public service announcements rightly affirm that "seeking help is a sign of strength" but in the "go to war" military, service members are expected be able to perform their mission. If someone is hearing voices telling them that Afghani villagers are actually Taliban or manically believes him/herself to be in charge of the world, they should not be carrying weapons or driving tanks.

In the almost two decades since September 11, 2001, there have been tensions between wanting to medically treat and restore service members and the practical necessity of deploying service members to the war zone. This is not new; similar ethical dilemmas existed in most wars.

Thus, for the military psychiatrist or psychologist, there are competing missions: to treat the patient and preserve the fit and healthy fighting force. A thorough description of these issues is covered in other publications [7]. It is worth adding the "dual master" theme here, to highlight some of the challenges facing military mental health personnel in reducing barriers to treatment.

Conclusion

We hope that this volume covers the most salient issues for providers treating the military and veterans. We realize that we do not discuss everything nor has every issue facing veterans yet been recognized and defined. Some topics, such as military sexual trauma, domestic violence, and evidenced-based treatment, are covered in more detail in other publications [7]. We hope to focus on themes that more military and less spoken of.

This volume alludes to both military and veteran experiences. The focus here is on those who are no longer on active duty, with some references to those who still are serving in the Armed Forces.

Nevertheless, we believe that this book will aid the clinician in caring for the brave men and women—America's sons and daughters—in their successful re-integration home.

References

1. Ritchie EC, senior editor. Combat and operational behavioral health. Textbook of military medicine, Borden Pavilion. Washington, DC: Office of The Surgeon General, US Department of the Army and Borden Institute; 2011.
2. Ritchie EC, senior editor. Forensic and ethical issues in military behavioral health. Textbook of military medicine, Borden Pavilion. Washington, DC: Office of The Surgeon General, US Department of the Army and Borden Institute; 2014.
3. Ritchie EC, Naclerio A, editors. Women at war. Oxford/New York: Oxford University Press; 2015.
4. Ritchie EC, editor. Post-traumatic stress disorder and related diseases in combat veterans: a clinical casebook. Cham: Springer; 2015.
5. Ritchie EC, editor. Intimacy post injury: combat trauma and sexual health. Oxford/New York: Oxford University Press; 2016.
6. Ritchie EC, Warner C, Mclay R, editors. Psychiatrists in war: personal experiences of clinicians in the combat zone. Cham: Springer; 2017.
7. Ritchie EC, Wise J, Pyle B, editors. Gay mental healthcare providers and patients in the military: personal experiences and clinical care. Cham: Springer; 2017.

Outline of Military Culture and Military and VA Health Systems

2

Elspeth Cameron Ritchie

Introduction

This chapter covers basic issues of military and veteran competence for providers, including a simple understanding of military culture. It then describes the basics of administrative separations and disability evaluations, the military and veteran's affairs health-care systems, and transitions to care. The information presented is a succinct version; enclosed references and websites cover many issues in more detail [1].

Most mental health providers, both in the civilian world and in the Veterans Health Administration, have not served in the armed forces. While many want to treat service members and veterans, they may feel unprepared.

For example, civilian mental health clinicians may or may not understand the importance of the service member's or veteran's military identity. While some veterans have a strong identity as service members and veterans, others are less identified with their military service, and still others may define themselves in opposition to aspects of that experience.

Some veterans wear articles of clothing—typically billed baseball hats or small pins—that identify the conflict in which they served wherever they go. These often serve as important signals for those who can decipher them and as subtle tests for those who observe but fail to ask about them. One key aspect of military culture is a concern that civilians don't understand their experience and aren't interested in hearing about it.

E. C. Ritchie (✉)
Department of Psychiatry, MedStar Washington Hospital Center, Washington, DC, USA

Georgetown University School of Medicine, Washington, DC, USA

George Washington University School of Medicine, Washington, DC, USA

Uniformed Services University of the Health Sciences, Silver Spring, MD, USA

© Springer Nature Switzerland AG 2019
E. C. Ritchie, M. D. Llorente (eds.), *Veteran Psychiatry in the US*,
https://doi.org/10.1007/978-3-030-05384-0_2

What is it like to actually serve in the armed forces? The short answer is that it varies dramatically, depending on when and where they served.

For some, their service was a brief period serving overseas in peacetime, perhaps in Germany or Japan when they were young, and without physical or psychological scars. Many who served more recently have physical or psychological wounds from training accidents, military sexual assault or combat, or all of the above. So the range of veterans' experience is quite varied. So are the expectations they have about their health-care providers.

The chapter lays the groundwork with some basic definitions. It also contains a discussion of the different types of discharges and the military and VA health-care systems.

Definitions

A few basic definitions are helpful as a starting point. Here the terms "armed forces" and "military" are used interchangeably. This chapter focuses on the United States military. Another term used is the Department of Defense. The military is comprised of the army, navy, air force, and marines. The coast guard has a unique structure, outlined in footnote.[1]

By "service member," we mean those who are currently serving in the US military: The term "veteran" usually refers to those who have been on active military duty but are no longer serving. Many in the National Guard and reserves go back and forth between serving on active duty and returning to civilian (but now a veteran) status.

The term "combat veteran" may apply to either active duty or those no longer serving, who have served in a combat theater. Recently (since 9/11/2001), those combat theaters have principally been Iraq and Afghanistan.

Other missions include operations other than war (OOTW), such as Bosnia, Somalia, and Haiti. Military members also commonly respond to natural disasters across the world. Civilian providers are often unaware of the special challenges faced by service members in peacekeeping, humanitarian, and other "non-combat" missions. Risks to life and limb are often significant. They may also be associated with important health liabilities such as physical injuries, exposure to tropical diseases, and psychological trauma.

---

[1] The *United States Coast Guard (USCG)* is a branch of the United States Armed Forces and one of the country's seven uniformed services. The coast guard is a maritime, military, multi-mission service unique among the US military branches for having a maritime law enforcement mission (with jurisdiction in both domestic and international waters) and a federal regulatory agency mission as part of its mission set. It operates under the US Department of Homeland Security during peacetime and can be transferred to the US Department of the Navy by the US President at any time or by the US Congress during times of war. As one of the country's five armed services, the coast guard has been involved in every US war from 1790 to the Iraq War and the war in Afghanistan.

The Importance of Time Periods

The major combat theaters in the past century include World Wars I and II, Korea, Vietnam, the first Gulf War, and the recent conflicts in Iraq and Afghanistan (known as Operation Enduring Freedom and Operation Iraqi Freedom and by other names). There have been numerous other conflicts, to include those in Panama, Haiti, Bosnia, Kosovo, Somalia, and other theaters in Africa. These conflicts have been termed Operations rather than Wars.

Each one has a different age group, a different cultural context, and their own stressors. For convenience, these conflicts and/or wars are often called by their most commonly used name, often the country where the conflict has taken place.

For example, whether the veteran was drafted or enlisted voluntarily affects their views of their service. In World Wars I and II and the Korean War, many service members were drafted. This meant that service members came from all sectors of American society. After the Vietnam War in 1973, the draft ended. Thus, recent service members were voluntary enlistees and tend to be proud of their service.

In World Wars I and II, service members were deployed as part of larger units and often remained with their cohorts overseas for 3 or more years. They returned together, leading to enhanced cohesion in their units and easier re-integration. In the Korean War (1950–1953) and the Vietnam War, service members usually deployed as individuals for 1 year.

The Korean War has often been called the "Forgotten War," coming so soon after World War II. In many ways, it was a proxy war between the superpowers during the Cold War. The return home of American veterans from Korea was further tainted by fears about "brainwashing," especially among those taken as prisoner of war (POW) by the Chinese. Thus, many veterans slipped quietly back in US society, without highlighting their veteran status [2].

In the Vietnam War (1964–1972), many were drafted and many volunteered to escape being drafted. Initially, that war was not unpopular but the Tet Offensive in 1968 led both to major offensives by the North Vietnamese and rejection of the war back in the United States. Massive antiwar protests erupted. Many service members experienced the brunt of the public negative sentiment upon returning home from war. Civilians would spit on them and call returning service members names, such as "baby killers" [3].

The first Gulf War in 1991 was considered a swift victory, but those on the ground faced stressful conditions including potential exposure to scud missiles and chemical weapons and witnessing the aftermath of highly effective artillery and missile barrages, resulting in mass casualties and widespread destruction. Many service members developed "Gulf War" syndromes. (This is covered in more detail in a later chapter in this volume, but of note, there was and remains considerable controversy over the contribution of psychological stress to that diagnosis.)

After 9/11, there was a tremendously positive attitude towards military members. But the wars in Iraq and Afghanistan have dragged on, without clear victories. The

American public learned from its mistakes with the Vietnam veterans and continues to recognize the important contribution and sacrifices of today's military, whether or not they are in agreement with current conflicts. Politicians today strive to outdo themselves in appreciating veterans.

Military Competence for the Provider

One cannot overstate how important it is for providers treating veterans to understand the military service of their veterans. Basic competence includes understanding (1) which service were they in (army, navy, air force, marines, coast guard), (2) what their job was, (3) where and when they deployed, (4) what their final rank was, and (5) what type of discharge they received from the service.

Asking about military services is also a good way to open an interview. I recommend asking about where they were in basic and advanced training, where they were stationed (I ask for the "brief version"), and when and where they have been deployed.

Recognizing the importance of the rank at discharge is another important part of military competence, as well as establishing some parameters as to the baseline functioning of the patient. In general, but not always, higher-ranking service members have done better in their career, have more assets, and have a better prognosis for life after the military.

The different services traditionally also have their own cultures, both of the larger service and within it. The infantries, both in the marines and army, are the "ground pounders," accustomed to Spartan living, such as sleeping on the ground rather than in air-conditioned tents. The air force is the newest service and the most technically sophisticated. Since they have planes, they usually can bring more and heavier equipment and live in relative luxury (or at least are perceived that way.)

Within the navy, there are the aviation, intelligence, submarine, and ship cultures. Special forces, whatever their service, have an elite culture, with frequent deployments which they are often not able to discuss. Many more examples abound of service-specific cultures.

Administrative Discharges and Retirement

There are several ways that a military member may leave the services. The preferred way is with an honorable discharge, either a routine administrative separation or retirement. Administrative separations may be for a variety of reasons from a scheduled ETS (end of time in service), for pregnancy, for psychiatric reasons, and for misconduct. The administrative separations are classified as honorable, other than honorable (often called "OTH"), dishonorable, and for bad conduct. (For further details, see [4].)

In general, honorable discharges offer access to the Veterans Health Administration (VHA) health care and may offer other financial benefits. Other than honorable or dishonorable discharges usually do not offer any benefits. There have been some recent changes as noted below.

Retirement may be after 20 years of military service or for medical reasons. Retirement from the military usually offers both VA care and access to the military health-care system, known as TRICARE. Access to the military health-care system is prioritized, with active duty first and then dependents and retirees. There is also a priority list for the VA, with priority given to recent veterans, those with service-connected disabilities, and those below a certain income level. The determination is a complex subject, covered further in other sources [5].

Other service members may be discharged for a variety of less favorable conditions. For example, in the past, many service members were discharged for personality disorders. In the army, these were termed "5-13s" for the applicable regulations (add ref). Although these are technically honorable discharges, they usually did not bring VA benefits, as the condition was considered existing prior to services (EPTS) [4].

Until 2005, service members could be discharged for being homosexual (Chap. 15). Other service members have been discharged under "other than honorable conditions" or OTH. Often, these discharges are related to drug offenses. Until recently, these veterans have had no access to VA care. Recently, this has been changed, allowing them to have emergency mental health care for up to 6 months [6].

Dishonorable or bad conduct discharges often followed allegations of misconduct, with or without judicial proceedings such as court martials. These are more punitive as veterans discharged this way are not historically eligible for VA benefits. In addition, the type of discharge is indicated on their discharge paperwork. Thus, it may follow them into the civilian word, making employment much harder to find, especially in the fields of law enforcement, which many veterans are attracted to.

All of those with the above negative discharges are at higher risk for problems with employment, homelessness, drug issues, and legal problems. Studies have shown that they are far more expensive to society as well because of the tremendous medical costs related to homelessness.

The Military Health-Care System (TRICARE) and the VA Health-Care System

The DoD or TRICARE system of health care offers both direct care through the military hospitals and clinics and purchased care through civilian networks. Together, these systems are called TRICARE. The military health-care system (MHS) normally refers to the direct health-care system.

The direct military health-care system includes hospitals like Walter Reed National Military Medical Center, Balboa Naval Medical Center, and Landstuhl in Germany, as well as hospitals and clinics on military bases throughout the world. Their primary focus is on active duty service members and their dependents (if space is available). Retirees also may access the MHS, if space is available.

The purchased care component of TRICARE is managed through a series of health-care companies. The DoD pays for care in the private sector, with a focus on retirees and dependents.

The Department of Veterans Affairs (DAV or VA) has three component sections: Veterans Health Administration (VHA), which provides health-care services through a continuum of care settings; Veteran Benefits Administration (VBA), which handles veterans' benefits, including compensation and pension, GI bill educational benefits, housing loans, and home construction; and the National Cemetery Administration (NCA), which handles cemeteries, burials, and decedent affairs.

The VA also has a purchased care system, previously known as "Choice" and now as Community Care. The Choice program has been politically sensitive, especially because of concerns that the care of veterans will be privatized. However, independent researches (RAND Ready to Serve [7] and RAND Ready or NOT [8]) indicate that community providers are significantly less competent in meeting the specific and essential cultural and clinical needs of service members, veterans, and their families. Funding is often dependent on politics.

Disability Evaluations

In the past, there were separate evaluations for the DoD and VA. The DoD evaluation was known as a medical board. Now, there is the Integrated Disability Evaluation System (IDES), intended to streamline the process between the two departments.

The VA still has the compensation and pension (C&P) evaluation, which determines whether a veteran has a disability, the level of the disability rating, and whether it is service connected. These exams may be done at a VA facility or through a contracted provider through the Veterans Benefit Administration (VBA).

Just being a veteran does not guarantee access to the VA's health system. Veterans must be eligible to receive VA services and must actively apply for them. As discussed above, eligibility is based on several factors, including type of discharge from military service, income, and service connection. For example, military retirees may be eligible for TRICARE and the VHA but, based upon their income, may make too much money to be eligible for VA health care or other benefits. Changes underway in the Transition Assistance Program (TAP) through which service members and their families are prepared for separation from the military are aimed at assisting better choices and fewer gaps in needed services.

Transition Issues

Traditionally, there are many gaps in care between the DoD and the VHA, which may lead to adverse outcomes, such as homelessness and suicide. There have been numerous efforts by both the DoD and VA to have a "seamless transition of care." In the authors' experience, these efforts work best for severely injured service members but less so for those who are simply leaving the service at the end of their enlistment.

Some of the barriers to a smooth transition include not being able to get a timely appointment at the VA upon discharge from the military and the need to get benefits established. Traditionally, the period between military discharge and entrance into the VHA is a high risk for suicides.

The chapter by Dr. Lowman describes some of the other efforts to develop smoother transitions from the military to the VA health system.

Conclusion

This chapter is intended to be a brief primer on military culture, discharges from the military, the military and VA health-care system and benefits, and transitions to care. All of these are enormous topics, with many regulations which outline them further. Other chapters in this volume will cover many more of these topics in greater detail.

References

1. Ritchie EC. The DoD and VA health care system overview. In: Cozza S, Goldenberg M, editors. Clinical manual for the care of military service members, veterans and their families. APPI; Feb 2014.
2. Ritchie EC. Psychiatry in the Korean War: perils, PIES and prisoners of war. Mil Med. 2002;67(11):898–903.
3. Camp NM US Army psychiatry in the Vietnam War: new challenges in extended counterinsurgency warfare. Borden Institute; 2014.
4. Army regulation 635–200 personnel separations active duty enlisted administrative separations, 6 Sept 2011. Available on the web at http://www.ansbach.army.mil/documents/RetVetAR635-200EnlSep.pdf.
5. https://www.va.gov/healthbenefits/. Accessed May 15, 2018.
6. https://www.va.gov/opa/pressrel/pressrelease.cfm?id=2923. Accessed May 15 2018.
7. Tanielian T, Farris C, Batka C, Farmer CM, Robinson E, Engel CC, Robbins M, Jaycox LII Ready to serve: community-based provider capacity to deliver culturally competent, quality mental health care to veterans and their families. Santa Monica: RAND Corporation, 2014. https://www.rand.org/pubs/research_reports/RR806.html. Also available in print form.
8. Tanielian T, Farmer CM, Burns RM, Duffy EL, Setodji CM. Ready or not? Assessing the capacity of New York state health care providers to meet the needs of veterans. Santa Monica: RAND Corporation, 2018. https://www.rand.org/pubs/research_reports/RR2298.html. Also available in print form.

Psychiatry in the United States Department of Veterans Affairs: A History and a Future

3

Harold Stephen Kudler

Introduction

How does a nation train and retain a high-capacity, highly experienced professional workforce to support the military-related mental health needs of service members, Veterans, and their families, and how does a nation respond to the broader mental health needs of all its citizens? History demonstrates that one goal cannot be fully accomplished without the other. This chapter traces the history of Veterans health care in the United States with a focus on how the development of American psychiatry informed the creation of the modern Veterans Affairs (VA) medical system and vice versa. This review demonstrates the singular and irreplaceable role which VA plays in American health care and sets the stage for recommendations for the future of mental health care for Veterans and for all Americans.

Historical Review

At the time of this writing, the nation is approaching the 100th anniversary of the armistice which ended World War I. World War I was a cataclysm which arguably ushered in what Henry Luce would dub "The American Century" [1]. It was also pivotal in the development of the modern Department of Veterans Affairs (VA) and,

Disclaimer The views expressed here are those of the author and do not represent those of the Department of Veterans Affairs.

H. S. Kudler (✉)
United States Department of Veterans Affairs Medical Center, Durham, NC, USA

Duke University School of Medicine, Psychiatry and Behavioral Sciences, Durham, NC, USA
e-mail: hkudler@duke.edu

© Springer Nature Switzerland AG 2019
E. C. Ritchie, M. D. Llorente (eds.), *Veteran Psychiatry in the US*,
https://doi.org/10.1007/978-3-030-05384-0_3

in a real sense, of American psychiatry. In fact, the history of American psychiatry, military medicine, population health, and VA health care are so inextricably intertwined that each continues to define and redefine the others. A brief historical review demonstrates that while we can trace VA's modern mission and methods to World War I, the nation has been defining and redefining its obligations to and services for Veterans and their families from its earliest colonial days [2].

The Plymouth Colony, established in 1620, was the first in English-speaking America to enact a law (in 1636) establishing pensions for those who were disabled in the colony's defense. Other colonies quickly followed suit, establishing the nation's ongoing commitment to support its Veterans. It is likely not a coincidence that this was the same year in which Massachusetts established the first militia regiments in North America in response to an armed conflict with the indigenous tribespeople which is remembered as King Philip's War. Those colonial militias were the predecessors of the National Guard which continues to recognize December 13, 1636 (the date the law established those regiments), as its birthday [3]. As will be seen, there is a close connection between the onset of new wars, the rapid mass induction of citizens into military service to fight in those wars, and the redefinition of services for Veterans and their families due to the specific circumstances of those wars and the evolving wisdom of each subsequent generation of Americans which can be followed through to the present day.

As the American Revolution began in full force in 1776, the Continental Congress enacted the first national benefits for military Veterans. These were disability pensions authorized as both an incentive and a recognized debt to those who were already waging the War of Independence. That first generation of United States Veterans was recognized again in 1811, when, as they approached old age, the nation opened the first federal Veterans facility, the Naval Asylum in Philadelphia. Of note, the Naval Asylum was reserved for regular Navy "lifers" who had served 20 years or more.

Was it a coincidence that the United States was on the verge of entering the War of 1812 (a war in which American naval forces would have to play a defining role) when this important new benefit was established? It's also important to note that the government only recognized an obligation to those who had completed a career in the military at that time. Army "lifers" only received parity in 1851 with the establishment of the US Soldiers Home in Washington, DC.

The end of the Civil War in 1865 saw the founding of the first federal facility for Union Army volunteer forces, the National Asylum for Disabled Volunteer Soldiers in Togus, Maine. This facility still renders services today as the Togus VA Medical Center. Perhaps 700,000 Americans died in that war (the equivalent of America losing 7 million warfighters today), and there were countless living casualties.

The Civil War spurred the coinage of new medical terms and popular idioms including "the basket case" (for quadruple amputees), "Soldier's Heart" (for those whose nerves were shattered during deployment), and "the Soldier's Disease" (for those who became addicted to the opiates so often used to treat combat injuries). Given the scope and severity of this medical and social impact, the United States was forced to recognize and attend to the needs of volunteer troops rather than restrict benefits to a much smaller cadre of professional service members as it had in previous conflicts. The nation also came to accept its responsibility to identify, report, and bury those who died in battle.

Both the modern "dog tag" and the military tradition of "the challenge coin" evolved from the grassroots development of identifying chips which Civil War combatants created for themselves and carried with them in case their bodies were rendered unidentifiable by the mechanized violence of modern warfare. The first national cemeteries were established in 1862 [4] after thousands died in the initial battles of the war. As early as 1868, there was a national call for a Decoration Day to be observed every May 30. According to tradition, this began as a spontaneous movement among widows and other survivors, family, and community members who decorated service members' graves (both Union and Confederate) with spring flowers [5].

After World War I, Decoration Day, set aside to specifically honor those who died in the Civil War, was expanded to honor those who had died in all American wars. Although it often continues to be referred to as Decoration Day, Congress renamed it Memorial Day in 1971 and designated it as a national holiday to be observed on the last Monday of May. Today, there are 149 national cemeteries. VA, through its National Cemetery Administration, administers 135 of them. In doing so, VA has defined a unique role for itself: the culturally sensitive support and counseling provided even after the death of the Veteran is far beyond that provided by other health-care systems but fully aligned with VA's essential mission of recognizing the special circumstances and sacrifice of those who have served their nation.

That mission was framed by President Lincoln in his second inaugural address: "To care for him who shall have borne the battle and for his widow and his orphan." These words frame the entrance to VA Central Office in Washington, DC, and the nation continues to explore and expand the scope, depth, and nature of that care.

Visitors to Washington, DC, who tour the National Building Museum are usually drawn by its informative and child-friendly exhibits dedicated to architecture, design, engineering, construction, and urban planning. Its spacious Great Hall, measuring 316 × 116 feet and supported by some of the largest Corinthian columns in the world (75 ft. tall and 8 ft. in diameter) [6], has hosted countless public events including inaugural balls. It is a delight as well as a significant challenge to the children who choose to race around its vast open space, but that vastness had a specific purpose which many visitors may not realize; the National Building Museum was originally designed to house the Pension Bureau for Civil War Veterans.

In the aftermath of the Civil War, Congress passed significant new laws meant to operationalize President Lincoln's vision by providing pension coverage for Veterans and their survivors and dependents. The number of these Veterans, the scope of the mission, and the 1500 staff members eventually required to administer it dictated the monumental scale and military theme of the Pension Bureau building. The brick structure was completed in 1887 and designed by Montgomery C. Meigs, the US Army quartermaster general. Among its most notable architectural features is the frieze, sculpted by Caspar Buberl, which stretches 1200 feet around its exterior and depicts over 1300 figures representing Civil War infantry, navy, artillery, cavalry, and medical components in stances and scenes reminiscent of the figures and processional scenes which cap the Parthenon.

The very architecture of the building speaks to the physical limitations of the injured and aging Veterans it was designed to serve: its massive height allowed the Veteran applicants to stay reasonably cool as they waited hours for their evaluation during hot, muggy Washington summers. The stone steps are fitted with unusually low risers suited to the disabled Veterans as they climbed to the upper floors to still more waiting rooms and to smaller offices where they submitted to examinations, administrative reviews and appeals hearings. The grandeur of this building, interior and exterior, clearly reflected the honor which their fellow citizens and government meant to bestow upon them. It was designed to be a beacon and a comfort to them as they and their families wrestled with the medical and social aftermath of war.

Nonetheless, this building, now repurposed for education and entertainment, remains one of the nation's most sobering if silent witnesses to the human cost paid by Civil War Veterans: the pathetic vision is realized if one leans across the grand banisters lining the upper galleries and dares to imagine the rows upon rows of benches upon which those Veterans sat and waited for recognition, care and compensation after having "borne the battle."

As Europe plunged into World War I (WWI) in 1914, Congress created the Bureau of War Risk Insurance (BWRI) to insure ships, cargoes, and merchant marine crewmembers traveling in the war zone. When the United States entered the war as a combatant nation in 1917, Congress authorized sweeping new benefits for WWI Veterans, including life insurance, medical and dental care, vocational and rehabilitative training, and prosthetics services. When the war ended in 1918, the BWRI did not have its own hospitals or clinics, so it networked with military hospitals, Public Health Service Marine Hospitals, the National Home for Disabled Volunteer Soldiers, and private civilian hospitals to provide additional medical support and services.

By 1921, the fragmentation of care and benefits which arose in these disparate medical systems, coupled with the rising frustration of WWI Veterans and their families, led Congress to consolidate three World War I programs into one independent agency known as the Veterans Bureau. Originally part of the Treasury Department, the Veterans Bureau was later authorized as an independent agency that answered directly to the President.

The Veterans Bureau oversaw the largest federal hospital construction program in American history as well as the largest life insurance program in the world at the time. By June 1930, the National Homes had 11 branches and secured approval to build 2–3 new branches the following year, while the Veterans Bureau had 49 hospitals with more underway. The Veterans Bureau exclusively served WWI Veterans but, in 1930, it was merged with the National Home for Disabled Volunteer Soldiers and the Bureau of Pensions to form the new Veterans Administration serving all Veterans and their dependents.

In 1945, General Omar Bradley took the reins at the Veterans Administration as roughly one in five American men became Veterans of World War II and steered its transformation into a modern organization with an expanded building program and a focus on affiliation with existing medical schools and major medical centers. He also helped develop VA's research programs on problems of special relevance to Veterans including spinal cord injury and physical and mental rehabilitation. In 1988, VA was elevated to a cabinet-level agency, the Department of Veterans Affairs. VA is now the second largest such agency with a budget of nearly $200 billion per year and a workforce of over 360,000.

The VA and American Psychiatry

As noted earlier, Soldier's Heart, which is now recognized as an earlier expression of post-traumatic stress disorder, was identified in American medicine in the aftermath of the Civil War. It was dubbed "Irritable Heart Syndrome" by J. M. Da Costa, the cardiologist who first described its symptoms in terms of a cardiac condition which bore many similarities to panic disorder (now classified as a mental health disorder) [7]. The neurologist, Silas Weir Mitchell, who was Da Costa's wartime colleague at Turner Lane Military Hospital in Philadelphia, understood the mental health problems of Civil War Veterans as a form of nervous exhaustion and developed the rest cure as a means to treat it [8].

It wasn't until World War I that American psychiatry had matured to the point where it was ready to play an essential role in defining and treating the medical sequelae of deployment stress among service members and Veterans. That effort was foundational to the modern Department of Veterans Affairs. It can also be argued that the national effort to meet the mental health needs of WWI Veterans helped unite a fragmented American psychiatry, gave birth to its modern nosology, and set the foundation for its national research and organizational efforts.

The years prior to WWI saw the birth of a number of different reforming forces in mental health-care and social interventions including psychoanalysis, the social work movement, and public health approaches to pressing clinical problems. Among the most prominent of these was the National Committee for Mental Hygiene. The Mental Hygiene movement grew out of Clifford Beers' lived experience as a psychiatric patient which he described in his best-selling 1908 autobiography, *A Mind that Found Itself* [9]. Beers crafted the book to inspire a national movement on behalf of the mentally ill and succeeded in engaging William James (the father of American psychology) and Adolph Meyer (the father of American psychiatry and promoter of public health research and advocacy) as his partners in founding the National Committee for Mental Hygiene. The organization was supported by the then new Rockefeller Foundation.

Mental Hygiene was designed to be a grassroots consumer movement which advocated a proactive approach on the understanding that mental illness was as much the province of the family member, the teacher, the employer, and the sufferer himself or herself as of clinicians, researchers, asylum owners, and policymakers. In addition to promoting more effective treatment, the Mental Hygiene movement was at least as interested in efforts leading to the prevention of mental illness through what would now be considered public or population health interventions including enhanced mental health literacy, early recognition of those at risk, confrontation of known or suspected causes of mental health problems, and facilitated access to support and care in schools, workplaces, and other social institutions.

Of key importance was Mental Hygiene's self-defined role as a consumer movement that partnered with the leaders in American mental health and American society to achieve its ends. The National Committee for Mental Hygiene evolved into the National Mental Health Association which now continues as Mental Health America, the nation's leading community-based nonprofit organization dedicated to addressing the needs of those living with mental illness and to promoting the overall mental health of all Americans [10].

Beers, James, and Meyer needed an executive officer to oversee the operations of the National Committee. They turned to a psychiatrist, Thomas Salmon. Salmon began his medical career as a general practitioner in rural New York but was unable to continue as the rigorous life of a "horse and buggy doctor" because of a debilitating bout of tuberculosis [11]. During his recuperation, he turned to tracking infectious diseases in state mental hospitals. This experience inspired him to become a psychiatrist. In 1903, Salmon joined the US Public Health Services and began examining new immigrants on Ellis Island for mental health problems. His bitter disagreement with the current standard for the assessment and management of these immigrants (which Salmon saw as a disservice to the mentally ill and a tragic mismanagement of the limited mental health resources of New York City) led to a brief suspension for insubordination in 1907. In all likelihood, it was Salmon's expertise with statistics coupled with his willingness to speak truth to power as an advocate for the mentally ill that led to his selection to direct the National Committee in 1913.

Although the United States didn't enter WWI until 1917, Salmon had been carefully tracking the toll taken by Shell Shock and other mental health problems since the European powers went to war in 1914. Shortly after America declared war, Salmon arranged a meeting with the US Army Surgeon General to advise steps that might prevent large numbers of American service members from succumbing to mental disorder under those same severe conditions of trench warfare. As a consequence, the Surgeon General recruited Salmon to become General Pershing's chief psychiatric consultant for the American Expeditionary Forces. As a first assignment, Salmon was sent to England in advance of American troops in order to develop preventative and treatment approaches.

Salmon's proactive engagement of the military as America entered the war was characteristic of the prevention-oriented, consumer-driven principles of the Mental Hygiene movement. The military's acceptance of Salmon's offer was based on the harsh realization that Shell Shock accounted for one-seventh of all discharges for disability from the British Army or one-third if discharges for wounds were excluded.

Salmon's preemptive visit to Great Britain resulted in his 1917 report, *The Care and Treatment of Mental Diseases and War Neuroses ("Shell Shock") in the British Army* [12]. With singular insight, this hastily prepared document defined the basic principles of what is now the international standard for combat stress control doctrine. Of particular importance was Salmon's recognition that, by 1917, twice as many hospital beds had been provided for British soldiers and sailors as had existed in the entire United Kingdom at the start of the war just 3 years earlier. He noted that "these almost incredible achievements" had been made possible by the "...deep sympathy which officials and the public alike bestow upon all those returning from the front who are in need of care or attention" ([12], p. 8). These observations contain the seed of the campaign on behalf of Veterans which Salmon was to champion after the war and for the rest of his life.

WWI ended on November 11, 1918, but its mental health effects continued to linger and even multiply. By war's end, Salmon was responsible for approximately 2000 "uncured" psychiatrically hospitalized American troops in France [11]. When he returned to the United States in 1919, he advocated for the creation of a presidential commission which would reconcile the conflicting policies and plans of the Army, the Navy, the Public Health Service and the Bureau of War Risk Insurance.

He laid out his concern in a letter to a colleague: "If any soldier who fought in France and received an invisible wound that has darkened his mind now lies in a county jail or almshouse or is for any reason deprived of the best treatment that the resources of modern psychiatry can provide, our national honor is compromised..." ([11], pp. 162–163). In 1920, he surveyed the nation's general hospitals, mental hospitals, and other care facilities where WWI Veterans were receiving mental health care and determined that there was an immediate need for 3200 new neuropsychiatric beds and that, within 1 year, there would be a need for 8000 such beds. History was to prove these predictions correct ([11], p. 175).

Salmon did his best to retain his carefully trained cadre of Army psychiatrists in the military and distribute them and their patients to a network of State Psychiatric Hospitals strategically sited across the nation where they would develop treatment programs specifically designed to meet the needs of Veterans and informed by the wartime experience of those psychiatrists ([11], pp. 165–166).

A major obstacle to this plan arose from military culture itself: Veterans and their relatives objected on the grounds that such institutions were public charities and that the federal government had a fundamental responsibility to provide for the treatment of mental health disorders among Veterans and the support of their families as a national obligation and an honorable, well-earned health benefit ([11] pp. 171–172). In his heart of hearts, Salmon could not but have agreed with this sentiment and he directed all his powers and his considerable influence to this cause.

Salmon's efforts on behalf of American service members and Veterans also included a groundbreaking project to establish a national nomenclature for mental illness. In 1918, the National Committee on Mental Hygiene, in partnership with the "Committee on Statistics" of what is now known as the American Psychiatric Association (APA), published the *Statistical Manual for the Use of Institutions for the Insane* [13] containing 22 standardized diagnoses. A nationally accepted nomenclature was a necessity if there were to be uniform diagnostics, appropriate treatment, and epidemiological tracking of thousands of neuropsychiatric war Veterans as they spread out across the nation. The Statistical Manual evolved into what was known as "the Standard Nomenclature" by the time WWII began.

History repeated itself when, in 1952, the APA adopted its first *Diagnostic and Statistical Manual of Mental Disorders* now known as DSM I [14] which was largely drawn from Medical 203, a classification system developed by a committee working under Brigadier General William Menninger and issued in 1943 as a "War Department Technical Bulletin" under the auspices of the Office of the Surgeon General. Menninger, like Salmon before him, was to become President of the American Psychiatric Association in the aftermath of his wartime service and to help reshape that organization and American psychiatric training programs, clinical organizations and member practices in order to better serve Veterans (and, ultimately, all Americans) by virtue of psychiatric lessons learned in war. As the introduction to DSM I notes, "Psychiatrists who had become accustomed to the revised nomenclature in the Army were unwilling to return to the Standard Nomenclature upon return to civilian life" ([14], p. viii).

The sixth edition of the *International Classification of Diseases* (ICD) was also drawn from General Menninger's Medical 203, demonstrating that military and Veteran psychiatry has repeatedly played a defining role in American psychiatry. Further, the establishment of Veterans Hospitals, the nation's largest network of psychiatric programs, has served as a driver for valid and consistently applied diagnostic systems and epidemiological tracking across the country and continues to advance this mission today thanks to VA's being the largest employer and trainer of psychiatrists, psychologists, psychiatric nurses, social workers and other mental health professionals in the United States.

Unfortunately, that national VA system was still a far-off dream in the immediate aftermath of WWI. Salmon was a leader in advocating for a coherent national plan for the redeployment of warfighters. Each military branch had its own psychiatric hospitals and its own approach. The 20 Public Health Service Hospitals set aside for the neuropsychiatric casualties of war were not coordinated with the military hospitals nor did they share the same diagnostic or treatment standards with the many public and private hospitals, asylums and rest homes to which Veterans were being sent.

The creation of the Veterans Bureau in 1921 didn't immediately solve that problem because the envisioned Veterans hospitals had yet to be built and that process became mired in a scandal so significant that it threatened to bring down the administration of President Harding [15]. Perhaps the greatest psychiatric lesson of WWI was that when the nation goes to war, it must think in very long terms and prepare well in advance for the mental health tail of the war. To illustrate, as of this writing, VA is still providing benefits to one dependent of a Civil War Veteran more than one and a half centuries after the end of that war.

Relevance of WWI History for the Present State and Future of VA

The Department of Veterans Affairs medical system is now the nation's largest integrated mental health system with the ability to screen for, assess, treat, and track mental health problems in Primary Care, in general and specialty Mental Health programs and through a broad spectrum of home-based and residential treatment programs organized around a progressive Recovery model. It is the nation's leading provider of telemental health and of evidence-based treatment for mental disorders including post-traumatic stress disorder (PTSD) and the mental health effects of traumatic brain injury (TBI).

Its extensive research program consistently targets deployment mental health concerns (which most other clinical institutions and pharmaceutical companies are not invested in), and its hundreds of academic affiliations across disciplines set it apart from other health systems. As noted, it employs and trains more mental health professionals than any other system in the nation and, although variability still remains across VA, it is arguably the nation's most influential and effective driver of high-quality clinical approaches to effective mental health care. As such, VA is a national resource which no other segment of American medicine could replace.

Further, any attempt to dismantle the VA health-care system would cripple the American medical education system across virtually all disciplines to an unthinkable degree and leave the future of research on deployment mental health to a national research infrastructure which has neither the mission, the clinical experience, nor the economic motivation required to succeed in addressing this national priority.

The value of VA has regularly been demonstrated independently. Of particular relevance are the findings of the 2014 RAND study, *Ready to Serve* [16], which found that while cultural competency may be the key factor in providing effective mental health care for Veterans and their families, clinicians who work primarily in a military or VA setting were significantly more likely to meet criteria for being culturally competent (70%) than providers who indicated they were registered within the military's TRICARE network (24%) and much more likely to be culturally competent than the average community provider (8%). Further, the authors found that only 13% of surveyed civilian providers met all the readiness criteria defined by RAND. Finally, those who did meet the threshold for cultural competency did not necessarily meet the threshold for providing evidence-based care. In summary, the RAND report found that providers who work primarily in a military or VA setting were significantly more likely to meet all criteria necessary to effectively treat Veterans than providers who did not.

A 2018 RAND study, *Ready or Not? Assessing the Capacity of New York State Health Care Providers to Meet the Needs of Veterans* [17], found that only 20% of licensed health-care professionals in New York State even screen their patients for military or Veteran affiliation on a routine basis and that only 2.3% met all criteria for effectively serving Veterans. To repeat an old medical aphorism, "If you don't take the temperature, you can't find the fever." RAND's recent findings suggest that the majority of licensed health-care professionals are not aware of whether or not the patient they are treating is a Veteran or someone close to a Veteran who might be significantly affected by deployment stress. If they were to simply ask the question "Have you or someone close to you served in the military?", there is a roughly one in five chances that the answer to this question would be "Yes" (considering that there are approximately 2.5 million Service Members, 22.5 million Veterans, and, conservatively estimated, 38 million dependents in the United States today).

VA exists to fill this gap in competency, but, perhaps more importantly, VA exists to insist on a basic awareness of the mental health cost of war among American health-care professionals, population health leaders, policymakers, and all citizens. Through its interactions with 6 million Veterans under care, 9 million enrolled Veterans, and millions of other Veterans and dependents who receive non-medical VA benefits and services, VA also has an opportunity to spark a renaissance of grassroots action on behalf of those who have served with the same scale and impact that Thomas Salmon and the Mental Hygiene movement achieved a century ago.

Conclusion

As we observe the 100th anniversary of the end of World War I and what may be the dawn of a Second American Century, we can best honor the past if we remember and build on its discoveries and its strengths. As this review demonstrates, much has been learned from the experience of WWI. Many of same lessons have had to be relearned with each subsequent war. VA is the repository of that learned experience. As the nation's largest educator of mental health professionals, it has played a major role in building upon and disseminating that experience across the nation, yet, as the RAND studies noted above demonstrate, unacceptably large gaps in knowledge persist across the rest of American psychiatry and American medicine. Recent professional, financial, and political debates over the wisdom of "privatizing" the care of Veterans need to be informed by these findings and this history.

In establishing VA as a national resource for Veterans mental health care, it is possible that the nation also precipitated the unintended consequence of making the distinct and significant mental health problems sometimes associated with military service "someone else's business." This may be the reason that the vast majority of professional schools and residency programs don't see the need to focus on these issues in their curricula or why professional organizations fail to promote either basic or continuing education about military or Veterans' mental health. These deficiencies underlie the gap demonstrated in the RAND reports noted above.

VA has an opportunity and an obligation to champion such awareness and training given the fact that, of the 22.5 million Veterans now living, only 6 million of these actually use VA health care in any given year. Further, even among those 6 million, many are simultaneously receiving at least some of their care in the community. Leaving aside the current problem of the fragmentation of both the medical record and the continuity of care across disparate systems, our current national system of mental health care for Veterans and those close to them would be greatly improved if all community providers were to ask, "Have you or someone close to you served in the military?" And, of course, they need to be trained and gain experience in order to respond effectively when that answer is "Yes."

These considerations define a path forward for VA and for American psychiatry. We need to apply the lessons of history in order to assure the best possible mental health outcomes for Veterans, for their dependents and for our nation as a whole.

References

1. Luce H. The American century. Life Magazine. 1941;10(7):61–5.
2. Department of Veterans Affairs. VA history in brief. https://www.va.gov/opa/publications/archives/docs/history_in_brief.pdf. Accessed 19 May 2018.
3. National Guard Bureau. How we began. http://www.nationalguard.mil/About-the-Guard/How-We-Began/. Accessed 19 May 2018.
4. Department of Veterans Affairs National Cemetery Administration. https://www.cem.va.gov/history/history.asp#GeneralHistory. Accessed 19 May 2018.
5. Department of Veterans Affairs Office of Public and Intergovernmental Affairs. Memorial Day history. https://www.va.gov/opa/speceven/memday/history.asp. Accessed 19 May 2018.
6. National Building Museum. https://en.m.wikipedia.org/wiki/National_Building_Museum. Accessed 19 May 2018.
7. Da Costa JM. On irritable heart; a clinical study of a form of functional cardiac disorder and its consequences. Am J Med Sci. 1871;61:17–52.
8. Mitchell SW. Fat and blood: and how to make them. Philadelphia: J.B. Lippincott & Co.; 1877.
9. Beers CW. A mind that found itself: an autobiography. New York: Longmans, Green; 1908.
10. Mental Health America: About Us. http://www.mentalhealthamerica.net/about-us. Accessed 19 May 2018.
11. Bond ED. Thomas Salmon, psychiatrist. New York: W.W. Norton & Co; 1950.
12. Salmon TW. The care and treatment of mental diseases and war neuroses ("shell shock") in the British army. Union Square, New York City: War Work Committee of the National Committee for Mental Hygiene; 1917.
13. Committee on Statistics, American Medico-Psychological Association, the National Committee for Mental Hygiene Bureau of Statistics. Statistical manual for the use of institutions for the insane. New York: National Committee for Mental Hygiene; 1918.
14. American Psychiatric Association. Diagnostic and statistical manual of mental disorders (DSM I). Washington, DC: American Psychiatric Association Mental Hospital Service; 1952.
15. Stevens R. A time of scandal: Charles R. Forbes, Warren G. Harding, and the making of the Veterans Bureau. Baltimore: Johns Hopkins University Press; 2016.
16. Tanielian T, Farris C, Batka C, Farmer CM, Robinson E, Engel CC, Robbins M, Jaycox LH. Ready to serve: community-based provider capacity to deliver culturally competent, quality mental health care to veterans and their families. Santa Monica: RAND Corporation; 2014. https://www.rand.org/pubs/research_reports/RR806.html. Accessed 20 May 2018.
17. Tanielian T, Farmer CM, Burns RM, Duffy EL, Setodji CM. Ready or not? Assessing the capacity of New York State health care providers to meet the needs of veterans. Santa Monica: RAND Corporation; 2018. https://www.rand.org/pubs/research_reports/RR2298.html. Accessed 20 May 2018.

Optimizing Clinical Outcomes in VA Mental Health Care

Cheryl A. Lowman

Introduction

The Department of Veterans Health Administration (VHA) system is the nation's largest provider of integrated health services, with a fiscal year (FY) 2017 operating budget of more than 72 billion for medical care [1]. Mission driven, its goal is to fulfill President Lincoln's promise "to care for him who shall have born the battle, and for his widow and his orphan," by serving and honoring the men and women who are America's Veterans. Many VA employees are veterans themselves, or have a veteran in the family, and are personally connected to the mission of the VA. Mental health care is a vital component of this promise, providing high-quality, evidence-based treatment, including state-of-the-art psychotherapies and psychopharmacological treatments, for the full range of mental health conditions, in a team-based setting.

Veterans receive comprehensive medical and mental health care, facilitated by an electronic medical record, the VA Computerized Patient Record System (CPRS). This system supports integrated care by allowing different providers, within the system and across the country, access to a patient's healthcare data, and facilitates the sharing of clinical care nationwide. This is a unique strength of the system as Veterans receive comprehensive health care in accordance with their treatment plan no matter where they travel throughout the United States, allowing them to receive care at any VA Medical Center.

There are multiple entry points for mental health care with 179 VA Medical Centers and 1061 Community-Based Outpatient Clinics (CBOCs), 300 Vet Centers, the Veterans Crisis Line, VA staff on college and university campuses, and other outreach efforts [1]. These sites of care are organized into 18 geographic regions called Veterans Integrated Service Networks (VISNs).

C. A. Lowman (✉)
VA Capitol Health Care Network, VISN 5, Linthicum, MD, USA
e-mail: Cheryl.Lowman@va.gov

© Springer Nature Switzerland AG 2019
E. C. Ritchie, M. D. Llorente (eds.), *Veteran Psychiatry in the US*,
https://doi.org/10.1007/978-3-030-05384-0_4

VA mental health care is advanced through national policy, research and funding. The foundation for the present-day system of integrated mental health care was established in 1999 with the advent of VHA Mental Health Program Guide 1103.3. This program guide required all enrolled Veterans to have access to a "comprehensive, integrated, continuum of high quality effective mental health services" [2].

Presently, the current VA strategic plan for FY 2018–2024 identifies several areas of mental health care as top priorities [3]. Specifically, these priority areas include reducing the Veteran suicide rate, ending Veteran homelessness, increasing access to care, and leading the nation in caring for Veterans with trauma-related mental health conditions. Former VA Secretary David J. Shulkin specifically identified preventing Veteran suicide as one of his top five priorities.

Integrating mental health care in medical settings has been the VA model since 2008 but is uncommon in the private sector. Coordinated, team-based care is designed to enhance access and treatment engagement, promote increased continuity of care, and lead to better outcomes than the fragmented, episodic model of community-based care.

Multiple reports and studies have compared VA care to the community sector and determined that VA care is as good as, or superior to, care in the community. Additionally, studies have found that community-based providers are unlikely to have the skills necessary to deliver high-quality evidence-based mental health treatment to Veterans, and that VA mental health care outperforms the community in terms of adhering to recommended guidelines [4–9].

In this way, VA is a national role model in providing coordinated care through programs such as Suicide Prevention, Primary Care-Mental Health Integration (PC-MHI), Behavioral Health Interdisciplinary Programs (BHIP), PTSD Clinical Team (PCL), Residential Rehabilitation Treatment Programs (RRTPs), and Substance Use Disorder Programs. VA has integrated mental health services into its geriatrics programs, embedding mental health professionals in the Home-Based Primary Care Program, Community Living Centers (nursing homes), and Palliative Care programs.

Tasked with caring for Veterans throughout their lifetime, VA incentivizes chronic disease management to keep patients healthy. To enhance prevention, VA is currently shifting to incorporate a more holistic approach to Veteran care. In March 2017, it began implementing a Whole Health model of patient care which utilizes complementary and integrative treatment methodologies.

The Whole Health initiative, disseminated by the Office of Patient Centered Care and Cultural Transformation, is a comprehensive model of care in which the patient is at the center. The model is an approach to healthcare that empowers Veterans to take charge of their health and well-being in partnership with medical providers. It incorporates a full range of conventional, complementary and integrative health approaches such as yoga, chiropractic, biofeedback, massage therapy, etc. These are available to all Veterans but are also prioritized for veterans suffering with chronic pain with the goal of providing nondrug alternatives in the treatment of chronic pain, in order to combat the national opioid epidemic.

VA is able to leverage its size and considerable resources to deliver many unique and exceptional mental health models of care that are not available in the private sector. The programs described in this chapter are a current focus of the VA strategic plan. They also meet the criteria initially conceptualized by the VHA Program Guide as being a "comprehensive, integrated, continuum of high quality effective mental health services." This chapter provides an overview of several of VA's exceptional mental health programs and should not be considered a complete description of every mental health service available throughout VA.

VA General Strong Mental Health Practices

VA develops clinical policies, disseminates national guidance for MH services, and provides system-wide oversight of MH services through its Central Office division, the Office of Mental Health and Suicide Prevention. Mental health services throughout the VA are defined and regulated by specific guidelines contained in the *Uniform Mental Health Services Handbook* (VHA handbook 1160.01) [10]. This handbook, published in 2008 and amended in November 2015, specifies the type of mental health services VA hospitals and clinics are required to offer to Veterans and their families. The requirements differ depending on the size and type of VA hospital or clinic but apply across the entire VA system.

In addition to the handbook, VHA mental health policy is guided by scientifically established protocols or clinical practice guidelines. Since 1998, VA and the Department of Defense (DoD) have partnered together through the Evidence-Based Practice Working Group to develop treatment guidelines. Clinical practice guidelines (CPG) are based upon a rigorous systematic review of the evidence and explicit processes aligned with the National Academy of Medicine's articulated set of standards. They are designed to optimize patient care by recommending evidence-based practices, create standard guidelines intended to reduce variations in care, and inform delivery of VA care. VA recognizes CPG guidelines as proven standards for clinical practice and policy. Currently, VA/DOD joint guidelines have been developed for a variety of physical health diagnoses and the following mental health diagnoses: PTSD, substance use disorder, major depressive disorder, and suicide prevention [11].

In order to monitor the implementation and quality of mental health care as prescribed by the handbook throughout its nationwide system, VA utilizes performance metrics. VA performance metrics gather data through the electronic medical record, providing a system of national quality review. The VA capability to analyze data nationally, as well as by facility, is unmatched within community medical settings.

Strategic Analytics for Improvement and Learning (SAIL) is a major VA initiative for measuring and benchmarking healthcare quality at its VA Medical Centers. Medical center performance is ranked or benchmarked against other VA Medical Centers. SAIL was developed in 2011 and originally measured the quality of medical care in medical domains such as acute-care mortality, length of stay, avoidable adverse events, etc.

In 2015, the VA added a set of 33 quality improvement measures for mental health. These measures collectively monitor population coverage, continuity of mental health care, and the experience of care from the patient and the provider perspective. The measures allow the facility to "drill down" to review individual cases. Unique to the VA, community mental health settings do not have an equivalent system to measure quality of mental health treatment on this scale.

Another quality improvement metric unique to VA is the Psychotropic Drug Safety Initiative (PDSI). Launched in 2013, this quality improvement initiative is designed to foster the highest quality of treatment with medications for Veterans with mental health problems. The national PDSI program office supports local quality improvement efforts by providing data, informatics tools, training and educational resources, and feedback and technical assistance. PDSI data include facility and national scores reported quarterly on prescribing metrics that address a variety of aspects of mental health treatment with psychiatric medications.

VA policy dictates that every Veteran must be screened for PTSD, major depression, suicide risk, and alcohol misuse, upon entry to the VA, on a yearly basis, and as clinically indicated. Evidence-based screening instruments are embedded into the Computerized Patient Record System (CPRS) as a templated note. To facilitate the screening, a clinical reminder system prompts the clinician to complete the screening tests that are appropriate for the patient based on their medical history and expressed symptoms. Positive results prompt in-depth assessment, and when problems are identified, the Veteran is referred to the appropriate mental health services.

Every Veteran who receives ongoing mental health care is assigned a Mental Health Treatment Coordinator (MHTC). This clinician and their contact information are clearly identified in the medical record as a point of contact. The MHTC provides continuity throughout the Veteran's mental health treatment and is included in the development of the Veteran's treatment plan. In this regard, the MHTC's role is to facilitate the overall mental health goals of the Veteran. The MHTC is responsible for ensuring the treatment plan is implemented and monitored, but does not need to be providing the actual treatment. Rather, the MHTC is designed to be a clinical resource and point of contact for the Veteran. Once assigned, it is intended that the MHTC will continue in this role as long as the Veteran receives mental health care in the VA.

Evidence-Based Psychotherapies

Exposure to military life, combat and multiple deployments creates stress for veterans and their families. Marital stress, substance misuse and PTSD are but a few of the sequelae of deployment. In order to meet their needs, VA mental health treatment has increasingly shifted to delivering high-quality, evidence-based treatments for the full range of mental health conditions. In this regard, VA is a national leader in the promotion of evidence-based psychotherapy (EBPs). EBPs are specific psychological treatments that have been consistently shown in controlled clinical research to be effective for mental or behavioral health conditions.

The VA Handbook requires that Veterans have full access to EBP services and that facilities maintain adequate staff capacity to provide these therapies. VA promotes the dissemination and implementation of EBPs, through the designation of an EBP Coordinator at each facility. The role of the EBP Coordinator is to educate patients and staff regarding the benefits of EBPs, work with facility and mental health staff for dissemination, assist in implementing clinical infrastructure to support the therapy (clinic structures and scheduling), track EBP delivery at the local level, and provide consultation support for clinicians [12].

To ensure the dissemination and utilization of EBPs, VA has implemented comprehensive clinician training programs in over 15 areas of intervention. Examples include evidence-based marital and family counseling (Integrative Behavioral Couples Therapy for Marital Distress, Behavioral Family Therapy for Serious Psychiatric Disorders, and Cognitive-Behavioral Conjoint Therapy for PTSD), as well as EBPs designed for the treatment of mental health conditions such as PTSD or depression. These include Prolonged Exposure, Cognitive Behavioral Therapy for Depression, Cognitive Processing Therapy, Motivational Interviewing, Motivational Enhancement Therapy, CBT for substance use disorder, CBT for insomnia and CBT for pain.

VA requires clinicians to utilize computerized note templates in CPRS for each of the EBP sessions, which are tracked nationally. VA has been monitoring the implementation and dissemination of evidence-based psychotherapies and in 2018 added additional performance metrics giving facilities additional credit for the therapies they have implemented. In a March 2018 email from the EBP program office, Kristine Day (Kristine.Day@va.gov) reported that VHA has provided EBP training to over 12,800 VA mental health staff as of February 28, 2018.

Distinctive VA Mental Health Programs

Comprehensive Suicide Prevention Programs

VA is unique across the nation in providing an integrative, comprehensive approach to suicide prevention. There is no equivalent private sector program in the United States that has the range and depth of coordinated, comprehensive suicide prevention programs that the VA delivers. VA suicide prevention initiatives include yearly screening for suicide risk, coordinated suicide prevention care, the Veterans Crisis Line, and REACH VET, a predictive analytics program.

These programs are overseen by the National Office of Mental Health Operations and Suicide Prevention. This office conducted an analysis of suicide mortality spanning 2001–2014, examining 55 million records from every state [13]. Results concluded that in 2014, an average of 20 Veterans died by suicide each day. Six of the 20 Veterans were users of VA health services in 2013 or 2014, and the other 14 were not currently enrolled with VA. The trend shows that veterans who receive their health care from VA have a significantly lower rate of suicide than veterans who do not receive VA care. In an effort to address the suicide rate, the VA Secretary prioritized suicide prevention as one of his top five priorities in 2017.

To broaden outreach to at-risk Veterans, all VA Medical Centers were directed to offer 90 days of emergency stabilization care for former service members with an Other Than Honorable Discharge (OTH) in March 2017. Specifically, former service members with an OTH administrative discharge may receive care for a mental health emergency for an initial period of 90 days, which can include inpatient, residential, or outpatient care. VA can authorize a 90-day extension, but if longer-term services are required, VA will coordinate a transition to community-based care, as it does not have the legal authority to provide ongoing care to OTH Veterans at the VA's expense.

In recognition that the first year of transition after separating from active duty is a difficult adjustment, President Donald J. Trump signed an Executive Order on January 9, 2018, enabling VA to provide one year of free mental health services to former service members in the year after separation from active duty military service. The Executive Order requires that VA and Department of Defense work together collaboratively in a joint advisory council to ensure coordinated approaches in meeting the needs of Service Members and Veterans.

Reach Vet

VA utilizes a predictive analytics program called Reach Vet (Recovery Engagement and Coordination for Health) [14]. The program is designed to identify the Veterans at the highest statistical risk, reach out to assess clinical risk, and proactively provide enhanced care if needed. Reach Vet was implemented in November 2016 and uses a multivariate analysis to identify enrolled patients in the highest risk category (0.1%), who are at risk of suicide, hospitalization, illness or other adverse events. This population tends to have multiple comorbidities, frequent mental health and primary care contacts, and high rates of polypharmacy.

The analysis is run monthly and distributed to the facility Reach Vet Coordinator, who is responsible for evaluating the Veteran's care, and notifying the medical team of the risk assessment. The clinicians are asked to contact the identified Veterans and collaboratively review their healthcare diagnoses and mental health conditions and ensure appropriate treatment is offered.

Veterans Crisis Line

VA's Veterans Crisis Line (VCL) (1-800-273-8255, press 1) was established in 2007. It has expanded to include chat and texting options for contacting the Crisis Line. The VCL is available 24/7 and employs trained responders, usually social workers or other mental health professionals, who are able to provide callers with immediate support and refer them to VA mental health services. If the caller is determined to be in imminent danger, the VCL will direct local emergency services to callers.

Since its launch in 2007 through March 2018, the Veterans Crisis Line has answered over 3.5 million calls and initiated the dispatch of emergency services to callers in imminent crisis nearly 93,000 times. Since launching chat in 2009 and text services in November 2011, the VCL has made over 397,000 chat connections and responded to nearly 92,000 requests for text services. The staff has forwarded more than 582,000 case referrals to local VA Suicide Prevention Coordinators to ensure continuity of care with the Veterans local VA providers [15].

Suicide Risk Management Consultation Program

VA also operates a Suicide Risk Management Consultation Program, which provides free consultation for any clinician, community or VA, who serves Veterans at risk for suicide. This program is housed in the Denver VA Mental Health Illness Education Research and Clinical Center (MIRECC) that specializes in research related to suicide prevention. Common consultation topics include risk assessment, lethal means safety counseling, strategies for how to engage Veterans at high risk, and clinician support after a completed suicide.

Suicide Prevention Teams

Each VA Medical Center is required to have a suicide prevention team, led by a Suicide Prevention Coordinator (SPC). The VHA Handbook specifies that the Suicide Prevention Coordinator has a full-time commitment to suicide prevention activities. Each VA Medical Center establishes a high risk for suicide list and a process to ensure that patients determined to be at high risk are provided with follow-up for all missed mental health and substance abuse appointments.

The Suicide Prevention Coordinators submit suicide behavior reports for all known suicide attempts and deaths into a centralized database, the VA Suicide Prevention Application Network (SPAN). Once the Veteran is entered into the SPAN, they are also placed on a VA high-risk list by establishing a Patient Record Flag (PRF) in the electronic medical record system. This enables any clinician throughout the nation working with the Veteran to identify their high-risk status and promotes tracking patients who are at high risk for suicide.

Patients who have been identified as being at high risk receive an enhanced level of care, including missed appointment follow-ups, telephone monitoring, safety planning, follow-up visits and care plans that directly address their suicidality. The suicide prevention team follows high-risk patients for at least 90 days and will continue to follow for longer periods as clinically indicated.

In addition to their clinical work with at-risk Veterans, Suicide Prevention Coordinators and their team function as consultants tasked with providing education about suicide prevention both in-house and in the community. They train all VA staff, both clinical and nonclinical, to provide effective interventions with patients in crisis. In addition, they: (1) collaborate with community organizations to provide training to their staff who have contact with Veterans; (2) provide general consultation to clinicians concerning resources for suicidal individuals; and (3) report on a monthly basis to mental health leadership and the National Suicide Prevention Coordinator on the Veterans who attempted or completed suicide.

Primary Care-Mental Health Integration (PC-MHI)

Primary care in the VA is arranged in Patient Aligned Care Teams (PACT). PACT teams are organized via the medical home model of healthcare, providing patient-centered, team-based, comprehensive, primary care. VA integrated mental health services into the PACT in 2008, deploying Primary Care-Mental Health Integration (PC-MHI).

The concept of PC-MHI is derived from the Institute of Medicine's definition: "Provides accessible, integrated biopsychosocial healthcare services by clinicians who are accountable for addressing a large majority of personal health care needs, developing a sustained partnership with patients and practicing in the context of family and community" [16]. Providing mental health treatment within the primary care clinic minimizes barriers and reduces stigma, which can discourage Veterans from seeking care. This allows Veteran's mental health needs to be recognized and treated early in the course of illness.

PC-MHI provides consultative advice, same-day assessment, time-limited treatment, and disease-specific care management. The mental health clinicians embedded in PACT teams ensure that common mental health conditions and other problems amenable to behavioral or psychopharmacological interventions presenting in primary care are addressed. Mild to moderate mental health conditions are managed within PC-MHI. PC-MHI staff and PACT team members collaborate to provide holistic treatment addressing the patient's medical and psychological concerns.

In addition, PC-MHI providers serve as a bridge between primary care and more specialized mental health services. They facilitate referral to services for Veterans who require longer-term or more intensive mental health care and coordinate referrals back to PACT following mental health treatment. Veterans treated within PC-MHI may have their needs addressed by two program components: Co-located Collaborative Care and Care Management.

A. Co-located Collaborative Care refers to mental health professionals who are physically embedded within primary care. These co-located staff provide brief (no longer than 30 min) evidence-based psychosocial treatment as needed for a wide variety of mental health conditions, typically focused on the impact of mental health concerns on functioning. They provide assessment, psychopharmacology and consultative support to the PACT providers. Co-located collaborative care operates on an open or same-day access basis. Typically, the mental health conditions that are treated within the primary care environment are mild to moderate in severity and include uncomplicated depression, anxiety, alcohol use disorders, adjustment disorders and other health-related behaviors or disorders.
B. Care Management is a disease-specific, protocol-driven telephone intervention that provides ongoing monitoring of patients treated for specific mental health conditions. Care Management focuses on monitoring adherence to treatment, medication side effects, decision support, patient education and behavioral activation, and referral management to more intensive mental health care if

needed. VA utilizes two models of care management: Behavioral Health Laboratory (BHL) and Translating Initiatives for Depression into Effective Solutions (TIDES) [10].

Behavioral Health Interdisciplinary Program (BHIP)

BHIP teams are interdisciplinary ambulatory mental health teams implemented at all VA facilities since their initial pilot in 2013. The BHIP team model is intended to promote continuous access to ongoing recovery-oriented, evidenced-based, outpatient mental health care for a panel of Veterans. This team-based staffing model is consistent with VA's focus on providing comprehensive, integrated mental health care. BHIP teams manage and coordinate services based on the treatment goals set by the Veteran. They are designed to provide the majority of mental health care necessary for a panel of assigned veterans and to coordinate care with other mental health and non-mental health providers. Treating Veterans through a team-based approach provides a proactive focus on the mental health needs and outcomes of each patient as well as improved treatment access, coordination, and continuity of care.

Each BHIP team has a weekly recurring interdisciplinary team meeting as well as daily huddles, which allow them to focus on Veteran needs and daily clinical operations. The services provided include triage, assessment, psychopharmacology, individual psychotherapy, group psychotherapy and case management services. For the most part, Veterans may participate in an episode of care until they are discharged or referred to a lower level of care. There are no time limits on an episode of care, so as to allow that some individuals may require treatment for an extended period of time.

Post-traumatic Stress Disorder (PTSD)

VA excels in the treatment of PTSD and is a national leader for PTSD research, treatment and education of VA and private sector providers on treatment of PTSD. To facilitate the dissemination of best practices for PTSD treatment, VA operates a National Center for PTSD (NCPTSD) created in 1984, whose mission is to "advance the clinical care and social welfare of America's Veterans who have experienced trauma, or suffer from PTSD, through research, education and training in the science, diagnosis and treatment of PTSD and stress related disorders" [17].

To accomplish its mission, NCPTSD created a national PTSD Mentoring program to facilitate the implementation of evidence-based psychotherapy for PTSD and to evolve PTSD treatment to an evidence-based, recovery-oriented model. PTSD Mentors, clinicians who are expert in the treatment of PTSD, are available to provide consultation and guidance to every VA facility PTSD treatment team.

In addition to mentorship for VA staff members, NCPTSD also established a PTSD Consultation Program in 2011 to support any provider who treats Veterans with PTSD. As research findings suggest that community providers are unlikely to have the skills necessary to deliver evidence-based mental health care to Veterans with PTSD, NCPTSD offers consultation to community providers. Clinicians can receive email or telephone consultation regarding the treatment of PTSD including assessment, referrals, and treatment in the interest of training and enhancing their skills. The NCPTSD created and operates a Web site which publishes research-based educational materials for Veterans and families, as well as for the providers who care for them [17].

The VA handbook and VA/DoD Clinical Practice Guidelines for PTSD guide and inform treatment for PTSD. VA policy dictates that every veteran must be screened for PTSD upon entry to the VA, on a yearly basis, and as clinically indicated. Treatments available for PTSD include evidence-based psychotherapy, residential treatment and pharmacotherapy. All VA Medical Centers and very large Community-Based Outpatient Clinics are required to provide either a PTSD Clinical Team (PCT) or a PTSD specialist, based on locally determined needs. In addition, programs must be able to address the care needs of Veterans with both PTSD and Substance Use Disorder by staff that have expertise in treating these co-occurring conditions.

Guidelines require that Veterans are offered evidence-based psychotherapy specifically researched for their effectiveness in treating PTSD: Cognitive Processing Therapy (CPT) and Prolonged Exposure (PE). Other evidence-based interventions may be offered dependent on staff resources and in accordance with Veteran preferences. Each VISN is required to offer at least one program that provides specialized residential or inpatient care programs to address the needs of Veterans with severe symptoms and impairments related to PTSD.

Military Sexual Trauma (MST)

Military sexual trauma (MST) refers to experiences of sexual assault or sexual harassment occurring during a Veteran's military service. It is VA policy that all Veterans treated in VA are screened for MST when enrolled, as many survivors of sexual trauma do not disclose their experiences unless asked directly. This screening is completed by using a MST clinical reminder within CPRS. VA Medical Centers and Vet Centers provide all MST-related care free of charge, and Veterans are able to receive this care even if ineligible for other VA care. This includes care of medical conditions that are related to the military sexual trauma.

Every VHA facility has a MST Coordinator who serves as a contact person for MST-related issues. The MST Coordinator oversees screening programs for MST, provides MST outreach, facilitates referrals for treatment, and ensures that necessary staff education and training is provided. All mental health and primary care staff are required to receive MST training. Lemle reports that VA's integrated MST care exceeds what is available in the community as "widespread screening and treatment programs do not exist in community based care, where mental health care providers are less likely to have relevant experience or recognize that it is important to ask Veterans about MST" [18].

Substance Use Disorders (SUD)

VA has been providing an integrated continuum of evidence-based SUD prevention and treatment since 1973. SUD care in VA is guided by the VA Handbook as well as the VA-DoD Clinical Practice Guidelines for the management of substance use disorders in January 2016 [19]. Treatment options are comprehensive and include screening and brief intervention for alcohol and tobacco use; Medication Assisted Treatment (MAT) for alcohol, opioid, and tobacco use disorders; psychosocial interventions; residential rehabilitation; and evidence-based psychotherapy.

Tobacco Use

Tobacco use is the most prevalent substance use disorder among Veterans, as approximately 1.42 million Veterans are current smokers [20]. Research has consistently shown that both Veterans in VA care and in the U.S. general population who are living with mental health disorders smoke cigarettes at a much higher rate than those without such disorders. For Veterans with these disorders in VA care, their rates of smoking range from 23% to almost 48% compared with a rate of less than 16% among Veterans without such disorders [21, 22].

VA services for tobacco-related disorders are provided in a manner that is consistent with the VA-DoD Clinical Practice Guidelines for Management of Tobacco Use [23]. VA policy requires that during new patient visits and at least annually, Veterans enrolled in primary care, medical specialty settings, and mental health care services must be screened for tobacco use, through a clinical reminder in CPRS.

Treatment options for Veterans who want to quit smoking include brief counseling in primary care, smoking cessation specialty clinics and/or at home through telehealth care. VA offers all FDA-approved smoking cessation medications on its national formulary. VA also operates a telephone quitline, 1-855-QUIT-VET, and a text messaging smoking cessation program called SmokefreeVet, both developed in collaboration with the National Cancer Institute.

Alcohol Misuse

VA policy requires that Veterans enrolled in primary care, medical specialty settings and mental health care services must be screened for alcohol misuse, through a clinical reminder in the CPRS, upon enrollment in the VA and annually. Veterans who screen positive for a substance use problem receive further diagnostic assessment and counseling. Veterans who continue to drink excessively are offered a range of treatments including brief motivational counseling, a referral to specialty providers or other interventions depending on the severity of the condition, and Veteran preference. Facilities must provide at least two empirically validated psychosocial interventions for all patients with SUD who need them, such as motivational counseling, cognitive behavioral therapy for relapse prevention, contingency management, 12-step facilitation counseling, and SUD-focused behavioral couples counseling.

The VA Handbook requires that each facility provides medically supervised withdrawal management (detoxification) in both an ambulatory and inpatient setting. After the veteran is detoxed, they are eligible for a range of coordinated outpatient SUD services, such as general outpatient treatment and intensive substance use treatment programs for all Veterans in early recovery. Intensive Outpatient Program (IOP) provides intense SUD treatment at least 3 hours a day over 3 days a week, delivered by an interdisciplinary clinical team with specialized training in substance use treatment. For those who are unable to take part in IOP due to logistics such as employment, lack of transportation, or other factors, VA provides intensive residential treatment specializing in SUD treatment within each Veterans Integrated Service Network (VISN).

Opioid Use Disorder

According to the Center for Disease Control, on average, 115 Americans die every day from an opioid overdose (including prescription and illicit opioids) [24]. VA is enhancing its efforts to address the opioid epidemic by employing four broad strategies which include education, enhanced pain management treatment, risk mitigation and increased access to SUD treatment. For those Veterans diagnosed with an opioid use disorder, VA offers pharmacotherapy with approved, regulated opioid agonists (buprenorphine and/or methadone) and antagonist medication such as naltrexone.

Opioid agonist treatment in VA is delivered through an opioid treatment program (OTP). VA OTPs are independently accredited by the Joint Commission as well as certified by Substance Abuse and Mental Health Services Administration). VA OTP programs provide evidence-based psychosocial interventions for SUD and opioid agonist maintenance treatment with either methadone or buprenorphine. Co-occurring mental health disorders are to be addressed and treated in the OTP.

Veterans may also be candidates for office-based buprenorphine treatment. Buprenorphine can be prescribed by a prescriber who has a DATA 2000 Waiver in non-specialty settings, such as primary care or general mental health clinics. The Drug Addiction Treatment Act of 2000 qualified prescribers to dispense buprenorphine in an office-based setting after completing 8 hours of training and applying for a waiver through SAMSHA. VA is currently implementing a stepped care model designed to broaden the availability of buprenorphine and naltrexone in non-specialty settings to improve access to SUD care.

Residential Rehabilitation Treatment Programs (RRTP)

The Domiciliary is the VA's oldest program, dating back to 1865 when President Lincoln established a national military and naval asylum for Union Veterans who had served in the Civil War. This was the first major Federal program to provide medical and rehabilitative services to America's Veterans. These programs were initially known as VA homes or Soldiers Homes before evolving into Domiciliaries [25].

The programs have evolved over the years from housing disabled Veterans, into therapeutic programs providing evidence-based clinical rehabilitation addressing mental health, substance abuse, medical and psychosocial needs for men and women. Residential care of this magnitude is unique to VA, and this level of care is not offered in the community sector (with the exception of community residential care for substance use disorder only).

Mental Health Residential Rehabilitation Treatment Programs (MH RRTP) provide a 24/7 therapeutic setting for Veterans with a wide range of problems, illnesses, or rehabilitative care needs that can include mental health, substance use disorder, PTSD, homelessness and co-occurring medical concerns. They provide rehabilitation, community integration, and evidence-based treatment for mental illness. Although these programs have different treatment modalities and eligibility policies, their clinical policies and clinical practices are set nationally and are uniform.

Each VISN is required to provide access to residential treatment and ensure that its programs are able to meet the needs of male and female Veterans diagnosed with serious mental illness, PTSD, military sexual trauma, substance use disorder, homelessness, and dual diagnosis either through special residential programs or specific tracks in residential care programs. To meet their needs, VA provides several types of programs that are either standalone programs or larger domiciliary programs (DOM) where specialty tracks are located in one location.

1. *Domiciliary Care for Homeless Veterans (DCHV)* – DCHVs provide 24/7 structured and supportive residential treatment environment for Veterans who are homeless.
2. *General Domiciliary (General Dom) or Psychosocial Residential Rehabilitation Treatment Programs (PRRTP)* – These programs provide 24/7 residential care for the general Veteran population, treating medical and psychiatric problems, substance use disorders, PTSD, and homelessness.
3. *Domiciliary PTSD (Dom PTSD) or Post-Traumatic Stress Disorder Residential Rehabilitation Treatment Program (PTSD-RRTP)* – These programs provide 24/7 residential care for Veterans with PTSD, including Military Sexual Trauma (MST). Both Dom PTSD and PTSD-RRTPs must provide evidence-based treatment for PTSD.
4. *Domiciliary SA (Dom SA) or Substance Abuse Residential Rehabilitation Treatment Program (SARRTP)* – These programs provide 24/7 residential care focused on specialized substance use disorder treatment to Veterans with substance use disorders.
5. *Compensated Work Therapy-Transitional Residence (CWT-TR)* – CWT-TR offers therapeutic work-based residential rehabilitation services designed to help Veterans return to their communities. Veterans participating in CWT-TR live in transitional housing and are enrolled in CWT working directly on employment goals. This program assists Veterans in finding community employment and building skills for independent living.

Comprehensive Continuum of Homeless Programs

VA's homeless programs, initiated in 1987, constitute the largest integrated network of homeless treatment in the country and are unmatched by private sector programs. The 2014–2020 VA strategic plan established ending Veteran homelessness as a key priority through the Eliminate Veteran Homelessness Initiative [26]. To this end, VA's homeless initiatives are designed to assist homeless Veterans to live as self-sufficiently and independently as possible. VA is the only Federal agency that provides substantial hands-on assistance directly to homeless persons [27].

VA works closely with state and local governments as well as the US Department of Housing and Urban Development (HUD) in its mission to prevent and end Veteran homelessness. VA also maintains and operates a National Call Center for Homeless Veterans (1-877-424-3838). This hotline is designed to assist homeless and at-risk Veterans and their families as well as clinicians and community agencies.

Veterans who are homeless or at risk of being homeless frequently have concurrent mental health conditions or substance use disorders. Therefore, homeless and mental health services at VA are closely coordinated in VA Medical Centers and clinics. Requirements for Homeless Program services are outlined in the Uniform Mental Health Services Handbook. Each VA must employ an Outreach Specialist to provide services to homeless Veterans. Each facility is expected to develop and maintain agreements with community providers for temporary housing, basic emergency services and placement. All facilities are also directed to provide homeless Veterans requiring mental health treatment and rehabilitation programs with care in programs offering the services.

All veterans are screened yearly for the risk of homelessness through a clinical reminder in the electronic medical record system and referred directly to homeless services if needed. VA Homeless Care programs fall into several categories: (1) programs which specifically focus on providing housing to Veterans in the VA and the community via a Housing First model, (2) programs providing biopsychosocial and medical services, and (3) outreach.

Housing First Programs

Housing First is an effective approach to ending homelessness for the most vulnerable and chronically homeless individuals. The Housing First model prioritizes housing and then assists the Veteran with access to healthcare and other supports that promote stable housing and improved quality of life.

Treatment is not required prior to securing housing. Instead, treatment and other support services are wrapped around Veterans as they obtain and maintain permanent housing. VA offers programs such as the Grant and Per Diem (GPD) and Housing and Urban Development-Veterans Affairs Supported Housing (HUD-VASH), that collaborate with federal and community agencies to provide housing. Specifically, the GPD program awards grants to community-based agencies to create transitional housing programs for Veterans. HUD-VASH, a collaboration between the US Department of Housing and Urban Development and VA provides rental assistance vouchers to homeless Veterans who are case managed by VA Homeless Program Staff.

Biopsychosocial Support

VA homeless programs providing biopsychosocial support and medical services include Community Resource and Referral Centers (CRRCs), Homeless Patient Aligned Care Teams (HPACTs), Supportive Services for Veteran Families (SSVF), and specific RRTP programs. CRRCs, strategically located in the community, provide biopsychosocial services to homeless Veterans on a walk-in basis. Veterans are referred to physical and mental health care resources, job development programs, housing options, and other VA and non-VA benefits.

H-PACTs provide a coordinated "medical home" with special expertise in homeless Veterans' needs. In addition to providing primary care, these teams include homeless program staff and others who offer case management, housing assistance, and social services. Supportive Services for Veteran Families provide services to very low-income Veterans and their families at risk of homelessness due to a housing crisis. Services include outreach, case management, assistance in obtaining VA benefits, and help in accessing and coordinating other public benefits. The program can also make time-limited temporary payments on behalf of Veterans to cover rent, utilities, security deposits and moving costs.

At VA Medical Centers, MH RRTP programs are open to any homeless Veteran who meets the eligibility criteria. RRTP programs that specifically address homeless Veteran's needs include Domiciliary Care for Homeless Veterans (DCHV), General Domiciliary or Psychosocial Residential Rehabilitation Programs (PRRTP) and Compensated Work Therapy-Transitional Residence Programs (CWT-TR).

Outreach VA programs providing outreach to the homeless population include the Healthcare for Homeless Veterans (HCHV) and the Veterans Justice Outreach Program (VJO). The HCHV program provides outreach in the community in order to connect homeless Veterans with health care and other services as needed. The program provides case management and has contracts with community-based programs for housing. This program is often the first step in offering homeless Veterans entry into VA care.

The Veterans Justice Outreach Program provides outreach to Veterans who are incarcerated. This program sends VJO specialists into the jails to provide outreach, assessment, and case management as well as provide a liaison with local justice system partners. Once Veterans are released from jail, the Health Care for Re-Entry Veterans Program helps incarcerated Veterans successfully rejoin the community through supports, including addressing their mental health and substance use needs.

Readjustment Counseling Services (Vet Centers)

The Vet Center Program was established by Congress in 1979 to meet the needs of a significant number of Vietnam era Vets who were experiencing readjustment problems and were not inclined to use VA services. Early on, Vet Centers were often located in storefronts and continue to be based in the community today. There are 300 Vet Centers throughout the United States, as well as a fleet of 80 Mobile Vet Centers which provide outreach to rural communities in need of their services.

Vet Centers offer counseling to Veterans who served in theater during any conflict, and their services are available to former active duty, National Guard, reserve service members, and their families, regardless of character of discharge. They provide counseling to any veteran who has experienced military sexual trauma even if they do not meet the other eligibility requirements of the Vet Center. Vet Centers are staffed by licensed mental health therapists and do not provide pharmacotherapy. The goal of the Vet Center program is to provide counseling, outreach, and referral services to eligible Veterans in order to help them make a successful post-war readjustment to civilian life.

Vet Centers also provide bereavement counseling services to surviving parents, spouses, children and siblings of service members who die while on active duty. Vet Centers operate a Combat Call Center; a 24/7 confidential call center where combat Veterans and their families can call for assistance. In FY 2015, the Vet Center Combat Call Center took over 113,000 calls from Veterans, service members, their families, and concerned citizens [28].

Although part of the U.S. Department of Veterans Affairs, Vet Centers are not administratively connected to the VA Medical Center organizational structure. Eligible Veterans or service members can use Vet Center services without being enrolled at VA Medical Centers and do not require a disability rating or service connection.

Vet Centers offer an added level of confidentiality for Veterans and their families, as they maintain a separate health record system from VA. Without the Veteran or service member's voluntary signed authorization, the Vet Centers will not disclose Veteran client information unless required by law. Vet Centers and VA Medical Centers have entered into a memorandum of understanding which defines how they interact to provide treatment for high-risk Veterans, and requires frequent collaboration on shared cases.

Comprehensive Use of Technology to Provide Mental Health Services

A strength of the VA has long been its adoption of technology to provide clinical care. It pioneered the electronic health record technology in the 1970s with the development of its Veterans Health Information System and Technology Architecture) system, and later implemented the computerized records system (CPRS) starting in 1997. Modernizing VA systems is one of the VA's top five priorities.

The former VA Secretary announced in 2017 that VA will improve its electronic medical record by upgrading to MHS Genesis, the same system operating in DoD. This will allow the VA EHR to have interoperability with DoD, enhancing coordinated medical care between DoD and VA. This will allow a seamless transition for service members discharging from the military, as their medical records will follow them electronically to VA.

VA incorporates access to technology throughout its medical system, offering an online portal for Veterans called My Healthe Vet. Through this portal, Veterans can communicate with their providers through secure messaging, track appointments and access health records. VA has launched an appointment request app (Veteran Appointment Request, VAR) that allows Veterans to view, schedule, and cancel primary care and mental health appointments on their smartphones or tablets. In recent years, VA has expanded its promotion of technology-assisted treatment by creating Internet-based resources for Veterans, family members, and clinicians, mobile apps, Facebook, YouTube, and web-based trainings.

VA has developed 15 mobile applications (apps) to support Veterans and their families with tools to help them manage emotional and behavioral concerns, available for cell phones and tablets. These are available online at the VA app store. These programs are designed to help patients track and manage symptoms associated with PTSD, depression, substance use and general mental health conditions. They are intended for self-help or to be used as an adjunct to therapy. These apps are available for both Android and IOS and include PTSD Coach, Act Coach for Depression, CPT Coach for PTSD, PE Coach for PTSD, CBT I Coach for Insomnia, Mindfulness Coach, Moving Forward, Mood Coach for Depression and PTSD Family Coach.

Telemedicine

VA is a national leader and early adopter of telemedicine and continues to use the modality to improve access to care, particularly in rural areas. Telemental Health technology was first used in the United States beginning in the 1950s at the University of Nebraska [29]. By the 1960s, the University of Nebraska was connected to the VA at Omaha, Lincoln and Grand Island to deliver Telemental Health services [30]. For large-scale adoption, however, Telemental Health technologies were too expensive and complex until desktop computers became widespread in the 1990s.

Beginning in 1997, the Veterans Administration implemented substantial startup funding for Telemental Health services nationally. Since then, Telemental Health within VA has expanded dramatically, and in FY 2017, VA delivered over 473,000 Telemental Health consultations to more than 151,600 Veterans [31]. Beginning in fiscal year 2017, VA has focused on expanding Telemental Health care by establishing 10 regional Telemental Health hubs across the VA health care system. These hubs are designed to enhance access to mental health care by connecting clinicians virtually to VA facilities where there is a need for more mental health resources.

Any state licensing barriers to this expansion have been removed with the publication of a new federal rule, "Authority of Health Care Providers to Practice Telehealth," effective June 11, 2018. This legislation allows VA health care providers to practice across state lines throughout the United States and into Veteran's homes, regardless of the state in which they are licensed as long as they hold a valid and unrestricted license to practice.

Clinical Video Technology (CVT) is the technology that allows VA providers from any location to virtually connect to Veterans at multiple sites of care, including

VA Medical Centers, CBOCS and Veteran's homes. Through this technology, VA connects clinical services to Veterans in need of care, providing evidence-based psychotherapy and psychopharmacology for nearly all diagnoses. Initially, CVT was deployed from one VA site to another through video conferencing equipment on its secured network but has now expanded to using a secure Internet-based application (VA Video Connect). This allows Veterans to receive services in their home on a smartphone, tablet, or laptop. Veterans who don't have the means to access this technology at home may receive loaner tablets provided by the VA to complete a course of evidence-based psychotherapy.

Summary

In summary, the Department of Veterans Affairs is the nation's largest provider of mental health services and offers an unparalleled range of programs and treatments. Drawing on its size, scope, and mission, VA provides a comprehensive, integrated continuum of mental health care. The VA healthcare system employs a wealth of clinical expertise, focused on the mission of providing timely, state-of-the-art care to all Veterans throughout their lifespan.

As a unified system, the VA is able to provide a high quality of care, utilizing its national resources to disseminate, implement, and monitor the quality of its clinical care. The National Academies of Science, Engineering, and Medicine 2018 comprehensive evaluation noted that "the VA healthcare system has tremendous mental health care expertise; many and diverse care delivery assets and substantial training and research capabilities." The report concluded that VA mental health care is "positioned to inform and influence how mental health care services are provided more broadly in the United States" [32].

The foundation to VA's success is related to its many strengths, such as national policies; strategic planning; the electronic medical record; expertise in and wide adoption of technology; encouragement of innovation and dissemination of best practices based on research; quality improvement with a focus on national standards, metrics, and outcomes; and collaboration with DoD and community partners. VA's greatest strength, however, are the talented and dedicated employees who make it their personal mission to fulfill President Lincoln's promise to our nation's Veterans.

References

1. US Department of Veterans Affairs. Fiscal year 2017 annual report: modernizing veteran health care. Washington, DC: Department of Veterans Affairs; 2017.
2. US Department of Veterans Affairs. VHA handbook 1103.3: mental health program guidelines for the new Veterans Health Administration. Washington, DC: Office of Patient Care Services, Department of Veterans Affairs; 1999.
3. US Department of Veterans Affairs. FY 2018–2024 strategic plan. Washington, DC: Office of Patient Care Services, Department of Veterans Affairs. Retrieved from: https://www.va.gov/performance/. Accessed 2 Dec 2017.

4. Tanielian, T, Farris C, Batka C, et al. Ready to serve: Community based provider capacity to deliver culturally confident, quality mental health care to veterans and their families. Rand Corporation. https://WWW.Rand.org/pubs/research_reports/RR806.HTML. Published November, 2014. Accessed 13 Jan 2018.
5. Association of VA Psychologist Leaders. The threat to veterans mental health care of renewing or expanding the choice program without supplemental funding; 2017. Retrieved from http://advocacy.avapl.org/pubs/AVAPL%20White%20Paper%20Veterans%20MH%20Care%20and%20Choice%20Program%20Renewal.pdf. Accessed 7 Apr 2018.
6. Longman P, Gordon S. VA health care: a system worth saving. Prepared for the American Legion; 2017. Retrieved from https://www.legion.org/publications/238801/longman-gordon-report-va-healthcare-system-worth-saving. Accessed on 13 Jan 2018.
7. Commission on Care. Commission on care: final report; 2016. Retrieved from https://s3.amazonaws.com/sitesusa/wp-content/uploads/sites/912/2016/07/Commission-on-Care_Final-Report_063016_FOR-WEB.pdf. Accessed on 31 Mar 2018.
8. Watkins KE, et al. The quality of medication treatment for mental disorders in the Department of Veterans Affairs and in private-sector plans. Psychiatr Serv (Wash). 2015;67(4):391–6. Epub.
9. Barry CN, Bowe TR, Suneja A. An update on the quality of medication treatment for mental disorders in the VA. Psychiatr Serv. 2016;67(8):930.
10. US Department of Veterans Affairs. VHA handbook 1160.01: uniform mental health services in VA medical centers and clinics. Washington, DC: Office of Mental Health and Suicide Prevention, Department of Veterans Affairs; 2008.
11. VA/DoD Clinical Practice Guidelines. VA/DoD clinical practice guidelines. Washington, DC: Department of Veterans Affairs and Department of Defense; 2010.
12. US Department of Veterans Affairs. VHA handbook 1160.05: local implementation of evidence-based psychotherapies for mental and behavioral health conditions. Washington, DC: Office of Mental Health and Suicide Prevention, Department of Veterans Affairs; 2012.
13. US Department of Veterans Affairs. Suicide among veterans and other Americans, 2001–2014. Office of Suicide Prevention. Updated August 2017. Accessed 24 Feb 2018.
14. McCarthy JF, Bossarte RM, Katz IR, et al. Predictive modeling and concentration of the risk of suicide: implications for preventative interventions in the US Department of Veterans Affairs. Am J Public Health. 2015;105(9):1935–42.
15. US Department of Veterans Affairs. Facts about veteran suicide. US Department of Veterans Affairs mental health factsheet. Washington, DC: Author; 2018.
16. IOM (Institute of Medicine). In: Donaldson MS, Yordy KD, Lohr KN, Vanselow NA, editors. Primary care: America's health in a new era. Washington, DC: National Academy Press; 1996.
17. PTSD: National Center for PTSD. http://www.ptsd.va.gov/about/divisions/index.asp. Updated February 11, 2016. Accessed 13 Jan 2018.
18. Lemle R. Choice program expansion jeopardizes high-quality VHA mental health services. Fed Pract. 2018;35(3):18–24.
19. VA/DoD Clinical Practice Guidelines. Management of substance use disorders (SUD). Washington, DC: Department of Veterans Affairs and Department of Defense; 2009.
20. US. Department Of Veterans Affairs. Factsheet: VHA mental health care. US Department of Veterans Affairs mental health factsheet; 2016. Retrieved from: https://www.va.gov/opa/publications/factsheets/April-2016-Mental-Health-Fact-Sheet.pdf.
21. SAMHSA (2017). Smoking and mental illness among adults in the United States. The CBHSQ report. Retrieved from https://www.samhsa.gov/data/sites/default/files/report_2738/ShortReport-2738.html.
22. Duffy SA, Kilbourne AM, Austin KL, Dalack GW, Woltmann EM, Waxmonsky J, Noonan D. Risk of smoking and receipt of cessation services among veterans with mental disorders. Psychiatr Serv. 2012;63(4):325.
23. VA/DoD Clinical Practice Guidelines. Management of Tobacco use disorders (SUD). Washington, DC: Department of Veterans Affairs and Department of Defense; 2009.
24. Centers for Disease Control and Prevention, National Center for Health Statistics. FastStats; 2017. https://www.cdc.gov/drugoverdose/epidemic/index.html.

25. Ploppert JR, Smits P. The history and origins of the VA's domiciliary care program. Washington, DC: Office of Mental Health Operations, US Department Of Veterans Affairs; 2014.
26. US Department of Veterans Affairs. FY 2014–2020 strategic plan. Washington, DC: Office of Patient Care Services, Department of Veterans Affairs; 2014.
27. US Department of Veterans Affairs. VA programs for homeless veterans. US Department of Veterans Affairs factsheet. Published January 2018. Washington, DC: Author.
28. Vet Center Program. US Department of Veterans Affairs. http://www.vetcenter.va.gov/. Updated January 17, 2018. Accessed 24 Feb 2018.
29. Wittson CL, Affleck DC, Johnson V. Two-way television group therapy. Ment Hosp. 1961;12:22–3.
30. Whitson CL, Benshoter R. Two-way television: helping the medical center reach out. Am J Psychiatr. 1972;129:136–9.
31. US Department of Veterans Affairs. Telemental health in the Department of Veterans Affairs. US Department of Veterans Affairs health factsheet. Published February 2018. Washington, DC: Author.
32. National Academies of Sciences, Engineering and Medicine. Evaluation of the Department of Veterans Affairs Mental Health Services. Washington, DC: The National Academies Press; 2018.

Part II
Clinical Issues—General

Military and Veteran Suicide Prevention

David A. Jobes, Leslie A. Haddock, and Michael R. Olivares

Case Example: One of four siblings from a single-parent home, a newly enlisted Soldier excitedly realized his lifelong dream to join the military. He had joined the Army National Guard as a Military Intelligence Analyst assigned to the 19th Special Forces Unit. To advance his career, he joined ROTC to commission as an officer, with aspirations of joining Special Forces. But military life was hard; he was challenged by juggling his career and his relationship with his wife, who was an active duty officer. Being in a relationship with another military service member created conditions of continuous tension; there was duty-location separation, various deployments, and school requirements. The relationship came under immense pressure and the related stress led to his developing suicidal thoughts. With the stigma of seeing a mental health provider and its possible impact on his military intelligence career, he rejected professional help and denied mental health issues or any suicidal intent. To all present, he appeared to be an intelligent, focused individual with high potential. He continued to socialize, work, and attend school. Paradoxically, he made plans with friends on the same day he took his life. On that day, he loaded his legally owned 0.40 caliber Glock, walked three miles to the local mountains, and shot himself in an isolated location. Located by smell of decay by local hikers a week later, the Soldier's body was too decomposed in the hot July weather to readily identify; an open casket at his funeral was simply not an option.

Overview

The Department of Defense (DoD) has made the health and well-being of all military service Veterans its top priority. Since the Global War on Terrorism started, over 2.5 million men and women have served in the military and over 2.7 million have

D. A. Jobes (✉) · L. A. Haddock · M. R. Olivares
Department of Psychology, The Catholic University of America, Washington, DC, USA
e-mail: jobes@cua.edu

deployed to either Afghanistan or Iraq [1, 2]. With advances in medical knowledge, training, and technology (i.e., tourniquets and hemostatic dressings), more service members have survived what would have previously been fatal wounds [3].

While this is a great accomplishment, it has created new thresholds for providing the appropriate healthcare for active duty service members and Veterans. Although physical wounds created from gunshots and explosions are visible and often medically treatable, psychological injuries have been dubbed the invisible wounds of war [4]. The potential consequences of these particular wounds are numerous. However, the consequence of greatest concern is suicide [4], which has been particularly true as suicide rates within the Armed Forces have drastically increased in the years following the attacks of 9/11 [5].

Given this drastic increase, the US Congress amended the 2009 National Defense Authorization Act and directed the Secretary of Defense to establish a Congressionally mandated Task Force within the Department of Defense to specifically examine suicide prevention within the military. The DoD Suicide Prevention Task Force was thus established after suicide rates reached a 28-year high among Armed Forces members in 2008, with each of the previous 4 years seeing a significant increase [6].

The DoD Task Force completed its initial report in 2010, after extensive review of the scientific literature and publicly available information, meetings with experts, and information gathering from military installations [7]. Since the report, suicide rates among service members have remained high—with some variation and slight decreases. But these stubbornly high rates continue to pose a major challenge to our Armed Forces' general health, wellness, and readiness to execute missions on behalf of the nation.

In recent years, more military service members have died from suicide than from combat-related mortality [8]. The US Department of Veterans Affairs, Office of Suicide Prevention has noted that post-service Veterans have shown a staggering 22% increase in suicides when compared to US non-Veteran adults [9]. The magnitude of this disparity in suicides between these populations poses a major concern for those who have served in the military.

In previous eras the data showed that serving in uniform was *protective*. But starting in 2008, suicide among service members exceeded the rates of age- and gendered-matched civilians for the first time in the nation's history, and these rates have not meaningfully decreased in the years since. Indeed, as of 2014, approximately 20 Veterans died per day by suicide, which is a 31.1% increase in Veteran suicide since 2001 [9]. Thus, it now seems that the moment a person enters military service they become a part of an organization with known higher risk of suicide perhaps impacting the rest of their life.

The scope of suicide across the Department of Defense can be measured, and broken down by active component (e.g., Army, Marine Corps, Navy, Air Force). While each of these active components can be combined into a singular entity, each also has a distinct mission and culture. In 2008, the Department of Defense began publishing annual Suicide Event Reports to provide up-to-date data on suicides within each service (Table 5.1). These reports display the severity of suicide within the military and are meant to help further prevention, research, and treatment efforts.

Table 5.1 Annual Suicide Rates in the Military by Active-Duty Service, 2011–2015 Suicide Rates per 100,000 by DoD Service [10–12]. These numbers do not include data on reserve and national guard components

Total yearly suicides by DoD Active Duty Service per 100,000					
DoD Service	2011	2012	2013	2014	2015
Air Force	12.9	15	14.4	19.1	20.5
Army	24.8	29.9	22.7	24.6	24.4
Marine Corps	15.4	24.3	23.6	17.9	21.2
Navy	15.9	18.1	12.7	16.6	13.1
Total	18.7	22.9	18.5	20.4	20.2

To understand the suicides in the military, multiple theories, hypotheses, and explanations have been offered. These theories have ranged from mental health issues (e.g., PTSD, depression, mood, disorders), physical health issues (traumatic brain injuries), combat and deployments, isolation, genetics, acquired capability, social support or social problems, financial and legal problems, and many, many more ideas have been presented [13–21]. While many of these studies are helpful and add to our understanding of the problem, they do not get to the heart of the challenge. Castro and Kintzle [22] have pointedly observed, "… the fact of the matter is that we do not know for certain why suicide rates were low in the 1990s and early 2000s, and we don't know why the suicide rates increased in the mid-2000s and continue to remain high." Despite all that is being done to prevent military suicides, the why's of military suicide remain unknown and the how's of military suicide prevention remain remarkably elusive.

A largely assumed explanation for the military suicide problem is the impact of combat. The Army has actively deployed Soldiers to combat zones since the start of the Global War on Terrorism. To this end, the Army is the primary ground force for the US Military and therefore has deployed at much higher rates and for longer periods of times when compared to its sister branches. Obviously, these on-ground deployments in various theaters subject Soldiers to direct and indirect combat engagements.

In turn, rates of PTSD and depression are higher in Soldiers who have been exposed to combat, which might suggest that suicidal ideation and behavior would also be higher in those who have been exposed to combat. Additionally, service member mental health has been shown to be adversely affected by increased exposure to combat [23]. But research shows that this presumed explanation does not hold up under scientific scrutiny. Indeed, a study conducted by Bryan et al. [24] determined that combat was *not* directly or indirectly related to suicidality. Moreover, research conducted under Leardman and colleagues [25] indicated that no deployment-related factors to include combat experiences were associated with increased suicide risk.

Nonetheless the US Army has persevered in their efforts to understand and prevent suicides within their forces. Following DoD directives, the Army has implemented policies, prevention and training programs, messaging campaigns, greater research funding, and more comprehensive medical and mental health services. Yet, even with these significant efforts to prevent suicide, rates have not meaningfully declined from recent high rates. Moreover, the Army is not the only service branch to struggle with this fatal challenge; each of its sister branches has also been struggling to understand the implications and consequences of suicide within their ranks.

For example, the US Air Force has implemented similar policies and prevention programs, but as of August of 2017 suicide is the leading cause of death for Active-duty Airmen [26]. In 2015, the Air Force experienced its highest suicide rate in 20 years [12]. Comparable statistics and trend are similarly seen in the US Navy and Marine Corp [7]. Each branch continues to implement and enhance their suicide-prevention policies and programs, but service member suicides continue to plague these branches.

Recognizing that each branch has their own unique attributes and culture—the Air Force flies and fights in air, space, and cyberspace; the Navy maintains freedom with the naval fleet from the sea; and the Marine Corps merges the gap between the Army and Navy with their amphibious capabilities to conduct both ground and water operations—they all require a level of dedication that asks a tremendous amount of their members. Regardless of branch, service members are asked to continue a rigorous training tempo to maintain readiness for current, future, and unexpected operations. As greater global involvement is demanded of the military, the impact trickles down to each individual Soldier, Airman, Sailor, and Marine.

Military service has long been considered a turning point for disadvantaged men and women. For instance, service during the Vietnam era resulted in setting these men up for success [27, 28]. Serving in the military was also considered a protective factor against suicide until 2005 because suicide rates were much lower in the military than among civilians [7]. Given the historic positive association of military service and lower suicide numbers, the need for military-specific research was not pressing. Consistent across the service branches is a lack of research in suicidology prior to the late 1990s. The 1996 high-profile suicide of Admiral Jeremy Boorda, the Chief of Naval Operations, gave pause to military leadership showing that no matter how high the rank, no service member is immune to suicide risk, which sparked the growth of formal suicide prevention programming [7]. But the dramatic increases of the past decade have prompted a major shift in policy and funding to allocate major resources in the pursuit of preventing these unnecessary and tragic deaths.

In 2011, the RAND corporation completed a major review of military suicide epidemiology and the various suicide-prevention programs and activities within the DoD [29]. Table 5.2 shows their listing of major program initiatives by service branch. These suicide prevention programs generally focus on raising awareness and identifying individuals who may be at risk for suicide, enabling those around them to help at-risk individuals seek medical treatment. The RAND report also noted that while there are suicide prevention programs, there is a lack of evidence supporting these programs' effectiveness [29]. Regardless, RAND identified 35 ongoing suicide prevention programs in the military (see Table 5.2), all of which aim to do the following: [1] raise awareness and promote self-care; [2] identify those at risk; [3] facilitate access to quality care; [4] provide quality care; [5] resist access to lethal means; [6] respond appropriately [29].

Table 5.2 Identified Military Suicide Prevention Initiatives collected by Ramchand and colleagues [29]

Identified Military Suicide Prevention Initiatives in 2011

Air Force	Army	Marine Corps	Navy
1. Air Force suicide-prevention program	1. Army suicide-prevention program	1. Annual suicide-prevention awareness training	1. Annual suicide-prevention awareness training
2. Assessing and managing suicide risk training for mental health clinical staff	2. Three-part training	2. Public information materials on suicide	2. Leadership messages and newsletters about suicide prevention
3. Landing gear	3. Strong bonds	3. Combat operational stress control	3. Reserve psychological health outreach program
	4. Ask, care, escort	4. Suicide-prevention module for the marine corps martial arts program	4. Command-level suicide-prevention program and suicide-prevention coordinator
	5. Resiliency training	5. Command-level suicide-prevention program, suicide-prevention program officers, and installation-level suicide-prevention program coordinators	5. Operational stress control
	6. Applied suicide intervention skills training	6. Operational stress control and readiness	6. Personal readiness summit and Fleet suicide-prevention conference and summit
	7. G-1 suicide-prevention website	7. Noncommissioned-officer suicide-prevention training	7. First-responder seminar
	8. Warrior adventure quest	8. Entry level training in suicide prevention	8. Returning warriors workshop
	9. Re-engineering systems of primary care treatment in the military	9. Assessing and managing suicide risk for mental health providers and chaplains	9. Front-line supervisor training
	10. The Army suicide-prevention task force	10. Are you listening?	
	11. Comprehensive soldier fitness program	11. Front-line supervisor training	
	12. Mental health advisory team		

Concurrent with the RAND report, the Congressionally mandated Suicide-Prevention Task Force also examined suicide in the military and then published their findings and recommendations to the Department of Defense [7]. The Task Force did a thorough investigation into the history of suicide within each branch and examined current suicide policies and prevention programming. First and foremost, the Task Force concluded that suicide *is preventable*. Therefore, considerable efforts and improvement within the Armed Forces is both necessary and urgent.

To help facilitate this effort, the Task Force organized their findings into four focus areas enabling the Department of Defense to utilize the information in the most effective way. These four focus areas are: (1) organization and leadership; (2) wellness enhancement and training; (3) access to, and delivery of, quality care; and, finally, (4) surveillance, investigation, and research [7]. Organizing suicide-prevention efforts into these four categories thus established a clear structure as to what, where, and for whom efforts should be applied to improve suicide prevention programs, policies, and treatments within the US military going forward.

Veteran-Specific Suicide Prevention

Alongside the work undertaken to understand and prevent suicide among active-duty service members, the military establishment has dedicated much effort to specifically addressing the troublingly high rate of Veteran suicide. Given that service members leave the military and are then outside the reach of military-specific prevention programming, the Department of Veteran Affairs (VA) has becoming increasingly active in "picking up" suicide prevention efforts for those who have served in uniform. In the last decade and a half, the VA has notably initiated several suicide prevention strategies, primarily centered on the following components:

1. Bolstering data collection on and evaluation of prevention efforts
2. Providing comprehensive training and education on best practices for Veteran Health Administration (VHA) staff
3. Establishing Suicide Prevention Coordinators (SPCs) across VHA facilities and tasking them with coordinating prevention programs and monitoring at-risk patients
4. Implementing varied-level interventions (e.g., the integration of mental health-care services and primary care, the tracking and targeted treatment of high-risk individuals)
5. Developing and augmenting, in collaboration with the National Suicide Prevention Lifeline, a suicide hotline specifically for Veterans (i.e., the Veteran Crisis Line)
6. Increasing the use and evaluation of contemporary evidence-based psychotherapeutic treatments for suicidality [30]

After evaluating these efforts, a Blue-Ribbon Work Group chartered by the Secretary of Veteran Affairs noted progress that the VHA had made, and further recommended several policy improvements to help reduce suicide risk among Veterans [30]. Many of these recommendations (e.g., enhanced suicide-screening and risk monitoring) have begun to be implemented [31], and will be reviewed below. Critically, the Work Group advocated for greater collaboration across federal agencies and non-VHA mental healthcare providers to facilitate the delivery of effective prevention strategies to all Veterans, irrespective of setting [30].

The expansion of evidence-based suicide-prevention practices for Veterans across non-VHA healthcare providers was seen as an imperative, as only 23% of Veterans receive mental healthcare through VHA medical facilities. Most Veterans do not access mental healthcare through the VHA [30]. For example, only 6 of the approximately 20 Veterans per day who die by suicide are current users of VHA services [32]. Thus, a reduction in suicide rates among the Veteran population will be in part contingent on broad nation-wide change. Indeed, as Bossarte et al. [33] noted in their review of Veteran suicide-prevention strategies, "the success of these efforts will depend, in part, on the ability… to identify and engage those at risk" (p. 462). The following section will thus focus on recent developments in the mission to advance the identification and engagement of suicidal Veterans across all treatment settings (not just VHA).

Identification of Veterans at Risk

Logically, the identification of at-risk individuals is usually a precondition to the delivery of effective and targeted interventions. Unfortunately, the reality is that suicidological science is imperfect. Given the low base-rate of suicide, it is inherently difficult, if not impossible, to predict with certainty whether an individual will take their life [34]. In fact, a recent meta-analysis of the last five decades of empirical work on suicide risk factors determined that suicidology lacked the capacity to adequately ascertain suicide risk [35].

Previously identified risk factors were barely better than chance at predicting suicide. At best, the methodologies used to assess the utility of extant risk factors have failed to prove their predictive value [35]. As such, the ability to connect specific psychological, environmental, or biological risk factors to precise probabilities of suicidal behavior is not presently feasible. Consequently, broad screening efforts may result in more harm than good (e.g., in false positives). In summarizing the state of risk assessment for the DoD and VA, the Assessment and Management of Risk for Suicide Working Group reported that "much of what constitutes best practice [for assessing risk] is a product of expert opinion, with a limited evidence base" [36].

However, as preventing suicide necessitates determining whom to engage, the Department of Defense and military establishment has dedicated much effort to expanding this evidence base and developing more effective methods of risk assessment. In the past half-decade, there has been a trend toward complementing traditional screening methods with alternative measures such as actuarial prediction and implicit markers of risk that do not rely on self-report.

Machine-Learning As the VHA maintains comprehensive data on its patients due to a uniform and integrated health administration system, a primary avenue of research has focused on harnessing machine learning-based algorithms to help better predict potential suicide risk. The first attempt to develop such an algorithm for a military population sought to predict suicide risk among VA patients by analyzing clinical notes contained in electronic medical records [37]. Through parsing the text of clinical notes for patients who had died by suicide, compared with those for psychiatric and non-psychiatric controls, Poulin and colleagues [37] were able to build models capable of identifying the words and phrases most highly associated with suicide risk. For example, words such as "agitation," "frightening," and "analgesia" were predictive of membership in the suicidal cohort. A machine-learning algorithm using these high-risk words and phrases was then able to retrospectively predict suicide risk according to the specific text contained in patients' clinical notes. Although based on a limited number of subjects, this classifier reached between 65% and 69% accuracy in discerning the risk level of a patient [37].

With these promising results, effort began to be directed toward utilizing machine-learning algorithms to predict and reduce post-hospitalization suicide risk among Army members [38]. Using data from the hospitalizations of over 40,000 soldiers, Kessler and colleagues [38] found that a machine-learning model with 68 individual predictor variables (narrowed down from 421) was able to retrospectively identify the individuals with highest suicide risk. The 5% of patients who comprised this highest stratum of risk accounted for 52.9% of post-hospitalization suicides. Kessler and colleagues [38] proposed that actuarial prediction of this nature could thus ensure that resource-heavy, intensive interventions are delivered to the highest-risk subpopulation with the direst need.

Following in the footsteps of a prior feasibility study [39], Kessler and colleagues [32] then developed a machine-learning algorithm capable of predicting high-risk patients among current users of VA healthcare services. To build their model, Kessler and colleagues [32] utilized 381 predictors from five variable domains (e.g., mental healthcare use, demographics, prior suicidal behavior). The researchers tested the fit of various algorithms using data on these predictors from fiscal year 2009–2010 and assessed these algorithms' differential ability to prospectively predict fiscal year 2011 data. These analyses determined that a penalized logistic regression model with only 61 of these predictors was necessary to establish a prediction model with adequate fit and sensitivity [32]. The Veterans who comprise the top 0.1% of risk, according to the prediction model, are 33 times more likely to die by suicide in the following month, 15 times more likely to die by suicide in the following year, and 81 times more likely to attempt suicide in the following year [40].

In 2017, the VHA began implementing this prediction model across all VA medical facilities to undergird a program entitled Recovery Engagement and Coordination for Health–Veterans Enhanced Treatment (REACH VET) [41]. Through REACH VET, high-risk Veterans are identified and then targeted for further care, the goal being to intervene before suicidality develops. Specifically, after a Veteran is selected by the actuarial prediction model, the Veteran's care provider reaches out to assess the Veteran's condition and ascertain whether "enhanced care" (e.g., skills-based training, safety planning, increased monitoring, greater access to care) is warranted. Thus far, at least 20,000 Veterans have been identified through REACH VET [40].

The REACH VET program is currently being evaluated, in comparison with "implementation as usual," as part of a three-year randomized clinical trial to examine the quality and cost of its implementation in 28 VA medical facilities. Given the promise of machine-learning models, efforts are currently underway to search for better predictors from other sources (e.g., online public records, wearable devices) and to examine the potential of using actuarial prediction to additionally determine which interventions to apply to specific patients [32]. While the efficacy of the prediction model powering REACH VET is in part based on the availability of comprehensive VHA data, its construction and findings could inform and enhance the development of machine-learning models for non-VHA settings [42].

Implicit Cognition Another novel method of determining suicide risk that has received much recent attention is the assessment of implicit cognition. As suicidal individuals may be unwilling or unable to convey their suicidality (e.g., due to fear of hospitalization, a lack of self-insight, or stigma), measures of implicit risk, such as the Death/Suicide Implicit Association Test (d/sIAT) [43], may be particularly useful. The d/sIAT assesses the differential strength of individuals' associations with life and death by measuring reaction times within a semantic categorization task; that is, comparing the time it takes to categorize constructs of death (e.g., "lifeless) versus constructs of life (e.g., "survive") with the construct of the self (e.g., "I") [44].

Research by Nock and colleagues [43] first established the ability of the d/sIAT to prospectively predict suicide attempt behaviors among a sample of civilian adolescents at an emergency department. Extending this work to a Veteran population for the first time, Barnes and colleagues [44] demonstrated that, among Veterans hospitalized in a VA inpatient facility, those with greater self-identification with suicide and death (per the d/sIAT) were almost twice as likely to attempt suicide in the following 6 months (irrespective of attempt history). However, as scores on the d/sIAT only predicted an additional 4.6% of variance in suicide attempts, the authors recommended the d/sIAT be used to augment other methods of risk assessment [44]. Further research will be needed to establish the role and utility of such implicit methods of assessment.

Crisis Intervention for Suicidal Veterans

Crisis Hotline and On-Line Chat In 2007, the VA collaborated with the Substance Abuse and Mental Health Services Administration (SAMHSA) and the National Suicide Prevention Lifeline (Lifeline) to create the VA National Suicide Hotline. It was later renamed as the Veterans Crisis Line (VCL) in 2011. As it is staffed by responders with knowledge of Veteran-specific concerns and VA services, the VCL can provide distressed or suicidal Veterans with beneficial coping strategies and skills as well as helpful referrals to further care (e.g., from Suicide Prevention Coordinators) [45]. Research has indicated that crisis lines staffed by paraprofessional responders can be remarkably effective in reducing callers' suicide risk. For instance, an evaluation of the effects of Lifeline contact found that suicidal callers experienced a substantial reduction in suicide risk (e.g., intent to die) throughout the duration of their call and a multi-week diminution in hopelessness and psychological pain after the call [46]. A separate study, in which interviews were conducted with a sample of callers who had utilized the Lifeline, found that suicidal callers followed through with healthcare referrals about 50% of the time [47]. Furthermore, of callers receiving follow-up care from Lifeline respondents (as part of a SAMHSA-funded program), a majority reported that the service stopped them from killing themselves and kept them safe [48].

Likewise, a recent study of the VCL found that approximately 30% of callers reported suicidal thoughts, and, overall, about 80% of callers reported "feeling better" by the end of the call [45]. In the course of this study's 6-month evaluation period, the VCL received 120,000 calls, 25% of which were from Veterans 60 years of age or older [45]. Given that the VCL may serve to mitigate crises before suicidality develops or worsens, media and messaging campaigns may be an effective and valuable mechanism for increasing crisis-line use by Veterans [49, 50].

Safety Planning An especially promising site of prevention may be emergency-care settings, as they represent a primary point of contact between suicidal Veterans and mental health services [30, 51]. This nexus creates an opportunity for identification, intervention, and preventive follow-up. As suicidal individuals who visit an emergency department (ED) are often unlikely to follow through with referrals and maintain treatment, an ED-based intervention that equips individuals to manage future suicidal crises on their own is warranted [52].

To this end, Stanley and Brown [52] developed the Safety Planning Intervention (SPI), a brief stand-alone intervention that involves the collaborative creation of a written list of resources and coping strategies that patients can utilize in the event of a suicidal crisis. Specifically, this list enumerates the steps that should be taken during, and leading up to, a suicidal crisis. These include recognizing warning signs, using predetermined coping strategies, contacting social support for distraction and crisis resolution, and reaching out to professionals and EDs [52]. The SPI additionally includes a discussion of lethal means reduction. Safety planning of this kind is premised on the notion that it is more effective to establish positive crisis-management strategies (with concrete steps) than it is to solicit agreement to keep "safe" and not engage in any suicidal behavior (i.e., with a contract for safety) [52].

The SPI has been recommended as a best practice by the Suicide Prevention Resource Center, the American Foundation for Suicide Prevention, and the Joint Commission [52, 53]. Additionally, the SPI has been adapted for use with Veteran populations and has become a component of standard care for suicidal individuals in the VHA [52, 54, 55]. Two emergent crisis interventions based on the safety-planning concept that have received increasing support are described below.

Crisis Response Planning A Crisis Response Plan (CRP) is a variant of the safety plan approach that has been used in cognitive behavioral therapy for suicidal individuals [56, 57]. Like the SPI, it involves the collaborative elaboration of concrete steps an individual can take in the midst of a suicidal crisis (i.e., utilizing coping strategies, accessing social support, engaging with formal mental healthcare) as well as individual-specific warning signs [53, 57]. This crisis-management action plan is written on a small card that an individual can carry on their person for quick reference when needed.

At its most basic, a CRP consists in a list of reasons for living (or a "survival kit" of hope-inducing objects), a commitment to restrict access to lethal means, contact information for an emergency resource (e.g., suicide hotline), and information regarding a specific ED that can be accessed [57]. In cognitive behavioral treatment for suicidality, the establishment of the CRP is accompanied by a request that the patient formally commit to using it when needed [57].

To date, two studies have analyzed the efficacy of the implementation of CRP as a stand-alone intervention. In the first, active-duty Army Soldiers presenting at an emergency behavioral health facility were randomly assigned to receive CRP, enhanced-CRP (i.e., CRP plus a discussion of reasons for living), or a contract for safety (CFS) [53]. Soldiers who received CRP (irrespective of type) were 76% less likely to attempt suicide in the following 6 months, spent a reduced number of days in inpatient units, and experienced a faster reduction in suicidal ideation [53].

A secondary data analysis of this randomized controlled trial (RCT) additionally examined the immediate impact on mood of each condition and found that both CRP conditions resulted in significantly greater improvement in most emotional states (including the urge to kill oneself) compared with the CFS condition [58]. Furthermore, Soldiers in the enhanced-CRP condition had a significantly lower likelihood of inpatient admission—despite no difference in risk, on average, as assessed by the attending clinician—and significantly higher ratings of calm and hopefulness [58]. In other words, the decision whether to admit a patient may be influenced by the immediate effect of the patient and their responsiveness to the crisis intervention. Bryan and colleagues [53, 58] conclude that crisis response planning could be an especially valuable tool, as its easy administration requires less expertise and time. As such, it may reduce the workload of overburdened service providers in both the short term and the long term (e.g., through reduced inpatient admissions).

SAFE VET The Suicide Assessment and Follow-up Engagement–Veteran Emergency Treatment (SAFE VET) is a brief behavioral intervention focused on crisis management and continuity of care [51]. Designed to enhance the Safety Planning Intervention [52] with structured follow-up, SAFE VET consists in safety planning in an emergency department or urgent care setting, and the subsequent facilitation and telephonic monitoring of suicidal individuals' transition to outpatient care [51]. SAFE VET is intended to create an alternative to hospitalization for moderate-risk patients, and simultaneously identify and coordinate care for high-risk patients [51].

A preliminary evaluation of SAFE VET implementation found that Veterans received it positively, with 93% of referred individuals following through with the program [51]. Furthermore, 80% of these Veterans completed at least one outpatient mental healthcare appointment in the following 6 months, and 60% received psychiatric care in the following 14 days [51]. A subsequent study demonstrated that, among Veterans who had been admitted at least twice to the ED for suicidality within a period of 6 months, SAFE VET resulted in increased treatment engagement (compared with treatment engagement during an equivalent 3-month period following individuals' prior ED admission) [59]. Additionally, both Veteran patients and ED staff have reported the SAFE VET intervention to be helpful in promoting safety and establishing connection to services [60, 61].

Although as designed SAFE VET relies on the position of the VA's Acute Services Coordinator (ASC) for the management and coordination of the intensive follow-up care [51], the role of the ASC could conceivably be translated into non-VHA settings. Like CRP, SAFE VET may reduce the burden on treatment providers at emergency departments and, in redirecting moderate-risk patients who would otherwise be admitted, assist overloaded inpatient facilities. A clinical trial is currently underway to further evaluate the effectiveness of SAFE VET and explore its effect on a variety of outcomes [62].

Clinical Treatments for Suicidal Veterans

Once a Veteran is identified as at-risk for suicide and further intervention is warranted, there should be a ready repertoire of effective treatments for use, according to the needs of the individual patient. While theories of and treatments for suicidality vary, some commonalities to effective suicide-specific interventions have been identified. Specifically, effective interventions tend to (1) employ an intelligible and relatable conceptual model of suicidality; (2) maintain the engagement and investment of the suicidal patient; (3) teach actionable skills for how to manage suicidal ideation and behavior; (4) foster in patients a sense of self-reliance, accountability, and purpose; (5) clarify and establish action plans for accessing emergency services and crisis support when necessary; and (6) retain detailed documentation of the plan and course of treatment [57]. However, there is often a disconnect between research findings and clinical practice, such that, even when an at-risk individual is identified, the most effective methods of intervention and treatment are not always employed [63]. Moreover, there are few evidence-based interventions—aside from hotlines and outreach programs—whose efficacy has been specifically established for use with Veterans in non-VHA settings [31].

While risk factors and correlates of suicidal ideation and behavior have been found to be mostly consistent across civilian and Veteran and military populations, Veterans and service members may differ in their needs and responsiveness to different interventions and treatments [64]. For example, Veteran and military populations may exhibit distinct post-trauma symptoms (e.g., combat-related), face unique patterns of emotion-regulation vulnerabilities [57, 65], suffer from distinct suicidal drivers (e.g., spirituality-based cognitive-affective states related to military experience) [64], and have greater access to and familiarity with weapons [66]. As such, there is a need for all providers to be competent in the delivery of Veteran-specific treatment for suicidal ideation and behavior.

Fortunately, in recent years there has been a surge in clinical studies evaluating the efficacy of suicide-specific treatments for military and Veteran populations specifically [65]. Many of these treatments appear to be effective due to their targeting "mechanisms of action" that are specific to Veteran and military populations (e.g., difficulties with certain aspects of emotion regulation and cognitive flexibility) [65]. The following is a review of the most substantiated and promising of these suicide-specific treatments. While there are a handful of effective treatments proven to work within randomized controlled trials (RCTs), for our purposes we are emphasizing proven treatments for suicidal risk that have been *replicated* with rigorous RCT research.

Cognitive Therapy for Suicide Prevention Developed by Greg Brown and Aaron Beck, a suicide-specific form of cognitive therapy called CT-SP has been shown to decrease repeat attempt behaviors in a community sample by 50% after 10 sessions at 18-month follow-up [67]. Patients in the experimental group also reported significantly less depression-severity at 6-, 12-, and 18-month follow-ups as well as less hopelessness at the 6-month follow-up [67]. This innovative study is a landmark investigation in the field of clinical suicidology. CT-SP involves helping the patient to recognize their "suicidal mode" and then using safety planning and other cognitive-behavioral coping strategies to enable the patient to manage difficult suicidal crises. Importantly, Brown and colleagues [67] developed a relapse-prevention protocol that involves in-session guided imagery exercises of patients' past attempt and their prospective future attempt. Additionally, an innovative intervention created in this study is the "Hope Box," which serves as a memory aid to remind the suicidal patient about reasons for living and objects that will instill hope in the context of a suicidal crisis (e.g., pictures of loved ones, prayer cards, poems, etc.) [67].

Brief Cognitive Behavioral Therapy Brief Cognitive Behavioral Therapy (BCBT) is a time-limited and phase-based version of Cognitive Behavioral Therapy that employs a directive, active, and skills-oriented focus to treat suicidal ideation and behavior [57]. Sessions are organized around three phases of treatment (i.e., orientation, skills focus, relapse prevention), through which patients pass according to their mastery of the particular set of skills associated with each phase [57]. As such, the course of BCBT proceeds differently for each patient, although it is designed to be completed within 12 clinical hours. Phase I involves the establishment of an agreed-upon conceptual model for treatment, the development of basic skills (i.e., in self-management and emotion regulation), and the fostering of investment in treatment. The latter is reified in a written commitment-to-treatment agreement (CTA), whose main components include an explicit list of patient responsibilities, an overview of treatment plans and goals, an actionable safety plan, and an intentional commitment to live (for a specific period of time). Phases II and III involve further development and refinement of skills taught in the orientation phase of treatment [56, 57].

The first study to investigate the efficacy of BCBT, and incidentally the first to study a suicide-specific treatment in a military population, was conducted in 1996 at outpatient, inpatient, and emergency clinics within a VA medical center [68]. In this initial investigation, BCBT, despite its brevity, resulted in comparable reductions in suicidal ideation and behavior to those associated with treatment as usual (TUA). More importantly, BCBT was significantly more effective at keeping high-risk patients with poor problem-solving skills in treatment [68].

Stronger evidence was provided by a recent study finding that, in a sample of active-duty Army Soldiers (with recent intent to die or suicide attempts), those receiving BCBT, compared with TUA, were 60% less likely to attempt suicide in the following 24-month period [69]. While BCBT and CT-SP differ in certain ways, both treatments emphasize precipitating cognitions and vulnerabilities and the development of adaptive functioning within a short timeframe. To this end, such time-limited interventions may be particularly effective within Veteran and military populations.

Dialectical Behavior Therapy Dialectical Behavior Therapy (DBT) [70] has perhaps received the most attention among suicide-specific interventions and treatments. Although it was originally designed to treat severely dysregulated individuals with borderline traits, DBT has repeatedly demonstrated efficacy in reducing suicidal risk through numerous studies and randomized controlled trials [71–75]. DBT involves individual psychotherapy, skills group meetings, telephonic coaching, and weekly consultation team meetings. Psychotherapy within DBT is alliance-centered and composed of techniques derived from CBT and blended with practices informed by Zen and the concept of dialectics (e.g., oscillating between acceptance and change) [76]. Skills taught include relational skills, mindfulness, emotion regulation, and distress tolerance [76].

However, the comprehensiveness of DBT, quite demanding on an already-impaired and distressed client's time and energy, can be a barrier to engagement in a full course of DBT [77]. This comprehensiveness, in conjunction with stringent requirements for therapist adherence, may be a cause of its relative underutilization [78]. Furthermore, much of the empirical support for DBT relies on mostly female samples [79]. Nonetheless, attempts have been made to adapt DBT for Veteran populations to improve treatment retention and accommodate Veteran-specific constraints [77, 78].

For example, to overcome possible barriers to engagement with DBT, Denckla and colleagues [77] proposed and evaluated a DBT-based skills-training group that could be attended on an as-needed basis. The group was structured such that sessions rotated in focus through four DBT-derived skills for tolerating distress and managing crises (i.e., ACCEPTS, IMPROVE the moment, self-soothing, Pros and Cons) [77]. Accordingly, every skill could be learned through attending four consecutive sessions, and relative understanding of one skill could be achieved in a single session. Furthermore, the group was not mandatory, referrals were not required for attendance, and no homework was assigned [77].

Of a cohort of Veterans at a VA medical facility who had refused prior referrals for care, Denckla and colleagues [77] conducted an exploratory evaluation of those who had attended at least eight sessions of this skills group. These Veterans experienced a significant reduction in crisis events (i.e., emergency department visits or inpatient admissions for suicidality) in the year following their joining the group compared with the prior year [77]. Although this study had low internal validity, it suggests that a drop-in, as-needed form of service delivery might be more effective for specific Veteran populations and may eliminate some barriers to care. The study authors further noted that, as some participants joined a full, traditional DBT group after attending the modified group, such a group might facilitate a transition to long-form treatment [77].

Collaborative Assessment and Management of Suicidality The Collaborative Assessment and Management of Suicidality (CAMS) [79] is a suicide-specific therapeutic framework that is compatible with multiple modalities of therapy. As its title suggests, CAMS is a collaborative exploration, elucidation, and treatment of a client's suicidality [79, 80]. The collaborative nature of CAMS extends beyond a simple focus on therapeutic alliance; in CAMS, the therapist and patient sit side-by-side during assessment and treatment planning, as the patient is engaged and encouraged to identify suicide-causing problems and participate in treatment planning. Treatment is thus oriented toward the "suicidal drivers" (i.e., what compels the patient to consider suicide) that the patient defines [63].

At the center of CAMS lies the Suicide Status Form (SSF), a collaborative assessment tool that tracks the nature and development of client-defined suicidal drivers, organizes treatment planning, and maintains a personalized stabilization plan. The SSF also includes a "Core Assessment," collaboratively assessed at the start of each session, which measures psychological pain, agitation, stress, hopelessness, self-hate, and overall risk [79]. Given the flexibility of the CAMS' framework, any intervention or technique, from any modality, may be employed in treatment. Through this approach to care, the patient, in essence, becomes a "member of the treatment team," motivated to understand and treat their suicidality [81]. CAMS concludes when three consecutive sessions occur in which the patient has successfully managed their suicidal thoughts, feelings, and behaviors through enhanced coping and a lowering of overall risk [63].

Evidence has consistently supported the effectiveness of CAMS for treating suicidal individuals. Currently, there are eight correlational clinical trials and three published randomized controlled trials in which CAMS has been shown to reliably lead to a decrease in suicidal ideation, overall symptom distress, depression, and hopelessness [63, 81–83]. Additionally, a superiority randomized controlled trial comparing DBT to CAMS showed CAMS performing comparably to DBT with respect to self-harm behavior and suicide attempts at 28 weeks [84]. Due to its demonstrated value in treating military populations [63, 85–87], CAMS has been continually promoted as a valuable approach to treating suicidal service members and Veterans [65].

Barriers to Treatment

As mentioned, it is necessary to be mindful of the unique contexts and needs of Veterans when translating suicide-prevention research into practice. Prevention strategies and interventions must be structured to address several barriers to Veterans' accessing care that research has identified. Firstly, certain aspects of military service may inculcate stigmatization of mental illness [88]. For example, a survey of OEF/OIF Soldiers and Veterans (62% of the sample) found high levels of self-stigma and perceived public stigma compared with a normed population [88]. Service members and Veterans report that concerns about stigma in the workplace, and its consequences for career advancement, are central barriers to accessing care [88, 89]. In the above-mentioned survey, career-related concerns were the strongest predictor of willingness to seek treatment and significantly associated with a lower likelihood of seeking treatment [88].

A separate, national survey of OEF/OIF Veterans found that negative beliefs about mental illness (e.g., "people with mental health problems cannot be counted on") and treatment (e.g., "meds for mental health problems have too many negative side effects") were significantly associated with a lower likelihood of seeking treatment [89]. In a review of research on military- and Veteran-specific barriers, Vogt [90] additionally noted that feeling deserving of services and as if one belongs in a VHA setting are associated with service use.

In order to address Veterans' negative mental health-related beliefs and concerns about stigma, prevention strategies should accommodate the cultural values in which Veterans were steeped through their military service [91]. For instance, throughout their tenure in the military, Veterans may have come to internalize values that, while undergirding military readiness, significantly impede help-seeking (e.g., collectivism, mental toughness, pain tolerance) [91]. After leaving the military, Veterans may become "trapped in their cultural identity" (p. 100), and have difficulty receiving treatment for suicidal ideation and behavior, when such treatment feels like an admission of weakness and dependency [91]. Accordingly, mental healthcare providers should strive to reframe suicide-specific treatments and prevention programs according to Veterans' values and worldviews (e.g., equating treating mental health to increasing overall strength and fitness) [86].

Conclusion

This chapter has reviewed the challenge of suicide prevention with active duty service members of the US military and Veterans who have left military life. We have reviewed the marked increases in suicidal risk within these populations and various policy initiatives that have been undertaken to decrease this risk. While commendable progress has been made, the rate of Veteran (and DoD) suicide has yet to meaningfully drop. As discussed above, more effort and public outreach needs to be made to disseminate and utilize, across all healthcare providers, the effective interventions and programs that have been identified. Broader implementation of

Veteran-specific suicide-prevention strategies may be assisted by, for instance, the formation of specific curricula at sites of clinical training (e.g., graduate programs) [31]. Additionally, experts could virtually train other providers in the provision of care for suicidal Veterans [31].

Identifying Veterans at-risk for suicide must be complemented by well-matched suicide-specific treatments. Ultimately, more research needs to be conducted to better understand what underlies, sustains, and prevents suicide risk in service members and Veterans. The vignette at the beginning of this chapter evokes the urgency and purpose behind suicide-prevention efforts, as well as the tragedy of ostensibly preventable suicides amongst our Veterans. Fortunately, as Jobes [73] commented, "there are no organizations in the world doing more to understand and prevent suicides than the United States Department of Defense and Veteran Affairs" (p. 130). We hope that this chapter helps convey this important work to providers who can help save the lives of the brave men and women who have served the nation in uniform and yet still too often die by suicide.

References

1. Department of Veterans Affairs. National center for Veteran's analysis and statistics. https://www.va.gov/vetdata/docs/SpecialReports/Post_911_Veterans_Profile_2016.pdf. Effective March 2018. Accessed 16 May 2018.
2. Sheppard SC, Malatras JW, Israel AC. The impact of deployment on U.S. military families. Am Psychol. 2010;65(6):599–609. https://doi.org/10.1037/a0020332.
3. Butler FK. Two decades of saving lives on the battlefield: tactical combat casualty care turns 20. Mil Med. 2017;182(3–4):e1563–8.
4. Holdeman TC. Invisible wounds of war: psychological and cognitive injuries, their consequences, and services to assist recovery. Psychiatr Serv. 2009;60(2):273.
5. Pickett T, Rothman D, Crawford EF, Brancu M, Fairbank JA, Kudler HS. Mental health among military personnel and Veterans. N C Med J. 2015;76(5):299–306. https://doi.org/10.18043/ncm.76.5.299.
6. Kuehn BM. Soldier suicide rates continue to rise. JAMA. 2009;301(11):1111. https://doi.org/10.1001/jama.2009.342.
7. Berman A, Bradley J, Carroll B, Certain R, Gabrelcik J. The challenge and the promise: strengthening the force, preventing suicide and saving lives: final report of the department of defense task force on the prevention of suicide by members of the armed forces. PsycEXTRA Dataset 2010. https://doi.org/10.1037/e660992010-001.
8. Pruitt LD, Smolenski DJ, Reger MA, et al. Department of Defense suicide event report: calendar year 2014 annual report. *National Center for Telehealth & Technology (T2) and Defense Centers of Excellence for Psychological Health & Traumatic Brain Injury (DCoE)*. http://t2health.dcoe.mil/sites/default/files/CY-2014-DoDSER-Annual-Report.pdf. Effective July 16, 2015. Accessed 16 May 2018.
9. Office of Suicide Prevention. Suicide among Veterans and other Americans, 2001–2014. *U.S. Department of Veteran Affairs*. https://www.mentalhealth.va.gov/docs/2016suicidedatareport.pdf. Effective August 3, 2016. Accessed 16 May 2018.
10. US Department of Defense. DoDSER Department of Defense Suicide Event Report: calendar year 2013 annual report; 2014. http://t2health.dcoe.mil/sites/default/files/DoDSER-2013-Jan-13-2015-Final.pdf. Accessed June 2, 2018.
11. US Department of Defense. DoDSER Department of Defense Suicide Event Report: calendar year 2014 annual report; 2015. http://t2health.dcoe.mil/sites/default/files/CY-2014-DoDSER-Annual-Report.pdf. Accessed 2 June 2018.

12. US Department of Defense. DoDSER Department of Defense Suicide Event Report: calendar year 2015 annual report; 2016. http://t2health.dcoe.mil/sites/default/files/DoDSER_2015_Annual_Report.pdf. Accessed 2 June 2018.
13. Baldessarini R, Hennen J. Genetics of suicide: an overview. Harv Rev Psychiatry. 2004;12(1):1–13. https://doi.org/10.1080/714858479.
14. Barnes SM, Walter KH, Chard KM. Does a history of mild traumatic brain injury increase suicide risk in Veterans with PTSD? Rehabil Psychol. 2012;57(1):18. https://doi.org/10.2139/ssrn.1988201.
15. Brenner LA, Gutierrez PM, Cornette MM, et al. A qualitative study of potential suicide risk factors in returning combat Veterans. J Ment Health Couns. 2008;30(3):211–25.
16. Bryan CJ, Rudd MD, Wertenberger E, et al. Improving the detection and prediction of suicidal behavior among military personnel by measuring suicidal beliefs: an evaluation of the suicide cognitions scale. J Affect Disord. 2014;159:15–22.
17. Conner KR, Bohnert AS, Mccarthy JF, et al. Mental disorder comorbidity and suicide among 2.96 million men receiving care in the Veterans health administration health system. J Abnorm Psychol. 2013;122(1):256–63. https://doi.org/10.1037/a0030163.
18. Lambert MT, Fowler DR. Suicide risk factors among Veterans: risk management in the changing culture of the department of Veterans affairs. J Ment Health Adm. 1997;24(3):350–8. https://doi.org/10.1007/bf02832668.
19. Schoenbaum M, Kessler RC, Gilman SE, et al. Predictors of suicide and accident death in the army study to assess risk and resilience in service members (Army STARRS). JAMA Psychiat. 2014;71(5):493. https://doi.org/10.1001/jamapsychiatry.2013.4417.
20. Wilson K, Kowal J, Henderson P, et al. Chronic pain and the interpersonal theory of suicide. J Pain. 2013;14(4):S98. https://doi.org/10.1016/j.jpain.2013.01.731.
21. Wisco BE, Marx BP, Holowka DW, et al. Traumatic brain injury, PTSD, and current suicidal ideation among Iraq and Afghanistan U.S. Veterans. J Trauma Stress. 2014;27(2):244–8. https://doi.org/10.1002/jts.21900.
22. Castro CA, Kintzle S. Suicides in the military: the post-modern combat Veteran and the Hemingway effect. Curr Psychiatry Rep. 2014;16(8):460.
23. Castro CA, McGurk D. The intensity of combat and behavioral health status. Traumatology. 2007;13(4):6.
24. Bryan CJ, Hernandez AM, Allison S, et al. Combat exposure and suicide risk in two samples of military personnel. J Clin Psychol. 2013;69(1):64–77.
25. Leardmann CA, Powell TM, Smith TC, et al. Risk factors associated with suicide in current and former US military personnel. JAMA. 2013;310(5):496. https://doi.org/10.1001/jama.2013.65164.
26. Grudo G. Suicide leading cause of death for active duty airmen. *Air Force Magazine*. 2017.
27. Sampson RJ, Laub JH. Socioeconomic achievement in the life course of disadvantaged men: military service as a turning point, circa 1940-1965. Am Sociol Rev. 1996;61(3):347. https://doi.org/10.2307/2096353.
28. Bryant RR, Samaranayake VA, Wilhite A. The effect of military service on the subsequent civilian wage of the post-Vietnam Veteran. Q Rev Econ Finance. 1993;33(1):15–31.
29. Ramchand R, Acosta J, Burns RM, et al. The war within: preventing suicide in the U.S. military. *PsycEXTRA Dataset*. 2011. https://doi.org/10.1037/e534112011-001.
30. Blue Ribbon Work Group. Report of the blue-ribbon work group on suicide prevention in the Veteran population. *Department of Veteran Affairs*. https://www.mentalhealth.va.gov/suicide_prevention/Blue_Ribbon_Report-FINAL_June-30-08.pdf. Effective June 2008. Accessed 16 May 2018.
31. York JA, Lamis DA, Pope CA, et al. Veteran-specific suicide prevention. Psychiatry Q. 2012;84(2):219–38. https://doi.org/10.1007/s11126-012-9241-3.
32. Kessler RC, Hwang I, Hoffmire CA, et al. Developing a practical suicide risk prediction model for targeting high-risk patients in the Veterans health administration. Int J Methods Psychiatr Res. 2017;26(3):e1575. https://doi.org/10.1002/mpr.1575.
33. Bossarte R, Claassen CA, Knox K. Veteran suicide. Mil Med. 2010;175(7):461–2.

34. Bagley SC, Munjas B, Shekelle P. A systematic review of suicide prevention programs for military or veterans. Suicide Life Threat Behav. 2010;40(3):257–65. https://doi.org/10.1521/suli.2010.40.3.257.
35. Franklin JC, Ribeiro JD, Fox KR, et al. Risk factors for suicidal thoughts and behaviors: a meta-analysis of 50 years of research. Psychol Bull. 2017;143(2):187.
36. U.S. Department of Veteran Affairs and U.S. Department of Defense. (2013). VA/DOD clinical practice guideline (CPG) for management of patients at risk for suicide. https://www.healthquality.va.gov/guidelines/MH/srb/VADODCP_SuicideRisk_Full.pdf. Effective June 2013. Accessed 16 May 2018.
37. Poulin C, Shiner B, Thompson P, et al. Predicting the risk of suicide by analyzing the text of clinical notes. PLoS One. 2014;9(1):1–7.
38. Kessler RC, Warner CH, Ivany C, et al. Predicting suicides after psychiatric hospitalization in US Army soldiers. JAMA Psychiat. 2015;72(1):49. https://doi.org/10.1001/jamapsychiatry.2014.1754.
39. McCarthy JF, Bossarte RM, Katz IR, et al. Predictive modeling and concentration of the risk of suicide: implications for preventive interventions in the US Department of Veterans affairs. Am J Public Health. 2015;105(9):1935–42. https://doi.org/10.2105/ajph.2015.302737.
40. Eagan A. REACH VET: predictive analytics for suicide prevention. Department of Veteran Affairs OR Defense Suicide Prevention Office. www.dspo.mil/Portals/113/Documents/2017%20Conference/Presentations/REACH%20VET%20August%20for%20DoD.VA%20Conf.pptx?ver=2017-08-10-132612-030. Effective August 2017. Accessed 16 May 2018.
41. Office of Public and Intergovernmental Affairs. VA REACH VET initiative helps save Veterans lives: program signals when more help is needed for at-risk Veterans. https://www.va.gov/opa/pressrel/pressrelease.cfm?id=2878. Accessed 16 May 2018.
42. Just MA, Pan L, Cherkassky VL, et al. Machine learning of neural representations of suicide and emotion concepts identifies suicidal youth. Nat Hum Behav. 2017;1(12):911–9. https://doi.org/10.1038/s41562-017-0234-y.
43. Nock MK, Park JM, Finn CT, et al. Measuring the suicidal mind. Psychol Sci. 2010;21(4):511–7. https://doi.org/10.1177/0956797610364762.
44. Barnes SM, Bahraini NH, Forster JE, et al. Moving beyond self-report: implicit associations about death/life prospectively predict suicidal behavior among Veterans. Suicide Life Threat Behav. 2016;47(1):67–77. https://doi.org/10.1111/sltb.12265.
45. Rasmussen KA, King DA, Gould MS, et al. Concerns of older veteran callers to the veterans crisis line. Suicide Life Threat Behav. 2016;47(4):387–97. https://doi.org/10.1111/sltb.12313.
46. Gould MS, Kalafat J, Harris-Munfakh JL, et al. An evaluation of crisis hotline outcomes part 2: suicidal callers. Suicide Life Threat Behav. 2007;37(3):338–52.
47. Gould MS, Munfakh JLH, Kleinman M, et al. National Suicide Prevention Lifeline: enhancing mental health care for suicidal individuals and other people in crisis. Suicide Life Threat Behav. 2012;42(1):22–35.
48. Gould MS, Lake AM, Galfalvy H, et al. Follow-up with callers to the National Suicide Prevention Lifeline: evaluation of callers' perceptions of care. Suicide Life Threat Behav. 2017;48(1):75–86.
49. Karras E, Stephens B, Kemp JE, Bossarte RM. Using media to promote suicide prevention hotlines to veteran households. Inj Prev. 2013;20(1):62–5. https://doi.org/10.1136/injuryprev-2012-040742.
50. Karras E, Lu N, Elder H, et al. Promoting help seeking to Veterans. Crisis. 2017;38(1):53–62. https://doi.org/10.1027/0227-5910/a000418.
51. Knox KL, Stanley B, Currier GW, et al. An emergency department-based brief intervention for Veterans at risk for suicide (SAFE VET). Am J Public Health. 2012;102(S1):S33. https://doi.org/10.2105/ajph.2011.300501.
52. Stanley B, Brown GK. Safety planning intervention: a brief intervention to mitigate suicide risk. Cogn Behav Pract. 2012;19(2):256–64. https://doi.org/10.1016/j.cbpra.2011.01.001.

53. Bryan CJ, Mintz J, Clemans TA, et al. Effect of crisis response planning vs. contracts for safety on suicide risk in U.S. Army soldiers: a randomized clinical trial. J Affect Disord. 2017;212:64–72.
54. Gamarra JM, Luciano MT, Gradus JL, et al. Assessing variability and implementation fidelity of suicide prevention safety planning in a regional VA healthcare system. Crisis. 2015;36(6):433–9.
55. Stanley B, Brown GK, Karlin B, et al. Safety plan treatment manual to reduce suicide risk: Veteran version. Washington, DC: Department of Veteran Affairs; 2008.
56. Rudd DM, Joiner T, Rajab MH. Treating suicidal behavior: an effective time-limited approach. New York: Guildford; 2004.
57. Rudd MD. Brief cognitive behavioral therapy (BCBT) for suicidality in military populations. Mil Psychol. 2012;24(6):592–603. https://doi.org/10.1080/08995605.2012.736325.
58. Bryan CJ, Mintz J, Clemans TA, et al. Effect of crisis response planning on patient mood and decision making: a clinical trial with suicidal U.S. soldiers. Psychiatr Serv Adv. 2018;1(4):108. https://doi.org/10.1176/appi.ps.201700157.
59. Stanley V, Brown GK, Currier GW, et al. Brief intervention and follow-up for suicidal patients with repeat emergency department visits enhances treatment engagement. Am J Public Health. 2015;105(8):1570–2.
60. Chesin MS, Stanley B, Haigh EA, et al. Staff views of an emergency department intervention using safety planning and structured follow-up with suicidal veterans. Arch Suicide Res. 2017;21(1):127–37.
61. Stanley B, Chaudhury SR, Chesin M, et al. An emergency department intervention and follow-up to reduce suicide risk in the VA: acceptability and effectiveness. Psychiatr Serv. 2016;6(76):680–3.
62. Currier GW, Brown GK, Brenner LA, et al. Rationale and study protocol for a two-part intervention: safety planning and structured follow-up among veterans at risk for suicide and discharged from the emergency department. Contemp Clin Trials. 2015;43:179–84. https://doi.org/10.1016/j.cct.2015.05.003.
63. Jobes DA. Clinical assessment and treatment of suicidal risk: a critique of contemporary care and CAMS as a possible remedy. Pract Innov. 2017;2(4):207–20. https://doi.org/10.1037/pri0000054.
64. Bryan CJ. Adjusting our aim: next steps in military and veteran suicide prevention. Spiritual Clin Pract. 2015;2(1):84–5.
65. Bryan CJ, Rozek DC. Suicide prevention in the military: a mechanistic perspective. Curr Opin Psychol. 2017;22:27–32.
66. Kaplan MS, Mcfarland BH, Huguet N, Valenstein M. Suicide risk and precipitating circumstances among young, middle-aged, and older male veterans. Am J Public Health. 2012;102(S1):S131. https://doi.org/10.2105/ajph.2011.300445.
67. Brown GK, Have TT, Henriques GR, Xie SX, et al. Cognitive therapy for the prevention of suicide attempts: a randomized controlled trial. JAMA. 2005;294(5):563–70.
68. Rudd MD, Rajab MH, Orman DT, et al. Effectiveness of an outpatient intervention targeting suicidal young adults: preliminary results. J Consult Clin Psychol. 1996;64(1):179–90. https://doi.org/10.1037//0022-006x.64.1.179.
69. Rudd MD, Bryan CJ, Wertenberger EG, et al. Brief cognitive-behavioral therapy effects on post-treatment suicide attempts in a military sample: results of a randomized clinical trial with 2-year follow-up. Am J Psychiatr. 2015;172(5):441–9. https://doi.org/10.1176/appi.ajp.2014.14070843.
70. Linehan MM. Cognitive behavioral treatment of borderline personality disorder. New York: Guilford Press; 1993.
71. Koons CR, Robins CJ, Tweed JL, et al. Efficacy of dialectical behavior therapy in women veterans with borderline personality disorder. Behav Ther. 2001;32(2):371–90. https://doi.org/10.1016/s0005-7894(01)80009-5.
72. Kliem S, Kroger C, Kosfelder J. Dialectical behavior therapy for borderline personality disorder: a meta-analysis using mixed-effects modeling. J Consult Clin Psychol. 2010;78(6):936–51.

73. Linehan MM, Comtois KA, Murray AM, et al. Two-year randomized controlled trial and follow-up of dialectical behavior therapy vs therapy by experts for suicidal behaviors and borderline personality disorder. Arch Gen Psychiatry. 2006;63(7):757. https://doi.org/10.1001/archpsyc.63.7.757.
74. Lynch TR, Trost WT, Salsman N, Linehan MM. Dialectical behavior therapy for borderline personality disorder. Annu Rev Clin Psychol. 2007;3(1):181–205. https://doi.org/10.1146/annurev.clinpsy.2.022305.095229.
75. Verheul R, Louise MC, Van Den Bosch LM, et al. Dialectical behaviour therapy for women with borderline personality disorder. Br J Psychiatry. 2003;182(02):135–40. https://doi.org/10.1192/bjp.182.2.135.
76. Linehan MM, Dexter-Mazza ET. Dialectical behavior therapy for borderline personality disorder. In: Barlow DH, editor. Clinical handbook of psychological disorders: a step-by-step treatment manual. 4th ed. New York: Guilford; 2008. p. 365–420.
77. Denckla CA, Bailey R, Jackson C, Tatarakis J, Chen CK. A novel adaptation of distress tolerance skills training among military veterans: outcomes in suicide-related events. Cogn Behav Pract. 2015;22(4):450–7. https://doi.org/10.1016/j.cbpra.2014.04.001.
78. Spoont MR, Sayer NA, Thuras P, et al. Adaptation of dialectical behavior therapy by a VA medical center. Psychiatr Serv. 2003;54(5):627–9. https://doi.org/10.1176/appi.ps.54.5.627.
79. Jobes DA. Managing suicidal risk: a collaborative approach. New York: The Guilford Press; 2016.
80. Jobes DA, Au JS, Siegelman A. Psychological approaches to suicide treatment and prevention. Curr Treat Options Psychiatry. 2015;2(4):363–70. https://doi.org/10.1007/s40501-015-0064-3.
81. Jobes DA. The collaborative assessment and Management of Suicidality (CAMS): an evolving evidence-based clinical approach to suicidal risk. Suicide Life Threat Behav. 2012;42(6):640–53. https://doi.org/10.1111/j.1943-278x.2012.00119.x.
82. Comtois KA, Jobes DA, O'Connor SS, et al. Collaborative assessment and management of suicidality (CAMS): feasibility trial for next-day appointment services. Depress Anxiety. 2011;28(11):963–72. https://doi.org/10.1002/da.20895.
83. Jobes DA, Comtois K, Gutierrez P, et al. A randomized clinical trial of the collaborative assessment and management of suicidality vs. enhanced care as usual for suicidal soldiers. January 2014. https://doi.org/10.21236/ada599270.
84. Andreasson K, Krogh J, Wenneberg C, et al. Effectiveness of dialectical behavior therapy versus collaborative assessment and management of suicidality treatment for reduction of self-harm in adults with borderline personality traits and disorder-a randomized observer-blinded clinical trial. Depress Anxiety. 2016;33(6):520–30. https://doi.org/10.1002/da.22472.
85. Jobes DA, Wong SA, Conrad AK, et al. The collaborative assessment and management of suicidality versus treatment as usual: a retrospective study with suicidal outpatients. Suicide Life Threat Behav. 2005;35(5):483–97. https://doi.org/10.1521/suli.2005.35.5.483.
86. Jobes DA. Reflections on suicide among soldiers. Psychiatry. 2013;76(2):126–31.
87. Jobes DA, Lento R, Brazaitis K. An evidence-based clinical approach to suicide prevention in the Department of Defense: the collaborative assessment and management of suicidality (CAMS). Mil Psychol. 2012;24(6):604–23.
88. Brown NB, Bruce SE. Stigma, career worry, and mental illness symptomatology: factors influencing treatment-seeking for operation enduring freedom and operation Iraqi freedom soldiers and veterans. Psychol Trauma. 2016;8(3):276–83.
89. Vogt D, Fox AB, Leone B. Mental health beliefs and their relationship with treatment seeking among U.S. OEF/OIF Veterans. J Trauma Stress. 2014;27(3):307–13. https://doi.org/10.1002/jts.21919.
90. Vogt D. Mental health-related beliefs as a barrier to service use for military personnel and Veterans: a review. Psychiatr Serv. 2011;62(2):135–42. https://doi.org/10.1176/appi.ps.62.2.135.
91. Bryan CJ, Jennings KW, Jobes DA, et al. Understanding and preventing military suicide. Arch Suicide Res. 2012;16:95–110.

Treatment for Trauma-Related Disorders: The "Three Buckets" Model

Elspeth Cameron Ritchie, Rachel M. Sullivan, and Kyle J. Gray

Introduction

Posttraumatic stress disorder (PTSD) is a complex disorder that involves several cognitive, emotional, and behavioral responses to an experienced or witnessed trauma that persist longer than 1 month and cause dysfunction in the patient's life. An estimated 6.8% of Americans will suffer from PTSD in their lifetime [1].

While PTSD continues to gain attention in the scientific literature and media, it is important to recognize that this is not just a disorder experienced by our military members. The patients who suffer from this disorder form a heterogeneous group and, not surprisingly, there is no silver bullet treatment. Practitioners treating this disorder are best served by having an array of treatment options.

This chapter develops the idea of the "three buckets" concept for PTSD treatment, focusing specifically on the "third bucket" that comprises "everything else." The "everything else" refers to treatments that have not yet been as rigorously tested (i.e., in large, well-controlled clinical trials) but are nevertheless very helpful in certain individuals. This definition includes complementary and alternative medicine (CAM) and emerging treatments.

E. C. Ritchie (✉)
Department of Psychiatry, MedStar Washington Hospital Center, Washington, DC, USA

Georgetown University School of Medicine, Washington, DC, USA

George Washington University School of Medicine, Washington, DC, USA

Uniformed Services University of the Health Sciences, Silver Spring, MD, USA

R. M. Sullivan
Psychiatry Residency Program, Tripler Army Medical Center, Behavioral Health, Honolulu, HI, USA

K. J. Gray
Walter Reed National Military Medical Center, Behavioral Health, Bethesda, MD, USA

While there are many therapies within the third bucket that deserve attention, we highlight the ones that we have found most useful in our practice. These include meditation, animal-assisted therapy, acupuncture, and transcranial magnetic stimulation (TMS).

Traumatic experiences span a wide variety. We will focus here on reactions to combat trauma. Another widely discussed trauma is sexual assault. There are some important differences in the epidemiology, etiology, and reactions to both combat versus sexual trauma, which will only briefly be discussed here.

Current Definition of PTSD

The *Diagnostic and Statistical Manual of Mental Disorders*, Fifth Edition (DSM-5) is the 2013 update to the *American Psychiatric Association's* classification and diagnostic tool, which, in the United States, serves as a universal authority for psychiatric diagnosis [2]. This manual describes the criteria for the diagnosis of PTSD.

DSM-5 criteria now identify the trigger to PTSD as exposure to actual or threatened death, serious injury, or sexual violation. The diagnosis of PTSD is currently based on eight criteria from the DSM-5.

The first four criteria pertain to the "actual event" and must result from one or more of the following scenarios, in which the individual:

1. Directly experiences the traumatic event
2. Witnesses the traumatic event in person
3. Learns that the traumatic event occurred to a close family member or close friend
4. Experiences first-hand repeated or extreme exposure to aversive details of the traumatic event

The disturbance, regardless of its trigger, causes clinically significant distress or impairment in the individual's social interactions, capacity to work, or other important areas of functioning. It is not the physiological result of another medical condition, medication, drugs, or alcohol.

Symptoms that accompany PTSD should be present for 1 month following the initial traumatic event and include reexperiencing, avoidance, negative cognitions and mood, and arousal, explained as follows:

- Reexperiencing covers spontaneous memories of the traumatic event, recurrent dreams related to it, flashbacks, or other intense or prolonged psychological distress.
- Avoidance refers to distressing memories, thoughts, feelings, or external reminders of the event.
- Negative cognitions and mood represent myriad feelings, from a persistent and distorted sense of blame of self or others, to estrangement from others or markedly diminished interest in activities, to an inability to remember key aspects of the event.
- Finally, arousal is marked by aggressive, reckless, or self-destructive behavior, sleep disturbances, hypervigilance, or related problems.

Common Comorbidities with PTSD

Trauma exposure can lead to a variety of negative mental and physical health sequelae beyond PTSD symptomatology and, as such, is commonly associated with at least one comorbidity. In fact, according to the National Comorbidity Survey data, 50% of patients with PTSD have three comorbid psychiatric diagnoses (16% and 17% have one and two additional psychiatric diagnoses, respectively) [3]. Substance use disorders, depressive disorders, and anxiety disorders appear to be the most common comorbid psychiatric conditions; prevalence rates of these disorders are two to four times higher in patients with PTSD than those without [3].

Among physical conditions, perhaps the most striking evidence is for comorbid TBI and chronic pain. Regarding the former, among the subpopulation of American soldiers returning from Iraq and Afghanistan who are diagnosed with mild TBI, 62% screened positive for PTSD. Only 11% of soldiers screened positive for PTSD overall in this study [4].

For chronic pain, studies show that up to one-half to three-quarters of patients with PTSD have a significant chronic pain condition. Scioli-Salter et al. provide an interesting review offering insight into some of the shared underlying neurophysiology of the conditions and their implications for treatment. Importantly, they note that patients who have both conditions experience greater pain, emotional distress, and disability than patients with either condition alone [5]. CAM for pain is covered in more detail elsewhere in this volume.

With this information in mind, it is key to consider a patient's comorbidities when prescribing treatment. For example, knowing that a patient suffers from chronic pain may lead a provider to consider acupuncture over other CAM modalities, as acupuncture is often commonly used to treat pain as well.

The "Three Buckets" Concept

One of the ideas that we believe is helpful to frame treatment options to patients is a concept termed by the first author as the "three buckets" of treatment for PTSD [6].

The first two buckets comprise the evidence-based therapies: medication and psychotherapy, respectively. Again, these therapies have demonstrated benefit in many large, randomized controlled trials and so are termed "evidence-based." These therapies have been covered extensively in other forums, so will only be summarized here.

The third bucket is "everything else" and is the focus of this chapter. While many of these therapies are starting to accumulate more rigorous academic study, most are still in the anecdotal phases of evidence accumulation. Some, such as meditation and acupuncture, have their roots established in thousands of years of tradition but little scientific theory. These comprise Complementary and Alternative Medicine (CAM) or integrative medicine, and often have their origins in ancient Asian medicine traditions. Others in this bucket, like transmagnetic cranial stimulation (TMS), are also rooted in Western medicine and scientific theory, but are just emerging as therapies for PTSD.

We encourage an open dialogue between patients and practitioners to help choose a regimen that works for them. Before delving deeper into the pros and cons of the third bucket, it is helpful to briefly review the first two and why patients may shy away from them.

Medications ("The First Bucket")

Medications can generally be very helpful for PTSD. Although only sertraline (Zoloft) and paroxetine (Paxil) are FDA approved for PTSD, many other antidepressants are used.

The first line of treatment is usually the antidepressant classes of SSRIs (selective serotonin reuptake inhibitors) or SNRIs (serotonin and norepinephrine reuptake inhibitors). The SSRIs are covered in more detail in the chapter on "Treatment Resistant Depression" in this volume by Lande.

Side effects are usually mild, such as dizziness and nausea. These usually go away in a few days. More problematic side effects are sexual ones, which include delayed or absent erections and decreased libido. If there are sexual side effects we can usually manage them, by switching medications, drug holidays or with phosphodiesterase inhibitors, such as sildenafil (Viagra). However, it is important to ask about these side effects, or risk nonadherence and the patient not returning.

Additional medication options include prazosin (Minipress), which is not yet FDA-approved for PTSD-related nightmares, but is frequently used for this purpose. The main limiting factor for this medication is orthostasis. Patients should be educated to get up slowly from lying down.

Many practitioners prescribe second-generation antipsychotics (usually quetiapine (Seroquel) or risperidone (Risperdal)) for refractory or partial response cases. The evidence for the use of these agents is not as strong and they carry significant health risks in their association with metabolic syndrome (i.e., weight gain, diabetes, and hyperlipidemia). Nevertheless, they are frequently used in clinical practice, probably because they seem to help in many patients.

Psychotherapy (The Second Bucket)

The second bucket includes psychotherapies, or as we say to our patients, "talking therapies." Evidence-based psychotherapy consists of trauma-focused cognitive-behavioral therapy such as exposure therapy (including virtual reality exposure therapy [7]), cognitive behavioral therapy (CBT), eye movement desensitization and reprocessing (EMDR), narrative treatments (narrative exposure and written exposure therapies such as Cognitive Processing Therapy), and cognitive behavioral therapy (CBT). In general, these processes include talking about the trauma and reducing the anxiety associated with it. These are all described in the 2017 VA/DOD Clinical Practice guidelines for the management of posttraumatic stress disorder and acute stress disorder, which can be found at the following link: https://www.healthquality.va.gov/guidelines/MH/ptsd/VADoDPTSDCPGClinicianSummaryFinal.pdf.

Traditionally, the trauma-focused therapies involve 12–20 sessions over many weeks. Recently, there have been efforts to shorten the time involved [8].

The main limiting factors specific to this trauma-based therapy are thought to be that patients cannot tolerate the increased anxiety during the sessions, or an inability to establish a good therapeutic alliance.

Understanding these limitations and the reasons our patients drop out of treatment can help us address this problem. Unfortunately, a recent study shows that only 52% of soldiers who screened positive for PTSD received minimally adequate care (four or more visits in 6 months), and 24% dropped out of care [9]. Of those who dropped out, 39% reported not liking the medication offered and two-thirds reported some form of discomfort with the mental health professional, such as that the practitioner was not adequately caring, communicative, or competent.

There have been efforts to minimize the anxiety with these therapies, including propranolol, and the use of calming agents, such as pets. Additionally, the Department of Defense (DoD) has developed the mobile app PTSD Coach, intended to provide psycho-education and self-management tools for trauma survivors with PTSD symptoms [7].

Understanding these limitations of the first two buckets, we endeavor to discuss how treatments from the third bucket can be incorporated into practice.

Complementary and Alternative Medicine or Integrative Medicine

First, it is important to clarify terms. According to the National Center for Complementary and Integrative Health (NCCIH) at the National Institutes of Health (NIH), "complementary" refers to non-mainstream practices that are used *together with* conventional medicine and "alternative" medicine is the term used when a practice is used *in place of* conventional medicine [10]. These practices are increasingly integrated into conventional medicine (prompting use of another related term, "integrative medicine").

CAM is commonly used by military members with PTSD (45% of active duty military versus 38% of civilians use CAM) [11]. The Veterans Affairs (VA) healthcare system reports that nearly 90% of their facilities offer CAM (mostly meditation), according to a 2011 survey [12]. Moreover, the VA has conducted a comprehensive literature review of CAM for PTSD and funded several ongoing clinical trials on meditation [13]. The review identified seven randomized controlled trials and two nonrandomized studies of CAM for PTSD [14]. They demonstrated there was strongest evidence (moderate) for benefit from acupuncture with recommendation for more rigorous study on this method and meditation.

This review will focus on three areas of CAM for PTSD in which we have the most experience and the most evidence is available: meditation, canine therapy, and acupuncture. Several other CAM techniques are used for PTSD and we encourage practitioners to read more in our book, *Posttraumatic Stress Disorder and Related Diseases in Combat Veterans* [15, 16].

Meditation

Meditation is the most widely used CAM for PTSD [12]. In addition to the advantages of all CAM therapies as stated above, it is a self-management approach that is safe, cost-friendly, portable, and easy-to-learn. This "self-management" aspect is often considered one of its greatest strengths in that it empowers patients to take an active role in their own healing process, and gives them a sense of control over their symptoms.

Meditation can be broadly conceptualized as a form of "mental training." It has a long history, rooted in ancient cultures and has evolved to take numerous styles. Most research on meditation for PTSD focuses on three broad types: mindfulness meditation, mantram repetition, and compassion meditation.

Mindfulness meditation has been the most well studied and has additional evidence that it may be useful in patients with comorbid conditions like depression, substance use disorders and sleep disturbance, and chronic pain [16]. Thus, it may be preferred in patients with these comorbidities. However, the best choice for the patient will largely depend on which practice most resonates with the patient (and they most likely will adhere to), availability, and teacher experience.

Regardless of type of meditation, there is evidence of activation of a common cognitive pathway wherein the benefits of meditation for PTSD may be derived. A recent quantitative meta-analysis of 10 neuroimaging studies across many different meditative practices showed activation of the left caudate body, the left entorhinal cortex, and the medial prefrontal cortex. While the significance of these findings is still being determined, we know that many of the symptoms of PTSD, such as hyperarousal and persistent fear states correlate with an overactivation of the amygdala. Activation of the prefrontal cortex can help regulate this response, leading to greater stress tolerance and self-acceptance [17, 18].

Mindfulness Meditation

Mindfulness meditation (MM) has a primary focus on breathing with an aim to achieve open, nonjudgmental awareness and acceptance. Research findings consistently demonstrate that this form of meditation produces improved health-related quality of life and well-being, as well as reduced avoidance, depression, and numbing symptoms. Importantly, and in contrast to some conventional treatments for PTSD, the practice is also associated with good treatment adherence, and meditation practice compliance at up to 6 months' follow-up [19].

Mantram Meditation

Mantram meditations are a group of meditations that include mantram repetition, transcendental meditation (TM), and relaxation response training which use the common technique of repeating a word, phrase, or sound. This process aims to redirect the person's attention from rumination and maladaptive thought patterns, instead creating a sense of peace and relaxation [20, 21]. Similar to MM, mantram meditations have been shown to decrease symptoms of PTSD such as hyperarousal [22, 23]. This decrease in symptoms is thought to be mediated through a physiologic relaxation response [22, 24].

Mantram repetition has also been associated with an increase in existential spiritual well-being that may contribute to its overall health and mental health benefits. Researchers cite importance in the spiritual meaning of the words selected by the individual and their potential power in eliciting feelings of well-being and self-confidence [23, 25].

Compassion Meditation

Compassion meditation, as the name suggests, emphasizes a sense of compassion or "loving-kindness" to all beings. It, too, takes many forms, but is primarily informed by Buddhist practice. Tonglen is one specific type of compassion meditation that is based on the Tibetan Buddhist tradition and involves the visualization of transforming another person's suffering into compassion [26].

Several studies suggest that compassion meditation has several positive outcomes that would benefit patients with PTSD. Like other meditative forms, compassion meditation has been shown to reduce hyperarousal. It additionally increases social connectedness measures, which can translate into improved social support and personal relationships that are key to recovery. Finally, compassion meditation has been shown generally to both increase positive emotions and decrease negative affect, which may, among other obvious benefits, improve the patient's capacity for resilience, making a case not just for its use in recovery but also in prevention of PTSD15 [25, 27–31].

Animal-Assisted Activities and Therapy

The two main categories of incorporating animals into healthcare and disability are animal-assisted activities, most commonly service dogs, and animal-assisted therapy (AAT).

Animal-Assisted Activities

The Americans with Disabilities Act (ADA) defines "service animals" as animals that have been individually trained to do work or perform tasks to aid a person with a disability [32]. The ADA specifically identifies calming a person with PTSD as one such specific task, but it is important to distinguish these kinds of highly trained dogs from pets whose sole function is to provide emotional support. The service dog designation allows for the dog to accompany the person with PTSD in all areas of facilities where the public is normally allowed to go. Service dogs of veterans may be qualified to receive veterinary care benefits through the VA. We recommend checking with your local VA.

Animal-Assisted Therapy

Scientific evidence demonstrating improvement in symptoms of PTSD from canine and equine therapy lags behind the remarkable growing interest and popularity of these programs. However, a growing body of evidence shows that the nurturing involved in this type of therapy provides positive sensory stimulation that can activate the antistress and pro-social neural and neurohormonal networks (e.g., increase oxytocin) in both humans and animals [33–37]. Furthermore, interactions with animals have been shown to decrease blood pressure and have a calming effect on individuals with dissociative disorder [38, 39].

Even just the presence of animals in a healthcare setting may be therapeutic. Studies have shown that their presence can increase the willingness to enter into therapy, facilitate therapeutic alliance, reduce the rate of attrition, and reduce symptoms of trauma [40–42]. One recent study found that adults who wrote about a recalled trauma in the presence of dogs found the exercise less distressing and had significantly reduced symptoms of depression at follow-up than those who completed the writing exercise without a dog [33].

Animal-assisted activities and therapy can be challenging to incorporate into practice; we recommend looking thoroughly into local resources, ensuring the program is reputable and will fit your patient's needs. When done correctly, this type of therapy appears to be particularly beneficial to patients who struggle with more of the avoidance and isolation symptoms of PTSD; the animals can help serve as a bridge to broader, healthier social interactions (Fig. 6.1).

Acupuncture

Acupuncture is an ancient treatment that utilizes thin, filament-like needles placed on the body to treat a variety of health (and even spiritual) problems. Its foundation is in traditional Chinese medicine (TCM) but since its first use thousands of years ago, it has been adopted by cultures all over the world leading to a multitude of different practice styles and philosophies. However, core aspects of the treatment remain the same.

Acupuncture was originally developed around a concept of a circulating life force known as *qi*. This concept elicits a great deal of skepticism and controversy and is not adopted as a framework by all practitioners. However, it is useful noting at least for historical reference.

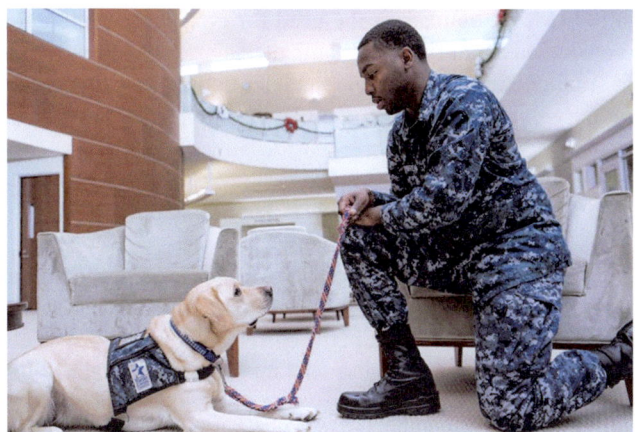

Fig. 6.1 Picture from National Intrepid Center of Excellence (NICoE) facebook page; picture uploaded 10MAR2016: https://www.facebook.com/NationalIntrepidCenterofExcellence/photos/a.10150163476202035.299199.156392117034/10153289164492035/?type=3&theater

Qi is thought to be conducted between the surface of the body and internal organs via 12 main and 8 secondary pathways called meridians. This normal flow can be disrupted by the opposing forces of yin and yang, influenced by environmental factors such as illness, trauma, and stress. Acupuncture targets points along the meridians in an effort to balance yin and yang and restore the normal flow of qi [43].

Modern scientists who may or may not subscribe to the above theory have attempted to explain some of the perceived benefits of acupuncture through other means. However, the clinical application of modern research on acupuncture is often limited by study design, sample size, selection of appropriate controls, and nonstandardized selection of points based on traditional methods of diagnosis and treatment [44].

While the specifics of this nascent research goes beyond the scope of this review, some of the research is starting to point to possible mechanisms such as: the release of endogenous opioids; modulation of neurotransmitters such as serotonin, norepinephrine, dopamine and GABA; effects on neurotrophins and cytokines to reduce inflammation; effects on the autonomic nervous system; regulation of the neuroendocrine system [45–47]. Each of these factors is known to be dysregulated to some degree in patients with PTSD.

In regard to how acupuncture fares against conventional treatments for PTSD (or waitlist controls), the evidence is again mixed, but seems generally favorable. A systematic review of four randomized controlled trials (RCTs) and two uncontrolled trials that met criteria for meta-analysis had several important findings. One high-quality RCT showed significant improvement (i.e., on posttraumatic symptom scale self-report and three other outcome measures) compared to waitlist controls but not significantly greater than the improvement seen with CBT. Two lesser quality studies, one of which had a high risk of bias, showed acupuncture plus moxibustion (another TCM technique) was superior to oral selective serotonin reuptake inhibitors (SSRI) therapy for PTSD [48].

As with all CAM, we emphasize the need for greater research before acupuncture can be considered as a first-line treatment. The existent literature is encouraging however. Acupuncture remains an excellent choice for adjunctive therapy for PTSD, particularly in patients with comorbid chronic pain.

Transcranial Magnetic Stimulation (TMS)

Transcranial magnetic stimulation (TMS) is a noninvasive brain stimulation technique that is FDA-approved for treatment of depression in patients who do not respond to at least one antidepressant in the current episode. Given its efficacy in the treatment of depression and its promise as a more benign, localized brain stimulation therapy alternative to electroconvulsive therapy (ECT), it continues to be vigorously researched and used off-label for a variety of additional uses. Despite its off-label use, at this time there is limited evidence in its use for this diagnosis, as PTSD treatment using TMS is an emerging area of research with additional study needed.

Without going into technicalities that are beyond the scope of this chapter, TMS devices use a coil placed near the patient's scalp to generate an electromagnetic current. This current stimulates a change in flow of the ionic current of the electrically conductive neuronal tissue, leading to neurotransmitter release. This local stimulation in turn can have downstream effects on additional neural networks leading to broader effects [49].

Researchers have successfully used TMS as a diagnostic technique to measure brain GABAergic and glutamatergic tone. Using a paired pulse technique, Rossi et al. [50] reported in 2009 that 20 drug-naïve patients with PTSD had reduced GABAergic tone in bilateral hemispheres and increased glutamatergic tone in the right hemisphere. Animal models have also demonstrated reduced GABA levels in the setting of chronic unpredictable mild stress, and that TMS reversed these neurochemical changes. These findings suggest stimulation of the left dorsolateral prefrontal cortex (DLPFC) and inhibition of the right DLPFC as a potential pulse sequence model for PTSD [51–54].

Currently, two manufacturers license TMS machines for use for major depression: MagVenture (the MagVita system) and Neuronetics (the Neurostar system). They offer training for practitioners considering incorporating this therapy into their practice. Treatment for depression typically involves treatment five times a week for 4–6 weeks; research is ongoing to see if similar durations are necessary for PTSD and other conditions (Fig. 6.2).

Yoga and Exercise Therapy

Yoga has become overwhelmingly popular in the United States, creating both a powerful cultural movement and a commercial industry built around fitness and wellness. Modern yoga traces its roots to ancient India, and is culled from varied teachings of

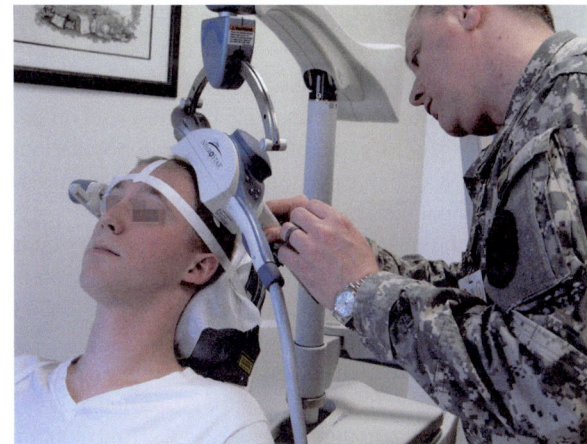

Fig. 6.2 Lt. Col. Geoffrey Grammer, chief of Inpatient Psychiatry, and Ensign James Decker, volunteer and medical student, demonstrate how to pinpoint the area of the brain responsible for mood regulation using the new technology. (Walter Reed photo by Kristin Ellis). Taken on March 29, 2009. https://www.flickr.com/photos/36255477@N06/3374935325

physical, spiritual, and mental practices that were developed and refined over the years. There are many different schools of yoga, ranging from full spiritual practice invoking the supernatural to simplifying it to simple exercise. In general, the principles that guide yoga practice can be highly valuable as an adjunct to traditional veteran PTSD treatment, and there is evidence to support its use [55–57].

One theory behind the benefits of yoga in veteran PTSD is that it modulates the parasympathetic nervous system, decreasing vagal tone and providing greater patient control over the stress response [58]. Another theory is that yoga improves psychological flexibility and set-shifting. One study showed that greater psychological flexibility was associated with lower PTSD and perceived stress, and that more yoga practice, before and during the study, was associated with greater psychological flexibility [55].

While the studies to date are not robust, there is data to support that the inclusion of a yoga program within a greater PTSD treatment program is feasible and effective for decrease in hyperarousal symptoms, improvement in sleep quality, and decrease in daytime dysfunction related to sleep [56]. Another study, specifically targeting a population with significant combat PTSD, found significant decreases in both biomarkers and pre- versus post-intervention subscale ratings for the veterans who participated [57].

It is not entirely clear if yoga as a specific modality is required for the benefits in the veteran population, as there are global benefits from exercise on psychiatric well-being. Other popular forms of exercise for PTSD in the veteran population include Tai Chi and water sports, but any exercise that a patient is willing to do may be beneficial.

There is evidence that any aerobic exercise can increase endocannabanoids in both healthy adults and those with PTSD, improving mood and psychobiological markers [59]. A recent review article supports that physical activity of any kind is an effective adjunct therapy to reduce PTSD symptom severity, though findings can be inconsistent when comparing objective data to subjective report, and studies thus far do not provide enough to identify the most effective dose and duration of any given type of exercise [60].

Emerging Therapies: ART and EFT

Currently emerging therapies include Accelerated Resolution Therapy (ART) and Emotional Freedom Technique (EFT). These and others show promise for the future direction of PTSD treatment in the veteran population, and may be useful for current patients who express interest in them or for patients who are not responding to more traditional therapies [61, 62].

These techniques are still not fully adopted as standard of care at most facilities, though they appear to be safe and effective. One reason adoption might be slow is the requirement of robust training by the practitioner. Another reason may be that some are quite costly due to the proprietary nature of the training (e.g., ART).

Others are more challenging to adopt due the technique's unorthodox methods and poorly understood mechanism of efficacy that is unlike anything else performed in a behavioral health clinic. For example, Emotional Freedom Technique is based on traditional Eastern medicine and may not be intuitively adopted by someone trained in Western medicine. It guides the patient to perform percussive tapping on theoretical acupressure points, combined with certain repeated phrases or mantras. This is thought to release blockages within the energy system that controls emotional functioning and may also have some mechanism akin to meditation or self-hypnosis. While not fitting traditionally into a Western model, EFT appears to be quite efficacious for at least some patients [8].

Though expensive and time-consuming to learn, ART has shown to be quite effective, and compares favorably to other standard practices such as Eye Movement Desensitization and Reprocessing (EMDR), as well as Cognitive Processing Therapy (CPT). It has been shown to be useful in the veteran population and is also helpful in improving provider satisfaction in clinics where large panels of patients with trauma might lead to burnout and compassion fatigue [63]. The practice combines eye movements with restructuring memory to replace distressing memory details with ones without traumatic content, thereby making the traumatic experience one that no longer triggers intense emotions or strong physical reactions.

Stellate Ganglion Block and Ketamine Infusion

Both stellate ganglion block (SGB) and ketamine infusion therapies are intriguing and novel options that involve psychiatrists collaborating with our Interventional Pain Management colleagues to provide more options for the most difficult to treat veterans with PTSD. These procedures are relatively safe when done by an appropriately trained interventionist and are already indicated for other diagnoses such as complex regional pain syndrome, phantom limb pain, and other chronic pain syndromes.

Benefits described in the literature are very impressive, with almost complete and immediate resolution of symptoms for many patients. Unfortunately, current available data studying this is not robust, and the one small randomized placebo-controlled study of SGB showed no increased benefit for the treatment arm participants. However, there were potentially significant limitations to the design and implementation of that study, and there are impressive case reports as well as a large body of anecdotal evidence that support the potential for significant benefit in PTSD symptoms, at least in the short term [64–70].

Significant limitations for these treatments include their short duration of efficacy (approximately 1–2 weeks of benefit per treatment for some patients), their labor- and resource-intensive nature, the fact that they are physically invasive compared to other treatments though only minimally so, and the fact that some physical pain is involved, though this should not be significantly more than the pain associated with blood draw or vaccine injection.

Cannabis and PTSD

Providers are increasingly asked about the use of marijuana for PTSD. Thus, whether or not providers opt to dip into the third bucket to treat PTSD, they should familiarize themselves with the available evidence regarding cannabis and PTSD. Approximately 15% of veterans treated in outpatient VA PTSD clinics report recent marijuana use and over a third of patients seeking cannabis for medical reasons list PTSD as the primary reason for the request [71, 72]. Unfortunately, that evidence is currently limited in both quantity and quality—in large part by marijuana's status as a schedule I drug, despite 31 states, the District of Columbia, Guam, and Puerto Rico all having state laws allowing for the medical use of marijuana [73].

As of publication of this volume, there are no completed randomized controlled trials (RCTs) studying the use of cannabis to treat PTSD. There has been one randomized controlled trial on nabilone, a synthetic cannabinoid, in the treatment of nightmares related to PTSD, which showed a significant reduction in nightmares but not other PTSD symptoms.

Three systematic reviews have evaluated the available evidence, primarily from observational studies and case reports as well as one small pilot study. The least rigorous of these noted the evidence suggested "potential benefit" [74] while the others assessed the evidence as either very low [75] or insufficient with high potential for bias [76].

Distinct from most of the therapies in the "everything else" bucket, cannabis use has been associated with some potentially serious harm. Foremost of these are the mental health and adverse cognitive effects, to include long-term and acute risk of psychosis and these risks would be important to mention in any shared decision-making discussion [76].

Fortunately, there are two forthcoming RCTs on the benefits and harms of cannabis for PTSD (Bonn-Miller, NCT02759185; NCT02517424). Meanwhile, there is growing evidence regarding the role of the endocannabinoid system in emotional memory processing, supporting the rationale for this research [77]. These developments will be important to follow as legal trends continue to support the availability of cannabis for medical use.

Conclusion

PTSD is a complex disease that can be difficult to treat. There are numerous barriers to adequate care including limitations to the more established, evidence-based treatments. Providing additional options, as adjuncts or alternatives can increase chances of successful treatment. We encourage providers to work with patients to find what is effective for them. We cannot yet predict which treatment modality works best for any one individual, though individual patient factors such as comorbidities and predominant symptoms can help guide treatment choices. The discussion among patients and providers should include what treatments are most accessible and affordable for the patient, and providers should be familiar with local resources that offer these services.

These therapies are wide-ranging; some of them require robust training by the practitioner (e.g., ART), some can be costly (e.g., CES), while others are low to no cost and are generally recommended by physicians to treat and prevent any health conditions (e.g., exercise). Thus, we almost always recommend the latter—exercise—to all patients unless there is some major contraindication, particularly given its demonstrated beneficial effects in many psychological conditions, including PTSD specifically [58, 78–81].

Multiple-Choice Questions

1. Which of the following criteria is necessary to diagnose PTSD:
    A. Hallucinations
    B. Hyperarousal
    C. Disorganized behavior
    D. Somatic symptoms
    Answer: B
2. The "three buckets" concept for PTSD refers to:
    A. A broad framework for the major categories of treatment modalities
    B. Three broad patient archetypes based on symptom clusters
    C. Complementary, alternative, and emerging treatments for PTSD
    D. Three main pharmacotherapies for PTSD (SSRIs, prazosin, atypical antipsychotics)
    Answer: A
3. Meditation appears to activate this brain region, which is also a target region for TMS?
    A. Hippocampus
    B. Frontal cortex
    C. Amygdala
    D. Prefrontal cortex
    Answer: D

4. We generally recommend the following to every patient:
   A. Fish oils
   B. Meditation
   C. More exercise
   D. Prazosin
   Answer: C

References

1. Kessler RC, Berglund P, Demler O, Jin R, Merikangas KR, Walters EE. Lifetime prevalence and age-of-onset distributions of DSM-IV disorders in the National Comorbidity Survey Replication. Arch Gen Psychiatry. 2005;62(6):593–602. https://doi.org/10.1001/archpsyc.62.6.593.
2. American Psychiatric Association. Diagnostic and statistical manual of mental disorders. 5th ed. Washington, DC: American Psychiatric Association Press; 2013.
3. Kessler RC, Sonnega A, Bromet E, et al. Posttraumatic stress disorder in the National Comorbidity Survey. Arch Gen Psychiatry. 1995;52:1048.
4. Schneiderman AI, Braver ER, Kang HK. Understanding sequelae of injury mechanisms and mild traumatic brain injury incurred during the conflicts in Iraq and Afghanistan: persistent postconcussive symptoms and posttraumatic stress disorder. Am J Epidemiol. 2008;167:1446.
5. Scioli-Salter ER, Forman DE, Otis JD, Gregor K, Valovski I, Rasmusson AM. The shared neuroanatomy and neurobiology of comorbid chronic pain and PTSD. Clin J Pain. 2015;31(4):363–74. https://doi.org/10.1097/ajp.0000000000000115.
6. Ritchie EC. Three buckets for treatment of PTSD [Web log post]. 2016, June 07. Retrieved August 18, 2016, from https://www.psychiatry.org/news-room/apa-blogs/apa-blog/2016/06/three-buckets-for-treatment-of-ptsd.
7. https://www.ptsd.va.gov/public/materials/apps/PTSDCoach.asp.
8. Waits WM, Kip KE, Hernandez DF. Accelerated resolution therapy. In: Ritchie EC, editor. Posttraumatic stress disorder and related diseases in combat veterans. New York: Springer; 2015. p. 105–22.
9. Cukor J, Gerardi M, Alley S, Reist C, Roy M, Rothbaum BO, Difede J, Rizzo A. Virtual reality exposure therapy for combat-related PTSD. In: Ritchie EC, editor. Posttraumatic stress disorder and related diseases in combat veterans. New York: Springer; 2015. p. 179–96.
10. Hoge CW, Grossman SH, Auchterlonie JL, Riviere LA, Milliken CS, Wilk JE. PTSD treatment for soldiers after combat deployment: low utilization of mental health care and reasons for dropout. PS Psychiatr Serv. 2014;65(8):997–1004. https://doi.org/10.1176/appi.ps.201300307.
11. NCCIH Homepage. 2016, August 4. Retrieved from https://nccih.nih.gov/health/integrative-health.
12. Goertz C, Marriott BP, Finch MD, Bray RM, Williams TV, Hourani LL, Hadden LS, Colleran HL, Jonas WB. Military report more complementary and alternative medicine use than civilians. J Altern Complement Med. 2013;19(6):509–17. https://doi.org/10.1089/acm.2012.0108.
13. VA Healthcare Analysis and Information Group. 2011 complementary and alternative medicine. Washington, DC: Department of Veterans Affairs; 2011.
14. Office of Research & Development. 2016, April 26. Retrieved August 18, 2016, from http://www.research.va.gov/topics/cam.cfm.
15. Strauss JL, Coeytaux R, McDuffie J, et al. Efficacy of complementary and alternative medicine therapies for posttraumatic stress disorder. Washington, DC: Department of Veterans Affairs; 2011.
16. Ritchie EC. Posttraumatic stress disorder and related diseases in combat veterans. Cham: Springer; 2015.

17. Khusid M. Meditation for combat-related mental health concerns. In: Ritchie EC, editor. Posttraumatic stress disorder and related diseases in combat veterans. New York: Springer; 2015. p. 133–5.
18. Creswell J, Way B, Eisenberger N, Lieberman M. Neural correlates of dispositional mindfulness during affect labeling. Psychosom Med. 2007;69(6):560–5.
19. Chiesa A, Serretti A. A systematic review of neurobiological and clinical features of mindfulness meditations. Psychol Med. 2010;40(8):1239–52.
20. Farb N, Anderson A, Segal Z. The mindful brain and emotion regulation in mood disorders. Can J Psychiatr. 2012;57(2):70–7.
21. Ospina M, Bond K, Karkhaneh M, Tjosvold L, Vandermeer B, Liang Y, et al. Meditation practices for health: state of the research. Evid Rep Technol Assess (Full Rep). 2007;155:1–263.
22. Vujanovic AA, Niles B, Pietrefesa A, Schmertz SK, Potter CM. Mindfulness in the treatment of posttraumatic stress disorder among military veterans. Prof Psychol Res Pract. 2011;42(1):24–31.
23. Bormann J, Thorp S, Wetherell J, Golshan S. A spiritually based group intervention for combat veterans with posttraumatic stress disorder: feasibility study. J Holist Nurs. 2008;26(2):109.
24. Bormann J, Liu L, Thorp S, Lang A. Spiritual wellbeing mediates PTSD change in veterans with military-related PTSD. Int J Behav Med. 2012;19(4):496–502.
25. Bormann J. Frequent, silent mantram repetition: a Jacuzzi for the mind. Top Emerg Med. 2005;27(2):163.
26. Lang A, Strauss J, Bomyea J, Bormann J, Hickman S, Good R, et al. The theoretical and empirical basis for meditation as an intervention for PTSD. Behav Modif. 2012;36(6):759–86.
27. Davidson RJ, Begley S. The emotional life of your brain: how its unique patterns affect the way you think, feel, and live—and how you can change them. New York: Plume Book; 2012.
28. Klimecki O, Leiberg S, Lamm C, Singer T. Functional neural plasticity and associated changes in positive affect after compassion training. Cereb Cortex. 2012;23(7):1552–161.
29. Lutz A, Brefczynski-Lewis J, Johnstone T, Davidson R. Regulation of the neural circuitry of emotion by compassion meditation: effects of meditative expertise. PLoS One. 2008;3(3):10.
30. Fredrickson B, Cohn M, Coffey K, Pek J, Finkel S. Open hearts build lives: positive emotions, induced through loving-kindness meditation, build consequential personal resources. J Pers Soc Psychol. 2008;95(5):1045–62.
31. Cohn M, Fredrickson B, Brown S, Mikels J, Conway A. Happiness unpacked: positive emotions increase life satisfaction by building resilience. Emotion. 2009;9(3):361–8.
32. Johnson D, Penn D, Fredrickson B, Kring A, Meyer P, Catalino L, et al. A pilot study of loving-kindness meditation for the negative symptoms of schizophrenia. Schizophr Res. 2011;129(2–3):137–40.
33. Service Animals. 2011, July 12. Retrieved August 07, 2016, from https://www.ada.gov/service_animals_2010.htm.
34. Hunt MG, Chizkov RR. Are therapy dogs like Xanax? Does animal-assisted therapy impact processes relevant to cognitive behavioral psychotherapy? Anthrozoös. 2014;27(3):457–69.
35. Olmert MD. Made for each other, the biology of the human-animal bond. Cambridge, MA: DaCapo Press; 2009.
36. Nuemann ID, Landgraf R. Balance of brain oxytocin and vasopressin: implications for anxiety, depression, and social behaviors. Trends Neurosci. 2012;35(11):649–59.
37. Beetz A, Uvnas-Moberg K, Julius H, et al. Psychological and psychophysiological effects of human-animal interactions: the possible role of oxytocin. Front Psychol. 2012;3:234. https://doi.org/10.3389/fpsyg.2012.00234.
38. Olff M. Bonding after trauma: on the role of social support and the oxytocin system intraumatic stress. Eur J Psycho-Traumatol. 2012;3:18597. https://doi.org/10.3402/ejpt.v3i0.18597.
39. Katcher AH. Interactions between people and their pets: form and function. In: Fogle B, editor. Interrelations between people and pets. Springfield: Charles C Thomas; 1987. p. 41–67.

40. Yount RA, Lee MR, Olmert MD. Service dog training program for treatment of posttraumatic stress in service members. US Army Med Dep J. 2012; 63–9.
41. Beck AM, Seraydarian L, Hunter F. Use of animals in the rehabilitation of psychiatric patients. Psychol Rep. 1986;58:63–6.
42. Wilkes JK. The role of companion animals in counseling and psychology: discovering their use in the therapeutic process. Springfield: Charles C. Thomas; 2009.
43. Earles JL. Equine-assisted therapy for anxiety and posttraumatic stress symptoms equine-assisted therapy. J Trauma Stress. 2015;28(2):149–52.
44. Hickey AH, Koffman R. Adding a face and the story to the data: acupuncture for PTSD in the military. In: Ritchie EC, editor. Posttraumatic stress disorder and related diseases in combat veterans. New York: Springer; 2015. p. 161–78.
45. Pillington K. Acupuncture therapy for psychiatric illness. Int Rev Neurobiol. 2013;111:197–216.
46. McDonald JK, Cripps AW, Smith PK. Mediators, receptors, and signaling pathways in the anti-inflammatory and antihyperalgesic effects of acupuncture. Evid Based Complement Alternat Med. 2015;2015:975632.
47. Yang J, Li Q, Li F, Fu Q, Zeng X, Liu C. The holistic effects of acupuncture treatment. Evid Based Complement Alternat Med. 2014;2014:10, Article ID 73978.
48. Manni L, Albanesi M, Guaragna M, Garbaro Paparo S, Aloe L. Neurotrophins and acupuncture. Auton Neurosci. 2010;157(1/2):9–17.
49. Kim Y, Heo I, Shin B, Crawford C, Kang H, Lim J. Acupuncture for posttraumatic stress disorder: a systematic review of randomized controlled trials and prospective clinical trials. Evid Based Complement Alternat Med. 2013;2013:12, Article ID 615857.
50. Rossi S, De Capua A, Tavanti M, Calossi S, Polizzotto NR, Mantovani A, Falzarano V, Bossini L, Passero S, Bartalini S, Ulivelli M. Dysfunctions of cortical excitability in drug-naïve post-traumatic stress disorder patients. Biol Psychiatry. 2009;66(1):54–61.
51. Grammer GG, Cole JT, Rall CJ, Scacca CC. Use of transcranial magnetic stimulation for the treatment of PTSD. In: Ritchie EC, editor. Posttraumatic stress disorder and related diseases in combat veterans. New York: Springer; 2015. p. 161–78.
52. Boggio PS, Rocha M, Oliveira MO, et al. Noninvasive brain stimulation with high-frequency and low-intensity repetitive transcranial magnetic stimulation treatment for posttraumatic stress disorder. J Clin Psychiatry. 2010;71(8):992–9.
53. Kim SY, Lee DW, Kim H, Bang E, Chae JH, Choe BY. Chronic repetitive transcranial magnetic stimulation enhances GABAergic and cholinergic metabolism in chronic unpredictable mild stress rat model: (1)H-NMR spectroscopy study at 11.7T. Neurosci Lett. 2014;572:32 7.
54. Karsen EF, Watts BV, Holtzheimer PE. Review of the effectiveness of transcranial magnetic stimulation for posttraumatic stress disorder. Brain Stimul. 2014;7(2):151–7.
55. Breit S, Kupferberg A, Rogler G, Hasler G. Vagus nerve as modulator of the brain–gut axis in psychiatric and inflammatory disorders. Front Psych. 2018;9:44. https://doi.org/10.3389/fpsyt.2018.0004.
56. Avery T, Blasey C, Rosen C, Bayley P. Psychological flexibility and set-shifting among veterans participating in a yoga program: a pilot study. Mil Med. 2018. https://doi.org/10.1093/milmed/usy045.
57. Staples JK, Hamilton MF, Uddo M. A yoga program for the symptoms of post-traumatic stress disorder in veterans. Mil Med. 2013;178(8):854–60. https://doi.org/10.7205/MILMED-D-12-00536.
58. Horowitz S. Transcranial magnetic stimulation and cranial electrotherapy stimulation: treatments for psychiatric and neurologic disorders. Altern Complement Ther. 2013;19(4):188–93. https://doi.org/10.1089/act.2013.19402.
59. McCarthy L, Fuller J, Davidson G, Crump A, Positano S, Alderman C. Assessment of yoga as an adjuvant treatment for combat-related posttraumatic stress disorder. Australas Psychiatry. 2017;25(4):354–7. https://doi.org/10.1177/1039856217695870. Epub 2017 Mar 1. PubMed PMID: 28747121.

60. Crombie KM, Brellenthin AG, Hillard CJ, Koltyn KF. Psychobiological responses to aerobic exercise in individuals with posttraumatic stress disorder. J Trauma Stress. 2018;31(1):134–45. https://doi.org/10.1002/jts.22253. Epub 2018 Feb 1. PubMed PMID: 29388710.
61. Oppizzi LM, Umberger R. The effect of physical activity on PTSD. Issues Ment Health Nurs. 2018;39(2):179–87. https://doi.org/10.1080/01612840.2017.1391903. Epub 2018 Jan 10. PubMed PMID: 29319376.
62. Kip KE, Rosenzweig L, Hernandez DF, Shuman A, Sullivan KL, Long CJ, Taylor J, McGhee S, Girling SA, Wittenberg T, Sahebzamani FM, Lengacher CA, Kadel R, Diamond DM. Randomized controlled trial of accelerated resolution therapy (ART) for symptoms of combat-related post-traumatic stress disorder (PTSD). Mil Med. 2013;178(12):1298–309. https://doi.org/10.7205/MILMED-D-13-00298. PubMed PMID: 24306011.
63. Church D, Yount G, Rachlin K, Fox L, Nelms J. Epigenetic effects of PTSD remediation in veterans using clinical emotional freedom techniques: a randomized controlled pilot study. Am J Health Promot. 2018;32(1):112–22. https://doi.org/10.1177/0890117116661154. Epub 2016 Aug 12. PubMed PMID: 27520015.
64. Hernandez DF, Waits W, Calvio L, Byrne M. Practice comparisons between accelerated resolution therapy, eye movement desensitization and reprocessing and cognitive processing therapy with case examples. Nurse Educ Today. 2016;47:74–80. https://doi.org/10.1016/j.nedt.2016.05.010. Epub 2016 May 21. PubMed PMID: 27250615.
65. Lynch JH, Mulvaney SW, Kim EH, de Leeuw JB, Schroeder MJ, Kane SF. Effect of stellate ganglion block on specific symptom clusters for treatment of post-traumatic stress disorder. Mil Med. 2016;181(9):1135–41. https://doi.org/10.7205/MILMED-D-15-00518. PubMed PMID: 27612365. Hanling SR, Hickey A, Lesnik I, Hackworth RJ, Stedje-Larsen E, Drastal CA, McLay RN. Stellate ganglion block for the treatment of posttraumatic stress disorder: a randomized, double-blind, controlled trial. Reg Anesth Pain Med. 2016;41(4):494–500. https://doi.org/10.1097/AAP.0000000000000402. PubMed PMID: 27187898.
66. McLean B. Safety and patient acceptability of stellate ganglion blockade as a treatment adjunct for combat-related post-traumatic stress disorder: a quality assurance initiative. Cureus. 2015;7(9):e320. https://doi.org/10.7759/cureus.320. PubMed PMID: 26487996; PubMed Central PMCID: PMC4601906.
67. Lipov E, Ritchie EC. A review of the use of stellate ganglion block in the treatment of PTSD. Curr Psychiatry Rep. 2015;17(8):599. https://doi.org/10.1007/s11920-015-0599-4. Review. PubMed PMID: 26073361.
68. Mulvaney SW, Lynch JH, Kotwal RS. Clinical guidelines for stellate ganglion block to treat anxiety associated with posttraumatic stress disorder. J Spec Oper Med. 2015;15(2):79–85. PubMed PMID: 26125169.
69. Mulvaney SW, Lynch JH, Hickey MJ, Rahman-Rawlins T, Schroeder M, Kane S, Lipov E. Stellate ganglion block used to treat symptoms associated with combat-related post-traumatic stress disorder: a case series of 166 patients. Mil Med. 2014;179(10):1133–40. https://doi.org/10.7205/MILMED-D-14-00151. PubMed PMID: 25269132.
70. Peterson K, Bourne D, Anderson J, Mackey K, Helfand M. Evidence brief: effectiveness of stellate ganglion block for treatment of posttraumatic stress disorder (PTSD). In: VA evidence-based synthesis program evidence briefs [Internet]. Washington, DC: Department of Veterans Affairs (US); 2017; 2011. Available From http://www.ncbi.nlm.nih.gov/books/NBK442253/ PubMed PMID: 28742302.
71. Bowles DW. Persons registered for medical marijuana in the United States. J Palliat Med. 2012;15(1):9–11.
72. Boden MT, Babson KA, Vujanovic AA, Short NA, Bonn-Miller MO. Posttraumatic stress disorder and cannabis use characteristics among military veterans with cannabis dependence. Am J Addict/Am Acad Psychiatr Alcohol Addict. 2013;22(3):277–84.
73. State Medical Marijuana Laws. National Conference of State Legislatures, 27 June 2018, www.ncsl.org/research/health/state-medical-marijuana-laws.aspx.

74. Shisko S, Oliveira R, Moore TA, Almeida K. A review of medical marijuana for the treatment of posttraumatic stress disorder: real symptom re-leaf or just high hopes? Ment Health Clin [Internet]. 2018;8(2):86–94. https://doi.org/10.9740/mhc.2018.03.086.
75. Wilkinson ST, Radhakrishnan R, D'Souza DC. A systematic review of the evidence for medical marijuana in psychiatric indications. J Clin Psychiatry. 2016;77(8):1050–64.
76. Kansagara D, O'Neil M, Nugent S, et al. Benefits and harms of cannabis in chronic pain or post-traumatic stress disorder: a systemic review [internet]. Washington, DC: Department of Veterans Affairs (US); 2017.
77. Bitencourt RM, Takahashi RN. Cannabidiol as a therapeutic alternative for post-traumatic stress disorder: from bench research to confirmation in human trials. Front Neurosci. 2018;12:502. https://doi.org/10.3389/fnins.2018.00502.
78. Lipov E. The use of stellate ganglion block in the treatment of panic/anxiety symptoms (including suicidal ideation) with combat-related posttraumatic stress disorder. In: Ritchie EC, editor. Posttraumatic stress disorder and related diseases in combat veterans. New York: Springer; 2015. p. 179–96.
79. Petruzzello SJ, Landers DM, Hatfield BD, Kubitz KA, Salazar W. A meta-analysis on the anxiety-reducing effects of acute and chronic exercise. Outcomes and mechanisms. Sports Med. 1991;11(3):143–82.
80. de Assis MA, de Mello MF, Scorza FA, Cadrobbi MP, Schooedl AF, Gomes da Silva S, de Albuquerque M, da Silva AC, Arida RM. Evaluation of physical activity habits in patients with posttraumatic stress disorder. Clinics (Sao Paulo). 2008;63(4):473–8.
81. Manger TA, Motta RW. The impact of an exercise program on posttraumatic stress disorder, anxiety, and depression. Int J Emerg Ment Health. 2005;7(1):49–57.

Treatment-Resistant Depression Among US Military Veterans

7

R. Gregory Lande

Introduction

Major depression is broadly defined as a 2-week period dominated by a pervasive and persistent depressed mood and loss of interest in pleasurable activities. The disorder is marked by negative cognitions and physical symptoms such as changes in sleep patterns, weight, and energy level, all of which combine to adversely affect a person's social and occupational functioning [1].

Among all mental disorders, major depression is one of the most common and, perhaps surprisingly, is responsible for the most disability. Prevalence data from a national epidemiologic survey found that 6.7% of adult Americans had at least one major depressive episode in the preceding year. In terms of prevalence by demographics, females (8.5%) and individuals between 18 and 25 years old (10.3%) constituted key groups with a major depressive episode in the past year [2].

Military veterans suffer major depressive episodes but the unique characteristics of military service influence the prevalence. Analyzing the prevalence of major depression in the military is limited by many methodological factors, but a meta-analysis reported a prevalence of 5.7% among service members never deployed, 12% among those currently deployed, and 13.1% among those with a prior deployment [3]. Gulf War veterans had twice the odds of major depression when compared to nondeployed civilians [4]. Lifetime depression among veterans who served in WWII and Korea were lower among veterans vs. nonveterans who served while the reverse occurred among veterans vs. nonveterans of the Vietnam War era [5].

The views expressed in this article are those of the author and do not reflect the official policy of the Department of Army/Navy/Airforce, Department of Defense, or US Government

R. G. Lande (✉)
Psychiatry Continuity Service, Walter Reed National Military Medical Center, Behavioral Health, Bethesda, MD, USA
e-mail: Raymond.G.Lande.civ@mail.mil

The Department of Veterans Affairs Health Care data between 2002 and 2008 identified 17.4% of Iraq and Afghanistan veterans with depression [6].

The Rand Corporation's Center for Military Policy Research undertook an extensive review addressing the psychological and cognitive injuries of service members deployed to Afghanistan and Iraq [7]. According to the report, major depression was not often considered a combat-related injury, with attention more commonly diverted to PTSD — this in spite of a reported equal 14% incidence rate for either major depression or PTSD among veterans of these two wars.

A different way of analyzing trends in military depression study examined nearly 3000 cases of service members with a disability discharge and retirement for a major depressive disorder [7]. The study authors report that hospital treatment for major depression among service members increased every year between 2004 and 2012, a pressure that significantly increased the incidence of medical disability discharges for major depression in the Army and Navy between 2007 and 2012. Rates were higher among females with at least one deployment [8].

Military service members certainly face unique challenges that increase the likelihood of a major depressive episode and these may linger years after leaving [9]. Voluntary service mitigates but does not eliminate core facets of military life. Perhaps the most fundamental is the omnipresent risk of injury or death in combat environments. Service members live on a risk precipice with imminent deployment to hostile environments pushing some over an emotional edge.

Military life also requires social adaptation and subordination of self to leadership and mission, both of which may create interpersonal conflicts. The list of potential destabilizing and dysphoria-inducing factors is long and includes frequent geographic assignments, marital and family problems, high stress work environments, deployment-related communication problems, and traumatic exposure.

Optimizing Depression Treatment Outcomes

Major depression is a complex biopsychosocial disorder that defies simple one-size-fits-all treatment approaches. Military service adds another complicating dimension that clinicians must consider in treatment planning. Clinical practice guidelines and seminal research studies help clinicians develop treatment plans that increase the likelihood of a best outcome.

The best treatment outcome for a major depressive disorder is remission, defined as minimal or no residual symptoms of depression following a course of treatment as measured by a standardized assessment instrument combined with the clinician's observations. Anything short of that increases the likelihood of recurrence and persistence of impairment in the person's social and occupational functioning [10].

Achieving remission is an obtainable goal but it requires a systematic approach that envisions echelons of intervention based on the individual's response to treatment. Just how many individuals could leave treatment for major depression in a state of remission awaited the results of research.

STAR * D Study

The Sequenced Treatment Alternatives to Relieve Depression study (STAR * D) conducted by the National Institute of Mental Health provided broad clinical guidance on the effectiveness of antidepressant treatment for major depressive disorder (MDD) [11, 12]. Subjects progressed through four levels of treatment based on treatment response. Level 1 participants included 2876 subjects who received an average dose citalopram above 40 mg daily with best reported remission rates of 33% after about 47 days of treatment. For the average subject in the Level 1 treatment, it took 7 weeks to achieve remission with a sizable 40% requiring 8 or more weeks [13].

Subjects not achieving remission entered Level 2 and could choose to switch to a group of specific antidepressant medications or opt for a medication augmentation approach. In Level 2, researchers randomly assigned subjects in the switch group to either venlafaxine-XR, bupropion-SR, or sertraline. Best remission rates and average medication doses for venlafaxine-XR was 25% at 193.6 mg, bupropion-SR was 26% at 282.7 mg, and sertraline-medicated subjects achieved 27% remission rate with an average dose of 135.5 mg. Subjects choosing the augmentation path in Level 2 were randomized to citalopram plus bupropion-SR or citalopram plus buspirone. An average dose of 267.5 mg bupropion-SR and 40.9 mg of buspirone led to best-reported respective remission rates of 39% and 33%.

Subjects progressing to Level 3 once again could choose between switching medications or augmenting their Level 2 medications. Remission rates for those randomized to an average 42.1 mg exit dose of mirtazapine and 96.8 for nortriptyline led to best reported remission rates of 12% and 20%, respectively. Researchers randomized subjects in the augmentation group to an average dose of 859.9 mg lithium or 45.2 µg triiodothyronine (T3), which led to best reported remission rates of 16% and 25%, respectively.

Level 4 subjects had failed three prior antidepressant trials and researchers switched them to a combination of mirtazapine plus venlafaxine-XR or tranylcypromine. In the combination medication group, an average dose of 35.7 mg of mirtazapine and 210.3 mg of venlafaxine-XR led to a best reported remission rate of 16%. An average dose of 36.9 mg tranylcypromine led to a 14% remission rate.

STAR * D identified what clinicians intuitively understood, that each subsequent failed intervention led to lower rates of remission. For all four levels, the overall remission rate was about 67%. This left roughly one-third of aggressively treated individuals still suffering with residual symptoms of major depression, a treatment resistant group that is the focus of this chapter.

Treatment Resistant Depression

Treatment-resistant depression (TRD) imposes a significant burden on society and its many sufferers. A meta-analysis of 62 studies examining the impact concluded that individuals with TRD had, on average, 3.8 depressive episodes over 4.4 years and underwent 4.7 unsuccessful medication treatments. The same study estimated that TRD added between 29 and 48 billion dollars in annual health care costs [14]. Another study underscored the morbidity of TRD by reporting the probability of remission at around 40% over the following 10-year period [15].

Many factors contribute to TRD including a lack of clinical consensus defining the condition. STAR * D emphasized measurement-based care that relied on the routine use of standardized screening instruments to assess treatment response and remission. Validated outcome-based instruments administered at regular intervals help clinicians monitor the results of their treatment plans and they may also detect changes patients are unaware of or neglect to mention. Other factors contributing to TRD include adherence, co-occurring disorders, and inadequate early medication trials, with the results of the STAR * D offering clinical guidance on dose and duration.

Measurement-Based Care

One of the main take-home points from the STAR * D study was the value clinicians should place on the regular use of standardized instruments to inform clinical practice. When combined with the clinician's observations and experience, such instruments help determine a person's remission, response, or nonresponse to a course of treatment.

In the STAR * D study, researchers relied on the results of the Hamilton Depression Scale (HAM-D) and the Quick Inventory of Depressive Symptomatology-Self-Report (QIDS-SR). The investigators used a score of 14 or greater on the (HAM-D) as a starting point for recommending pharmacologic treatment for major depression [16]. The HAM-D is a clinician administered instrument available in the public domain that enjoys a record of good test-retest reliability [17]. Clinicians can expect the average HAM-D encounter to take about 12 minutes and with scores of 7 or less following a course of treatment signaling remission while a 50% reduction from the baseline pre-treatment score is a clinically significant response [18].

STAR * D investigators also used the Quick Inventory of Depressive Symptomatology-Self-Report (QIDS SR) that is a freely available 16-item instrument completed by the patient. Clinicians can use the validated instrument after beginning treatment to gauge the treatment's effectiveness. Scores of 9 or greater indicate no response, 6–8 some response, and 5 or less equals remission [18–20]. Researchers validated the QIDS SR among military veterans adding further value to this instrument [21].

There are many notable competitors to the HAM-D and QIDS SR. The Patient Health Questionnaire (PHQ-9) is a validated instrument that can also be used to assess response to treatment [22, 23]. Zung's Self-Rating Depression Scale (SDS) is another option clinicians might consider [24]. An extensive meta-analysis examined a number of screening instruments for adult depression including the Hospital Anxiety and Depression Scales (HADS) and the Geriatric Depression Scale (GDS) before recommending no specific single instrument, suggesting that practitioners should make choices based on their patient population, ease of administration, and clinical experience [25]. The Hamilton Depression Rating Scale, long considered a standard assessment instrument, may not be the best choice based on a recent analysis [26].

Factors Contributing to TRD

Adherence

Screening instruments combined with the clinician's observations and experience help determine a person's response to treatment. This is an important first step in practicing outcome-based clinical practice, but it does not describe factors that make remission elusive. Failure to achieve remission may be due to many factors but clinicians should always consider treatment adherence [27].

This may be particularly relevant in the early course of treatment for major depression when the symptoms of the disorder such as distrust, doubt, and despondency predominate, all of which should be countered by the clinician encouraging the patient to stay the course. Medication side effects, pessimism, lower socioeconomic status, and a poor clinician-patient rapport are among a long list of factors that impede adherence. Estimating the incidence of nonadherence is difficult to ascertain with certainty although one study suggested that 70% of depressed patients did not completely follow complicated medication trials [28].

Co-occurring Disorders

Failure to achieve remission could be the result of a co-occurring disorder complicating recovery. An initial comprehensive psychiatric evaluation, and if necessary a reevaluation, as part of a systematic assessment of a less than optimum treatment outcome guards against this possibility. A thorough assessment takes into account other plausible diagnoses, as well as the potential for suicide and homicide, functional impairments, and motivation for recovery. Patient care is dynamic, and requires the clinician also to remain vigilant to new information that may amend the original conclusions.

Among veterans, PTSD and MDD constitute one of the more common co-occurring complexes. Military service may expose an individual to traumatic experiences that may subsequently develop into PTSD. Focusing solely on PTSD may miss the co-occurrence of major depression, a presentation that effects more than half of the individuals with military-related PTSD [29]. The overlap between the two disorders is partly a function of the diagnostic criteria with PTSD's dysphoric elements clustering around the negative cognitions that both disorders share [30].

Not surprisingly, a bidirectional relationship probably exists between military-related PTSD and MDD reinforcing the importance of considering both disorders [31]. In fact, according to a large study, 43.2% of veterans with PTSD had concomitant depression while 20.6% of veterans with depression met the diagnostic criteria for PTSD [32]. The presence of depression significantly retards PTSD treatment [33]. Of even more concern is the heightened risk of suicide among veterans with both disorders that nearly double the rate for each disorder by itself [34].

Personality disorders with their associated chronic maladaptive response to psychosocial stressors contribute to relapse and TRD [35]. Among veterans, personality disorders are the principle co-occurring disorder with PTSD, even slightly edging out depression. A nonmilitary but nationally representative survey of individuals with MDD reported that TRD aligned most closely with borderline personality disorder [36]. From a more descriptive perspective, pervasive anger and hostility are common features of many personality disorders, which contribute to TRD [37]. The constellation of depression and personality disorder may contribute to aggression, a factor that may inhibit therapeutic acceptance, alliance, and adherence [38].

Another significant factor to consider among veterans is substance misuse, particularly alcohol. Occult substance use disorders significantly complicate treatment for MDD and left untreated can be wrongly classified as TRD [39]. Estimating alcohol and drug use disorders among veterans varies depending on the sampling method and diagnostic criteria applied to the analysis. A large epidemiologic review based on a research meta-analysis encompassing studies extracted between 1995 and 2013 found that the use of traditional diagnostic criteria led to higher reported rates of both alcohol use disorders (32% versus 10%) and drug use disorders (20% versus 5%) compared to studies using administrative data culled from ICD-9 codes [40]. Another large study using diagnostic criteria reported a lifetime prevalence of alcohol use disorders of 42.2% and a past year probable rate of alcohol use disorders at 14.8% [41]. Surveys conducted post deployment suggest that the combat experience increases the risk of binge drinking [42].

Military suicide among active duty service members and veterans led researchers to examine the Behavioral Risk Factor Surveillance Survey for clues that would help clinicians and healthcare planners provide more focused interventions. Among the correlates with suicide, depression, binge drinking, and smoking were prominent [43]. A nonmilitary but international meta-analysis also reported that severe depression and substance use disorders heightened the risk for suicide [44].

Emerging evidence suggests that a cannabis use disorder among veterans from Iraq and Afghanistan may be associated with higher suicide attempt rates [45]. Veterans with pain and subsequent opioid use greater than 30 days increase the risk of TRD, with risk rising even more as a function of longer duration of use [46, 47].

Individuals with a tobacco use disorder are four times more likely to have depression and less likely to quit: a dysfunctional bidirectional relationship [48, 49]. Quitting tobacco is difficult, part of which is related to nicotine's addictive properties but another, cognitive resistance is rooted in an erroneous belief that cessation will worsen a person's depression. Emerging evidence would suggest otherwise as demonstrated in a study involving veterans whose depression improved after quitting tobacco [50]. Similar studies among nonveterans also suggest that measures of both physical and mental well-being improve with smoking cessation [51–53].

Authors of a meta-analysis reported that unrecognized bipolar disorder was another factor contributing to TRD [54]. Anxiety disorders also frequently complicate the treatment of major depression [55]. Lifestyle choices such as a poor diet and limited exercise can reduce recovery rates from MDD [56]. Not surprisingly, physical problems such as a severely compromised cardiovascular system and cerebrovascular injuries carry a higher risk of TRD [57].

Sleep Issues

Unremitting sleep disorders can complicate recovery. A cursory sleep history may not be sufficient with accumulating evidence suggesting that sleep problems independently impair recovery [58]. Among service members returning from a combat deployment, one of the most frequently cited complaints is persistent sleep problems [59]. Obstructive sleep apnea compounds the problem since this breathing disorder often goes undetected and is more prevalent in veterans, a possible confluence of combat-related PTSD and an alcohol use disorder [60]. Elevated levels of alcohol biomarkers, specifically ethyl glucuronide and ethyl sulfate, pointed toward obstructive sleep apnea in a study of active duty service members [61]. Tobacco use also disrupts a service member's sleep architecture and contributes to breathing problems while asleep [62].

The constellation of symptoms associated with obstructive sleep apnea mimic many of the symptoms associated with major depression. Fatigue, irritability, poor concentration, mood lability, and a lower quality of life are common accompaniments of both major depression and sleep apnea [63]. Studies suggest that the treatment of sleep apnea improves depressive symptoms, and in a similar finding researchers reported that among veterans with PTSD, a disorder commonly co-occurring with major depression and contributing to TRD also improved with positive airway pressure treatment [64, 65].

Sleep and mood pivot in a different direction with bipolar disorder. The manic phase of the disorder is characterized by a decreased need for sleep. During the more frequent depressive cycles, a person with bipolar disorder typically displays hypersomnia. While not pathognomonic, the presence of hypersomnia in a person with TRD should alert the clinician to the possibility of a bipolar disorder [66].

Medical Comorbidities

Medical comorbidities can substantially reduce treatment remission: a burden that grows with each additional organ system impacted by illness or injury [67]. Pain and depression have a bidirectional relationship and are commonly comorbid, with estimates suggesting that nearly two-thirds of individuals with depression experience pain; a situation that contributes to treatment-resistant depression [68].

A long list of physical disorders complicates the treatment and recovery from major depression [69]. In very broad terms, these physical disorders can be grouped as endocrine, neurological, malignant, and cardiac disorders. More specifically, thyroid disorders, demyelinating diseases, and pancreatic cancer are examples of potentially undetected conditions that adversely impact depression treatment.

Depression and cardiovascular disease are interrelated [70]. In some cases, depression heralds the onset of occult cardiac disease while in other cases preexisting depression worsens with known cardiovascular disease. Estimates would suggest that about 15% of patients with cardiovascular disease have co-occurring major depression.

Neurocognitive Disorders

Depression has a bidirectional relationship with dementia as evidenced by longitudinal studies and meta-analyses that consistently demonstrate that chronic depression increases the risk of dementia [71]. Individuals with preexisting mild cognitive impairment or dementia experience increased rates of depression [72]. Identifying the contributions of mild cognitive impairment or dementia to a clinical picture appearing as treatment-resistant depression requires careful assessment: an important distinction since antidepressant medications are less effective for neurocognitive disorders [73].

Treatment Dose and Duration

One of the principle factors contributing to a lack of remission is an inadequate duration or dose of antidepressant medication. Researchers highlighted the importance of an adequate duration of treatment in a meta-analysis that primarily examined studies involving 12 months of antidepressant treatment by reporting a two-thirds reduction in the risk of relapse [74].

What constitutes an adequate duration of antidepressant medication is still unsettled, but with both remission and relapse prevention as goals of treatment, clinical guidelines suggests 6–9 months of continuous treatment, with the longer time span preferred for optimal outcomes [75]. Many factors affect medication adherence: broadly grouped as patient factors such as medication side effects, beliefs about medications, and premature discontinuation along with clinician factors such as limited medication education and poor follow-up [76].

Defining an adequate medication dose depends on many factors such as the medication choice, variations in metabolism, other prescribed and nonprescribed medications, physical health, and individual responsiveness. With all of these factors in mind, initial treatment for major depression often begins with a selective serotonin uptake inhibitor (SSRI). As a group, these medications are safe, well tolerated, and effective, particularly in relation to their tricyclic antidepressant predecessors [77].

The minimally effective dose of an SSRI can be conceptualized as balancing the medication's effectiveness, safety, and tolerability. For example, the minimally effective dose for paroxetine is 20 mg/day, sertraline 50 mg/day, and citalopram 20 mg/day [78].

Raising the SSRI beyond the minimally effective dose is the subject of extensive and still unsettled research. A large meta-analysis concluded that higher doses of SSRIs slightly improve the outcome in major depression but carry the risk of increased side effects and treatment adherence [79].

Part of the debate about SSRIs involves their flat dose response efficacy. Accumulating but still not fully conclusive evidence would suggest that SSRIs have a narrow therapeutic range, implying that most individuals will not benefit from raising the dose above the minimally effective dose. Conversely, the incidence of SSRI adverse drug events is dose dependent creating a potential for misdiagnosis. For example, increasingly elevated doses of SSRIs can produce anxiety, insomnia, suicidal ideation, and sexual dysfunction, all of which might be misinterpreted as treatment-resistant depression instead of underlying adverse drug events [80].

The timing of the dose increase above the minimally effective dose is yet another factor affecting the person's response to an SSRI. As demonstrated in the STAR * D study, subjects who achieved remission required at least 6 weeks of SSRI treatment [81]. Another study reported that 8 weeks of antidepressant treatment best predicted remission [82].

Clinical Vignette

A retired lieutenant colonel presented to a Veterans Affairs (VA) clinic for a new onset depression. His symptoms started 3 months ago after the death of a close friend. The clinician did a brief assessment, was satisfied that he was not suicidal, and after discussing the treatment with the patient prescribed 50 mg of sertraline. At his next appointment that was 2 weeks later, the patient complained about not sleeping, feeling moody, and irritable. The clinician increased his sertraline to 100 mg and scheduled another appointment in 1 week. On his return, he looked even more depressed and voiced concerns about the lack of progress. After assuring his safety, the clinician increased the sertraline to 200 mg. One week later, the patient was hospitalized for severe insomnia, anxiety, and irritability that concerned his wife. During his brief stay, the dose of sertraline was lowered to the minimally effective dose of 50 mg resulting in a marked decrease in symptoms. The patient was discharged with a recommendation to maintain that dose for at least 6 weeks.

Management of Treatment-Resistant Depression

The first principle in the management of TRD is prevention. Optimum treatment of major depression can decrease the likelihood of its progression to TRD. Clinical practice guidelines emphasize a thorough assessment, evaluation of safety, monitoring progress, promoting adherence, and the use of standardized assessment instruments [13, 83, 84]. Mild to moderate depression benefits from antidepressant medications and/or cognitive behavior and interpersonal psychotherapies. Severe depression primarily benefits more from medication management and as envisioned in the STAR * D study, increasing echelons of medication intervention based on responsiveness.

Echelons of intervention or stepped care as practiced in the STAR * D study is based on the premise that the treatment of depression unfolds in a systematic fashion starting with the least intensive intervention and subsequent adjustments based on treatment response [85]. This is a valid approach adopted in practice guidelines and by professional consensus [13, 86, 87]. Despite its widespread clinical application there are critics contending that the scientific basis for the therapeutic model is lacking [88, 89].

Integrated care is another important factor to consider in reducing TRD. This approach is multifaceted and includes pairing primary care providers with mental health care specialists to improve outcomes [90]. Authors of a meta-analysis cited collaborative care that provides a range of interventions, such as telephone calls encouraging adherence, to more structured psychosocial activities as one of the most effective strategies in managing depression.

Medication Management

STAR * D both initiated treatment for major depression with citalopram and preserved its role through Level 2. While that remains a reasonable choice, escitalopram offers advantages in terms of its minimal effective dosing that is effective, safe, and well tolerated making its use a suitable if not superior alternative [91, 92]. In terms of next steps, venlafaxine is effective but more side effects make it a better Level 2 choice [93].

Failure of two successive medication trials or Level 3 in the STAR * D paradigm is a reasonable definition for TRD with entry into Level 4 representing an even more intractable depressive state [94]. The continuing morbidity associated with both Level 3 and 4 argues for more aggressive evidence-based interventions. This includes consideration of newer medications, evidence-based psychotherapy, and nonpharmacological interventions.

Newer pharmacologic strategies involve the use of second-generation antipsychotics for purposes of augmenting antidepressants. Aripiprazole and quetiapine had more robust augmentation efficacy than olanzapine and risperidone but all had worse tolerability [95]. On a more fundamental level, combination antidepressant pharmacotherapy appears more efficacious than monotherapy for TRD although once again the rate of adverse events is a factor clinicians should consider [96].

The United States Veterans Health Administration launched a large-scale study examining the augmentation and switching treatments for improving depression outcomes (VAST-D). Investigators of the multisite VAST-D designed a study exploring next-step pharmacologic strategies among subjects not achieving remission from a major depressive episode who were currently taking a selective serotonin reuptake inhibitor, selective serotonin norepinephrine reuptake inhibitor, or mirtazapine. The next step involved one of three randomized options: a switch to bupropion-SR or augmenting the current antidepressant with either bupropion-SR or aripiprazole [97].

Results from the VAST-D were mixed. Augmentation with aripiprazole produced a modest, but statistically significant likelihood of remission during the 12-week study as compared to bupropion-SR monotherapy or the bupropion-SR augmentation. These next-level treatment interventions were not without side effects — bupropion-SR increased anxiety and aripiprazole contributed to weight gain and sedation. The findings in the VAST-D are limited in terms of generalizability by the preponderance of male subjects with posttraumatic stress disorder (PTSD) [98, 99].

Lithium augmentation appears to be equally effective with tricyclic antidepressants and their second-generation successors, suggesting this as a viable option [100, 101]. Triiodothyronine (T3) is a time-tested augmentation choice for depression that requires careful implementation and periodic monitoring; an efficacy that may extend to newer generation antidepressants but its long-term safety is still uncertain [102–104]. Tranylcypromine is an effective intervention for TRD but its tyramine diet restrictions requires patient vigilance and the risk of serotonergic toxicity when combined with other similar acting drugs makes it reasonable as, at best, a Level 4 choice for the most treatment refractory cases [105]. Tricyclic and tetracyclic antidepressants are also effective treatments for depression but their use must weigh the risk of overdose and side effects that impinge on tolerability [106, 107].

Psychotherapy

Results for psychotherapy are mixed. A systematic review of behavioral therapies versus psychodynamic, humanistic, and integrative therapies reported low to moderate quality evidence that were all equally effective for acute depression while acknowledging overall study design limitations [108]. Another meta-analysis concluded that cognitive behavior therapy (CBT) was an effective treatment for the acute phase of major depression [109].

In terms of TRD the literature is mixed. A randomized controlled trial examining the benefit of 20 sessions of short-term psychotherapy reported improved remission rates [110]. Another randomized controlled trial reported that antidepressant augmentation with CBT reduced depression [111]. Alternatively, the provision of interpersonal psychotherapy for augmentation in TRD was not supported in a smaller RCT [112].

Neuromodulation

The previously mentioned, the Rand report explored barriers to care among veterans seeking mental health care with the top concern voiced by nearly half of the respondents being medication side effects. This provides both an opportunity and the rationale for nonpharmacologic treatments [7]. Included among this group are neuromodulation interventions such as transcranial magnetic stimulation (TMS), transcranial direct current stimulation (TDCS), deep brain stimulation, and electroconvulsive therapy [113].

TMS is an intervention that relies on the principle of magnetic induction to produce subconvulsive levels of neuronal stimulation. A magnetic coil is placed on the patient's forehead and depending on location either depolarizes or hyperpolarizes cortical neurons. TMS begins with the electrical stimulation of a coil, which is transformed to magnetic pulses, which allows unimpeded passage through the skull after which the magnetic energy once again becomes electrical. Repetitive delivery of magnetic pulses modulates cortical and subcortical regions, which through an internal cascade affect synaptic activity.

For example, it is theorized that TMS applied to the left dorsolateral prefrontal cortex depolarizes subcortical neurons with stimulation reaching the limbic system and modulating neurotransmitter activity favorable for treating depression. As a focal treatment, TMS has nonsystemic side effects, the most common being scalp discomfort, headaches, and the rare occurrence of seizures. The FDA approved TMS for TRD, defined as failing one antidepressant trial, in 2008 [114].

The efficacy, tolerability, safety, and indications for TMS are a continuing focus of many clinical investigations but based on systematic reviews, randomized controlled studies, and observational studies the novel approach is a promising intervention for depression [115]. TMS may also be a suitable choice for older adults with TRD [116]. Researchers reported a 45% remission rate among veterans and 59% among a sample of active duty service members [117, 118]. For TRD, TMS is roughly twice as effective as sham treatment and is well tolerated with manageable side effects [119]. Practice guidelines provide additional empiric support while promoting standards for treatment and documentation [120]. In a head-to-head comparison between electroconvulsive therapy (ECT) and TMS, authors of a systematic review and meta-analysis concluded that while ECT was more effective than TMS for TRD it was less well tolerated leaving TMS with a better balance between efficacy and tolerability [121]. Using STAR * D terminology, TMS could be conceptualized as a Level 3 or 4 augmentation strategy.

Clinical Vignette

A retired master sergeant presented with a history of chronic depression that did not respond to three prior antidepressant medication trials of adequate dose and duration. The patient was not eager to try another medication and was hoping for nonpharmacologic options. After reviewing the patient's medical record, the clinician suggested TMS, a suggestion readily agreed to. After obtaining the patient's consent, the treatment began and over the course of the next 6 weeks of daily TMS her self-assessment instruments showed a steady improvement. At the end of TMS the patient was in remission.

Glutamate Receptor Modulators

Researchers looking for alternative treatment options for depressions are targeting the glutamate system where ample evidence suggests its role in the pathogenesis of the mood disorder. The majority of that attention is focused on ketamine, an N-methyl-D-aspartate (NMDA) antagonist. A systematic review of published research on 11 glutamate receptor modulators examined ketamine, memantine, D-cycloserine, and several investigational compounds. Only intravenous ketamine surpassed placebo and that effect was fleeting, diminishing rapidly after 1 week and completely gone in 2 weeks. Ketamine's side effects were confusion and emotional blunting [122].

Anticonvulsants

Although more commonly used for bipolar disorder, anticonvulsants may also have a role in TRD. Carbamazepine, lamotrigine, phenytoin, and topiramate may have an adjunctive role with antidepressants. Less certain evidence suggests a role for anticonvulsants when irritability or agitation forms a prominent part of the major depression [123].

Inflammation

Co-occurring depression is common among individuals with inflammatory diseases such as rheumatoid arthritis, inflammatory bowel disease, and hepatitis, observations which now suggest that abnormal activation of inflammatory pathways may contribute to TRD [124]. Research suggests that increased levels of pro-inflammatory cytokines correlate with depression [125].

Among older adults, research suggests that elevated C-reactive protein and Interleukin-6 levels contribute to depression [126]. Pharmacologic management of TRD with the use of anti-inflammatory medications is an emerging area of clinical interest and research, providing an opportunity to tailor treatment consistent with mood and physical disease [127].

Exercise and Nutrition

Clinicians commonly recommend exercise as part of a healthy lifestyle, but as a treatment for depression it appears more effective than no treatment, but in terms of TRD its role as an adjunctive intervention seems very limited, although further research is warranted [127]. The scientific base for adding nutritional supplements to improve mood remains embryonic and in need of further research but the limited evidence suggests such a role [128]. In terms of specific supplements, limited evidence suggests folate added to an antidepressant may be helpful [129]. Vitamin D supplementation may also reduce depressive symptoms but, like folate, it requires additional research [130].

Conclusion

The goal of treatment for major depressive disorder is remission, an outcome achieved by roughly two-thirds of the cases. Among those who do not achieve remission, mood disorder becomes chronic as it waxes and wanes and contributes to a significant deterioration of the person's quality of life.

For active duty service members, the transition from an acute episode to one with a chronic course may impair the individual's fitness for duty, an outcome that may culminate in a medical discharge. In the broadest terms, "unfit for duty" implies the service can no longer perform the basic aspects of their job, meet physical fitness standards, and be world-wide deployable. Rating the degree of impairment for disability determinations follows instructions provided in the Veteran Affairs Schedule for Rating Disabilities (VSARD) that requires an assessment focused on "the frequency, severity, and duration of psychiatric symptoms, the length of remissions, and the veteran's capacity for adjustment during periods of remission." [131]

Optimizing treatment for active duty service members with major depressive disorder increases the likelihood of their remaining fit for duty. But even with the most aggressive treatment at least one-third will follow a chronic course leading to TRD.

TRD offers the opportunity to provide a truly personalized level of care that considers the unique factors that complicate a veteran's recovery. A complete diagnostic reassessment may uncover co-occurring disorders, a wide range of possibilities from PTSD to neurocognitive disorders.

The good news is that clinicians have more diverse treatment options, both pharmacologic and nonpharmacologic. The relatively nascent field of neuromodulation is linking clinical research with device manufacturers and producing interventions such as transcranial magnetic stimulation. Experimental interventions using novel medications also offer the promise of new pathways.

TRD is a debilitating disorder and one that may justify separate diagnostic consideration. For veterans suffering with this chronic disorder, their hope for remission should be sustained by the continuing clinical and research efforts to relieve their burden.

References

1. Association AP. Diagnostic and statistical manual of mental disorders (DSM-5®). 5th ed. Arlington: American Psychiatric Publishing; 2013.
2. Quality. CfBHSa. 2015 National survey on drug use and health: detailed tables. Rockville: Substance Abuse and Mental Health Services Administration. p. 2016.

3. Gadermann AM, Engel CC, Naifeh JA, et al. Prevalence of DSM-IV major depression among U.S. military personnel: meta-analysis and simulation. Mil Med. 2012;177(8 0):47–59.
4. Blore JD, Sim MR, Forbes AB, Creamer MC, Kelsall HL. Depression in Gulf War veterans: a systematic review and meta-analysis. Psychol Med. 2015;45(8):1565–80.
5. Boakye EA, Buchanan P, Wang J, Stringer L, Geneus C, Scherrer JF. Self-reported lifetime depression and current mental distress among veterans across service eras. Mil Med. 2017;182(3–4):e1691–6.
6. Seal KH, Metzler TJ, Gima KS, Bertenthal D, Maguen S, Marmar CR. Trends and risk factors for mental health diagnoses among Iraq and Afghanistan veterans using Department of Veterans Affairs Health Care, 2002–2008. Am J Public Health. 2009;99(9):1651–8.
7. Tanielian TL, Jaycox LH, editors. Invisible wounds of war: psychological and cognitive injuries, their consequences, and services to assist recovery. Santa Monica: RAND Corporation; 2008. https://www.rand.org/pubs/monographs/MG720.html. Also available in print form.
8. Packnett ER, Elmasry H, Toolin CF, Cowan DN, Boivin MR. Epidemiology of major depressive disorder disability in the US military: FY 2007–2012. J Nerv Ment Dis. 2017;205(9):672–8.
9. Lande RG. Stress in service members. Psychiatr Clin. 2014;37(4):547–60.
10. Kelsey JE. Achieving remission in major depressive disorder: the first step to long-term recovery. J Am Osteopath Assoc. 2004;104(3 Suppl 1):S6–S10.
11. Health NIoM. Sequenced Treatment Alternatives to Relieve Depression (STAR*D) Study. 2017.
12. A. John Rush, Madhukar H. Trivedi, Stephen R. Wisniewski PD, et al. Acute and longer-term outcomes in depressed outpatients requiring one or several treatment steps: a STAR * D report. Am J Psychiatr 2006;163(11):1905–1917.
13. Hales DJ, Rapaport MH, Moeller K. FOCUS Major depressive disorder maintenance of certification (MOC) workbook. American Psychiatric Publishing; 2012.
14. Mrazek DA, Hornberger JC, Altar CA, Degtiar I. A review of the clinical, economic, and societal burden of treatment-resistant depression: 1996–2013. Psychiatric services (Washington, D.C.). 2014;65(8):977–87.
15. Fekadu A, Wooderson SC, Markopoulo K, Donaldson C, Papadopoulos A, Cleare AJ. What happens to patients with treatment-resistant depression? A systematic review of medium to long term outcome studies. J Affect Disord. 2009;116(1):4–11.
16. Cain RA. Navigating the Sequenced Treatment Alternatives to Relieve Depression (STAR*D) study: practical outcomes and implications for depression treatment in primary care. Prim Care. 2007;34(3):505–19, vi.
17. Trajkovic G, Starcevic V, Latas M, et al. Reliability of the Hamilton Rating Scale for Depression: a meta-analysis over a period of 49 years. Psychiatry Res. 2011;189(1):1–9.
18. Baer L, Blais MA. Handbook of clinical rating scales and assessment in psychiatry and mental health. New York: Humana Press; 2009.
19. Trivedi MH, Daly EJ. Measurement-based care for refractory depression: a clinical decision support model for clinical research and practice. Drug Alcohol Depend. 2007;88(Suppl 2):S61–71.
20. Reilly TJ, MacGillivray SA, Reid IC, Cameron IM. Psychometric properties of the 16-item Quick Inventory of Depressive Symptomatology: a systematic review and meta-analysis. J Psychiatr Res. 2015;60:132–40.
21. Surís A, Holder N, Holliday R, Clem M. Psychometric validation of the 16 Item Quick Inventory of Depressive Symptomatology Self-Report Version (QIDS-SR16) in military veterans with PTSD. J Affect Disord. 2016;202(Supplement C):16–22.
22. Fowler JC, Patriquin M, Madan A, Allen JG, Frueh BC, Oldham JM. Early identification of treatment non-response utilizing the Patient Health Questionnaire (PHQ-9). J Psychiatr Res. 2015;68(Supplement C):114–9.
23. Kocalevent R-D, Hinz A, Brähler E. Standardization of the depression screener Patient Health Questionnaire (PHQ-9) in the general population. Gen Hosp Psychiatry. 2013;35(5):551–5.

24. Dunstan DA, Scott N, Todd AK. Screening for anxiety and depression: reassessing the utility of the Zung scales. BMC Psychiatry. 2017;17(1):329.
25. O'Connor E, Rossom RC, Henninger M, et al. U.S. Preventive Services Task Force Evidence Syntheses, formerly Systematic Evidence Reviews. *Screening for Depression in Adults: An Updated Systematic Evidence Review for the U.S. Preventive Services Task Force*. Rockville: Agency for Healthcare Research and Quality (US); 2016.
26. Bagby RM, Ryder AG, Schuller DR, Marshall MB. The Hamilton Depression Rating Scale: has the gold standard become a lead weight? Am J Psychiatry. 2004;161(12):2163–77.
27. Association AP. American Psychiatric Association Practice Guidelines for the Treatment of Psychiatric Disorders: Compendium 2006: American Psychiatric Association; 2006.
28. Souery D, Amsterdam J, de Montigny C, et al. Treatment resistant depression: methodological overview and operational criteria. Eur Neuropsychopharmacol. 1999;9(1–2):83–91.
29. Rytwinski NK, Scur MD, Feeny NC, Youngstrom EA. The co-occurrence of major depressive disorder among individuals with posttraumatic stress disorder: a meta-analysis. J Trauma Stress. 2013;26(3):299–309.
30. Elhai JD, Contractor AA, Tamburrino M, et al. Structural relations between DSM-5 PTSD and major depression symptoms in military soldiers. J Affect Disord. 2015;175(Supplement C):373–8.
31. Stander VA, Thomsen CJ, Highfill-McRoy RM. Etiology of depression comorbidity in combat-related PTSD: a review of the literature. Clin Psychol Rev. 2014;34(2):87–98.
32. Hepner KA, Sloss EM, Roth CP, et al. Quality of care for PTSD and depression in the military health system: phase I report. Rand Health Q. 2016;6(1):14.
33. Richardson JD, Contractor AA, Armour C, St Cyr K, Elhai JD, Sareen J. Predictors of long-term treatment outcome in combat and peacekeeping veterans with military-related PTSD. J Clin Psychiatry. 2014;75(11):e1299–305.
34. Ramsawh HJ, Fullerton CS, Mash HBH, et al. Risk for suicidal behaviors associated with PTSD, depression, and their comorbidity in the U.S. Army. J Affect Disord. 2014;161(Supplement C):116–22.
35. Newton-Howes G, Tyrer P, Johnson T. Personality disorder and the outcome of depression: meta-analysis of published studies. Br J Psychiatry J Ment Sci. 2006;188:13–20.
36. Skodol AE, Grilo CM, Keyes KM, Geier T, Grant BF, Hasin DS. Relationship of personality disorders to the course of major depressive disorder in a nationally representative sample. Am J Psychiatry. 2011;168(3):257–64.
37. Fisher LB, Fava M, Doros GD, et al. The role of anger/hostility in treatment-resistant depression: a secondary analysis from the ADAPT-A study. J Nerv Ment Dis. 2015;203(10):762–8.
38. Dutton DG, Karakanta C. Depression as a risk marker for aggression: a critical review. Aggress Violent Behav. 2013;18(2):310–9.
39. Kornstein SG, Schneider RK. Clinical features of treatment-resistant depression. J Clin Psychiatry. 2001;62(Suppl 16):18–25.
40. Lan C-W, Fiellin DA, Barry DT, et al. The epidemiology of substance use disorders in US Veterans: a systematic review and analysis of assessment methods. Am J Addict. 2016;25(1):7–24.
41. Fuehrlein BS, Mota N, Arias AJ, et al. The burden of alcohol use disorders in US military veterans: results from the National Health and Resilience in Veterans Study. Addiction. 2016;111(10):1786–94.
42. Lande RG, Marin BA, Chang AS, Lande GR. Survey of alcohol use in the U.S. army. J Addict Dis. 2008;27(3):115–21.
43. Thomas KH, Turner LW, Kaufman EM, et al. Predictors of depression diagnoses and symptoms in Veterans: results from a national survey. Mil Behav Health. 2015;3(4):255–65.
44. Hawton K, Casañas i Comabella C, Haw C, Saunders K. Risk factors for suicide in individuals with depression: a systematic review. J Affect Disord. 2013;147(1):17–28.
45. Kimbrel NA, Newins AR, Dedert EA, et al. Cannabis use disorder and suicide attempts in Iraq/Afghanistan-era veterans. J Psychiatr Res. 2017;89(Supplement C):1–5.

46. Scherrer JF, Salas J, Sullivan MD, et al. The influence of prescription opioid use duration and dose on development of treatment resistant depression. Prev Med. 2016;91:110–6.
47. Scherrer JF, Salas J, Copeland LA, et al. Prescription opioid duration, dose, and increased risk of depression in 3 large patient populations. Ann Fam Med. 2016;14(1):54–62.
48. Prochaska JJ, Das S, Young-Wolff KC. Smoking, mental illness, and public health. Annu Rev Public Health. 2017;38:165–85.
49. Weinberger AH, Kashan RS, Shpigel DM, et al. Depression and cigarette smoking behavior: a critical review of population-based studies. Am J Drug Alcohol Abuse. 2017;43(4):416–31.
50. Paul K, Erin R, David S, Steven F, Binhuan W, Scott S. Relationship between tobacco cessation and mental health outcomes in a tobacco cessation trial. J Health Psychol. 2016. https://doi.org/10.1177/1359105316644974.
51. Kahler CW, Spillane NS, Busch AM, Leventhal AM. Time-varying smoking abstinence predicts lower depressive symptoms following smoking cessation treatment. Nicotine Tob Res. 2011;13(2):146–50.
52. Morozova M, Rabin RA, George TP. Co-morbid tobacco use disorder and depression: a re-evaluation of smoking cessation therapy in depressed smokers. Am J Addict. 2015;24(8):687–94.
53. Secades-Villa R, Gonzalez-Roz A, Garcia-Perez A, Becona E. Psychological, pharmacological, and combined smoking cessation interventions for smokers with current depression: a systematic review and meta-analysis. PLoS One. 2017;12(12):e0188849.
54. Correa R, Akiskal H, Gilmer W, Nierenberg AA, Trivedi M, Zisook S. Is unrecognized bipolar disorder a frequent contributor to apparent treatment resistant depression? J Affect Disord. 2010;127(1–3):10–8.
55. Souery D, Oswald P, Massat I, et al. Clinical factors associated with treatment resistance in major depressive disorder: results from a European multicenter study. J Clin Psychiatry. 2007;68(7):1062–70.
56. Lopresti AL, Hood SD, Drummond PD. A review of lifestyle factors that contribute to important pathways associated with major depression: diet, sleep and exercise. J Affect Disord. 2013;148(1):12–27.
57. Iosifescu DV, Bankier B, Fava M. Impact of medical comorbid disease on antidepressant treatment of major depressive disorder. Curr Psychiatry Rep. 2004;6(3):193–201.
58. Gupta MA, Simpson FC. Obstructive sleep apnea and psychiatric disorders: a systematic review. J Clin Sleep Med. 2015;11(2):165–75.
59. McLay RN, Klam WP, Volkert SL. Insomnia is the most commonly reported symptom and predicts other symptoms of post-traumatic stress disorder in US service members returning from military deployments. Mil Med. 2010;175(10):759.
60. Lande RG. Sleep problems, posttraumatic stress, and mood disorders among active-duty service members. J Am Osteopath Assoc. 2014;114(2):83–9.
61. Lande RG, Gragnani CT, Pourzand M, Hangemanole D. Alcohol biomarkers associated with obstructive sleep apnea. Subst Use Misuse. 2018;53(5):867–72.
62. Lande RG, Gragnani CT. Tobacco use & sleep problems among active duty service members. Osteopath Fam Phys. 2017;9(4):10.
63. Moyer CA, Sonnad SS, Garetz SL, Helman JI, Chervin RD. Quality of life in obstructive sleep apnea: a systematic review of the literature. Sleep Med. 2001;2(6):477–91.
64. Edwards C, Mukherjee S, Simpson L, Palmer LJ, Almeida OP, Hillman DR. Depressive symptoms before and after treatment of obstructive sleep apnea in men and women. J Clin Sleep Med. 2015;11(9):1029–38.
65. Orr JE, Smales C, Alexander TH, et al. Treatment of OSA with CPAP is associated with improvement in PTSD symptoms among veterans. J Clin Sleep Med. 2017;13(1):57–63.
66. Krystal AD. Psychiatric disorders and sleep. Neurol Clin. 2012;30(4):1389–413.
67. Iosifescu DV, Nierenberg AA, Alpert JE, et al. The impact of medical comorbidity on acute treatment in major depressive disorder. Am J Psychiatr. 2003;160(12):2122–7.
68. Bair MJ, Robinson RL, Katon W, Kroenke K. Depression and pain comorbidity: a literature review. Arch Intern Med. 2003;163(20):2433–45.

69. Cosci F, Fava GA, Sonino N. Mood and anxiety disorders as early manifestations of medical illness: a systematic review. Psychother Psychosom. 2015;84(1):22–9.
70. Hare DL, Toukhsati SR, Johansson P, Jaarsma T. Depression and cardiovascular disease: a clinical review. Eur Heart J. 2014;35(21):1365–72.
71. Cherbuin N, Kim S, Anstey KJ. Dementia risk estimates associated with measures of depression: a systematic review and meta-analysis. BMJ Open. 2015;5(12):e008853.
72. Snowden MB, Atkins DC, Steinman LE, et al. Longitudinal association of dementia and depression. Am J Geriatr Psychiatry. 2015;23(9):897–905.
73. Morimoto SS, Kanellopoulos D, Manning KJ, Alexopoulos GS. Diagnosis and treatment of depression and cognitive impairment in late life. Ann N Y Acad Sci. 2015;1345(1):36–46.
74. Geddes JR, Carney SM, Davies C, et al. Relapse prevention with antidepressant drug treatment in depressive disorders: a systematic review. Lancet (London, England). 2003;361(9358):653–61.
75. Ballenger JC. Clinical guidelines for establishing remission in patients with depression and anxiety. J Clin Psychiatry. 1999;60(Suppl 22):29–34.
76. Sansone RA, Sansone LA. Antidepressant adherence: are patients taking their medications? Innov Clin Neurosci. 2012;9(5–6):41–6.
77. Mandrioli R, Mercolini L, Saracino MA, Raggi MA. Selective serotonin reuptake inhibitors (SSRIs): therapeutic drug monitoring and pharmacological interactions. Curr Med Chem. 2012;19(12):1846–63.
78. Caley CF, Kando JC. SSRI efficacy—finding the right dose. J Psychiatr Pract. 2002;8(1):33–40.
79. Jakubovski E, Varigonda AL, Freemantle N, Taylor MJ, Bloch MH. Systematic review and meta-analysis: dose-response relationship of selective serotonin reuptake inhibitors in major depressive disorder. Am J Psychiatr. 2015;173(2):174–83.
80. Safer DJ. Raising the minimum effective dose of serotonin reuptake inhibitor antidepressants: adverse drug events. J Clin Psychopharmacol. 2016;36(5):483–91.
81. Rush AJ. STAR* D: what have we learned? Am J Psychiatr. 2007;164(2):201–4.
82. Uher R, Mors O, Rietschel M, et al. Early and delayed onset of response to antidepressants in individual trajectories of change during treatment of major depression: a secondary analysis of data from the Genome-Based Therapeutic Drugs for Depression (GENDEP) study. J Clin Psychiatry. 2011;72(11):1478–84.
83. Group MoMW. VA/DoD clinical practice guideline for management of major depressive disorder (MDD). Washington, DC: Department of Defense and Department of Veterans Affairs; 2009.
84. Hepner KA, Farris C, Farmer CM, et al. Delivering clinical practice guideline-concordant care for Ptsd and major depression in military treatment facilities. Santa Monica: RAND Corporation; 2017.
85. O'Donohue W, Draper C. Stepped care and e-Health: practical applications to behavioral disorders. New York: Springer New York; 2010.
86. Trivedi MH, Lin EH, Katon WJ. Consensus recommendations for improving adherence, self-management, and outcomes in patients with depression. CNS Spectr. 2007;12(8 Suppl 13):1–27.
87. Health NCCfM. Depression: the treatment and management of depression in adults (updated edition). 2010.
88. van Straten A, Hill J, Richards DA, Cuijpers P. Stepped care treatment delivery for depression: a systematic review and meta-analysis. Psychol Med. 2014;45(2):231–46.
89. Firth N, Barkham M, Kellett S. The clinical effectiveness of stepped care systems for depression in working age adults: a systematic review. J Affect Disord. 2015;170:119–30.
90. Katon W, Von Korff M, Lin E, et al. Collaborative management to achieve treatment guidelines: impact on depression in primary care. JAMA. 1995;273(13):1026–31.
91. Cipriani A, Santilli C, Furukawa TA, et al. Escitalopram versus other antidepressive agents for depression. The Cochrane Library. 2009.
92. Cipriani A, Purgato M, Furukawa TA, et al. Citalopram versus other anti-depressive agents for depression. Cochrane Database Syst Rev. 2012;(7):Cd006534.

93. de Silva VA, Hanwella R. Efficacy and tolerability of venlafaxine versus specific serotonin reuptake inhibitors in treatment of major depressive disorder: a meta-analysis of published studies. Int Clin Psychopharmacol. 2012;27(1):8–16.
94. Conway CR, George MS, Sackeim HA. Toward an evidence-based, operational definition of treatment-resistant depression: when enough is enough. JAMA Psychiat. 2017;74(1):9–10.
95. Komossa K, Depping AM, Gaudchau A, Kissling W, Leucht S. Second-generation antipsychotics for major depressive disorder and dysthymia. The Cochrane Library. 2010.
96. Rocha FL, Fuzikawa C, Riera R, Hara C. Combination of antidepressants in the treatment of major depressive disorder: a systematic review and meta-analysis. J Clin Psychopharmacol. 2012;32(2):278–81.
97. Mohamed S, Johnson GR, Vertrees JE, et al. The VA augmentation and switching treatments for improving depression outcomes (VAST-D) study: rationale and design considerations. Psychiatry Res. 2015;229(3):760–70.
98. Mohamed S, Johnson GR, Chen P, et al. Effect of antidepressant switching vs augmentation on remission among patients with major depressive disorder unresponsive to antidepressant treatment: the VAST-D randomized clinical trial. JAMA. 2017;318(2):132–45.
99. Fava M. Lessons learned from the VA augmentation and switching treatments for improving depression outcomes (VAST-D) study. JAMA. 2017;318(2):126–8.
100. Nelson JC, Baumann P, Delucchi K, Joffe R, Katona C. A systematic review and meta-analysis of lithium augmentation of tricyclic and second generation antidepressants in major depression. J Affect Disord. 2014;168:269–75.
101. Bauer M, Adli M, Ricken R, Severus E, Pilhatsch M. Role of lithium augmentation in the management of major depressive disorder. CNS Drugs. 2014;28(4):331–42.
102. Abraham G, Milev R, Lawson JS. T3 augmentation of SSRI resistant depression. J Affect Disord. 2006;91(2):211–5.
103. Aronson R, Offman HJ, Joffe RT, Naylor C. Triiodothyronine augmentation in the treatment of refractory depression: a meta-analysis. Arch Gen Psychiatry. 1996;53(9):842–8.
104. Morin AK. Triiodothyronine (T3) supplementation in major depressive disorder. Ment Health Clin. 2015;5(6):253–9.
105. Ricken R, Ulrich S, Schlattmann P, Adli M. Tranylcypromine in mind (Part II): review of clinical pharmacology and meta-analysis of controlled studies in depression. Eur Neuropsychopharmacol. 2017;27(8):714–31.
106. Linde K, Kriston L, Rücker G, et al. Efficacy and acceptability of pharmacological treatments for depressive disorders in primary care: systematic review and network meta-analysis. Ann Fam Med. 2015;13(1):69–79.
107. Undurraga J, Baldessarini RJ. Direct comparison of tricyclic and serotonin-reuptake inhibitor antidepressants in randomized head-to-head trials in acute major depression: systematic review and meta-analysis. J Psychopharmacol. 2017. https://doi.org/10.1177/0269881117711709.
108. Shinohara K, Honyashiki M, Imai H, et al. Behavioural therapies versus other psychological therapies for depression. The Cochrane Library. 2013.
109. Butler AC, Chapman JE, Forman EM, Beck AT. The empirical status of cognitive-behavioral therapy: a review of meta-analyses. Clin Psychol Rev. 2006;26(1):17–31.
110. Abbass AA. Intensive Short-Term Dynamic Psychotherapy of treatment-resistant depression: a pilot study. Depress Anxiety. 2006;23(7):449–52.
111. Wiles N, Thomas L, Abel A, et al. Cognitive behavioural therapy as an adjunct to pharmacotherapy for primary care based patients with treatment resistant depression: results of the CoBalT randomised controlled trial. Lancet. 2013;381(9864):375–84.
112. Souza LH, Salum GA, Mosqueiro BP, Caldieraro MA, Guerra TA, Fleck MP. Interpersonal psychotherapy as add-on for treatment-resistant depression: a pragmatic randomized controlled trial. J Affect Disord. 2016;193:373–80.
113. Holtzheimer PE, Mayberg HS. Neuromodulation for treatment-resistant depression. F1000 Med Rep. 2012;4:22.

114. Holtzheimer PE, McDonald W. A clinical guide to transcranial magnetic stimulation. New York: Oxford University Press; 2014.
115. Janicak PG, Dokucu ME. Transcranial magnetic stimulation for the treatment of major depression. Neuropsychiatr Dis Treat. 2015;11:1549–60.
116. Conelea CA, Philip NS, Yip AG, et al. Transcranial magnetic stimulation for treatment-resistant depression: naturalistic treatment outcomes for younger versus older patients. J Affect Disord. 2017;217:42–7.
117. Kozel FA, Hernandez M, Van Trees K, et al. Clinical repetitive transcranial magnetic stimulation for veterans with major depressive disorder. Ann Clin Psychiatry. 2017;29(4):242–8.
118. Lande RG, Pierce J. Efficacy of transcranial magnetic stimulation for treatment resistant depression among active duty service members. Gen Hosp Psychiatry. 2017;45:99–100.
119. Leggett LE, Soril LJJ, Coward S, Lorenzetti DL, MacKean G, Clement FM. Repetitive transcranial magnetic stimulation for treatment-resistant depression in adult and youth populations: a systematic literature review and meta-analysis. Primary Care Companion CNS Disord. 2015;17(6) https://doi.org/10.4088/PCC.4015r01807.
120. McClintock SM, Reti IM, Carpenter LL, McDonald WM, Dubin M, Taylor SF, Cook IA, O'Reardon J, Husain MM, Wall C, Krystal AD, Sampson SM, Morales O, Nelson BG, Latoussakis V, George MS, Lisanby SH, National Network of Depression Centers rTMS Task Group, American Psychiatric Association Council on Research Task Force on Novel Biomarkers and Treatments. Consensus recommendations for the clinical application of repetitive transcranial magnetic stimulation (rTMS) in the treatment of depression. J Clin Psychiatry. 2018;79(1). pii: 16cs10905. https://doi.org/10.4088/JCP.16cs10905.
121. Chen J-j, Zhao L-b, Liu Y-y, Fan S-t, Xie P. Comparative efficacy and acceptability of electroconvulsive therapy versus repetitive transcranial magnetic stimulation for major depression: a systematic review and multiple-treatments meta-analysis. Behav Brain Res. 2017;320:30–6.
122. Caddy C, Amit BH, McCloud TL, et al. Ketamine and other glutamate receptor modulators for depression in adults. Cochrane Database Syst Rev. 2015;(9):Cd011612.
123. Vigo DV, Baldessarini RJ. Anticonvulsants in the treatment of major depressive disorder: an overview. Harv Rev Psychiatry. 2009;17(4):231–41.
124. Shariq AS, Brietzke E, Rosenblat JD, Barendra V, Pan Z, McIntyre RS. Targeting cytokines in reduction of depressive symptoms: a comprehensive review. Prog Neuro-Psychopharmacol Biol Psychiatry. 2018;83:86–91.
125. Wohleb ES, Franklin T, Iwata M, Duman RS. Integrating neuroimmune systems in the neurobiology of depression. Nat Rev Neurosci. 2016;17(8):497–511.
126. Smith KJ, Au B, Ollis L, Schmitz N. The association between C-reactive protein, Interleukin-6 and depression among older adults in the community: a systematic review and meta-analysis. Exp Gerontol. 2018;102:109–32.
127. Köhler O, Krogh J, Mors O, Benros ME. Inflammation in depression and the potential for anti-inflammatory treatment. Curr Neuropharmacol. 2016;14(7):732–42.
128. Harbottle L, Schonfelder N. Nutrition and depression: a review of the evidence. J Ment Health. 2008;17(6):576–87.
129. Taylor MJ, Carney SM, Geddes J, Goodwin G. Folate for depressive disorders. The Cochrane Library. 2003.
130. Shaffer JA, Edmondson D, Wasson LT, et al. Vitamin D supplementation for depressive symptoms: a systematic review and meta-analysis of randomized controlled trials. Psychosom Med. 2014;76(3):190.
131. Register OotF. Code of Federal Regulations, Title 38, Pensions, Bonuses, and Veterans' Relief, Pt. 0–17, Revised as of July 1 2010. U.S. Government Printing Office; 2010.

Psychotic Disorders and Best Models of Care

8

Philip M. Yam, Dinesh Mittal, and Ayman H. Fanous

Introduction

Schizophrenia is uncommon in the active duty military, partly due to pre-screening and accession standards. However, when military members present with psychotic symptoms, a plethora of challenges arise. Behavioral health providers must balance patient-centered care, confidentiality of treatment, public safety, and fitness for duty.

This chapter is a review and discussion on psychotic disorders and their impacts on active duty military members and veterans. Psychotic disorders significantly affect a military member's career, health, and family. This chapter will explore stages of psychosis from pre-symptom social withdrawal, to hospitalizations and treatments, and to becoming a veteran. Antipsychotic treatments and side effects are discussed, notably the effects of metabolic syndrome. Barriers to care exist including stigma, which is also reviewed. The etiology of schizophrenia and psychotic disorders is complex. This chapter also presents a summary of the genetic research on this topic relevant to veterans. Lastly, further innovations in outreach and treatment are discussed.

The views expressed in the article are those of the authors and do not necessarily reflect the official policy or position of the Department of the Navy, Department of Defense, nor the U.S. Government.

P. M. Yam (✉)
Naval Branch Health Clinic Belle Chasse, Department of Behavioral Health,
Belle Chasse, LA, USA
e-mail: Philip.m.yam.mil@mail.mil

D. Mittal
G. V. (Sonny) Montgomery VA Medical Center, Department of Mental Health,
Jackson, MS, USA

A. H. Fanous
SUNY Downstate Medical Center, Psychiatry and Behavioral Sciences, Brooklyn, NY, USA

Presentation of Psychosis in the Military

The presentation of psychosis may range from mild to severe, however all forms may create challenges for the clinical team. A member with mild or subtle symptoms of psychosis will likely continue to maintain their ability to stay outpatient, seek voluntary evaluation and treatment, and even stay at work in a limited capacity. The medical team may not have the clinical indication to pursue involuntary hospitalization. Building trust and rapport with the member is critical at every stage to improve the clinical outcome for the member. Psychotic symptoms may or may not be mood-congruent, and insight of illness of the member also may be impaired.

Social withdrawal (83%) was the most common prodromal symptom experienced by eventual service members diagnosed with schizophrenia [1]. Military members are young, and as such, mild psychotic symptoms should not be untreated due to the risk of developing a significantly disabling schizophrenia or schizoaffective disorder.

In the case of a severely psychotic service member, treatment and evaluation is necessary in a hospital-based setting. The service member in a psychotic state may be deemed to lack capacity to make their own decisions, thus requiring the treatment team to proceed with the emergency hospitalization, without the patient's consent, for the purpose of the health and safety of the member and public.

Military members serve worldwide, hence evaluations must be thorough and consider a wide range of causes and differential diagnoses. Designer drug abuse, dissociative disorders, personality disorders, conversion disorder, and malingering must also be explored. Best results occur when there is established trust, open communication, and adherence to treatment.

A presentation of psychosis will greatly impact a service member's career. These members predominantly transition out of active duty to become veterans and retirees. This process necessitates an organized clinical team, a working relationship with the member's command, and an established rapport with the patient. Goals include building strengths, family connection, and community function. Early interventions are important as young veterans were much more likely to have worse mental health quality of life than non-veterans of the same age [2] (Fig. 8.1).

Active Duty Military Epidemiology and Prevalence

The first onset of psychotic disorders usually occurs in young persons. Therefore, an understanding of psychosis in veterans warrants discussion of the prevalence of psychosis in active duty populations. While all-cause prevalence of psychosis has not been explored, studies have reviewed schizophrenia in the military. In the United States military, first time schizophrenia hospitalization occurred in 1.6/10,000 person-years. This rate of hospitalization was similar to other studies outside the military in 25 nations. There was no difference in males vs females. African-American military members had higher rates of schizophrenia admissions with relative risk of 1.5 [3].

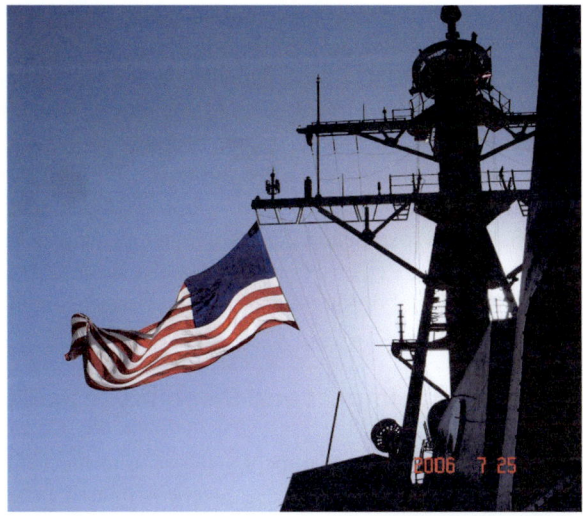

Fig. 8.1 US flag aboard a navy destroyer. (Photograph by Philip Yam, MD)

Schizophrenia and schizoaffective disorders are not conducive to continued service and therefore the vast majority are referred for a medical evaluation board, which may result in a medical discharge from military service. Between 1992 and 2001, there were 1291 discharges for schizophrenia through the disability system, or an average of 129.1 service members per year covering all military branches [4]. In the same study, the time of initial symptoms to referral to medical board was 1.6 years. Prodromal symptoms will be further discussed in this chapter.

Veterans and Serious Mental Illness, Population Data from SMITREC Data

Serious Mental Illness Treatment Resource and Evaluation Center (SMITREC) categorizes psychotic disorders in veterans into schizophrenia spectrum, bipolar spectrum, and other psychotic disorders [5]. Psychotic disorders constitute a group of serious mental illnesses that can affect the functionality of the brain to varying degrees.

Serious mental illness (SMI) is defined as any psychotic spectrum diagnosis of schizophrenia, delusional disorders, and severe affective disorders like bipolar and major depressive disorder causing substantial interference with activities of daily living (ADLs), instrumental activities of daily living (IADLs), and functioning in social, family, and vocational contexts [6, 7]. Serious mental illness also includes persistent and disabling mental health conditions [8].

Prevalence

According to Veterans Health Administration (VHA) SMITREC's National Psychosis Registry [5], FY15, a total of 2,58,662 VHA patients were suffering from psychosis, 60.8% of the users were between 35 to 65 years of age, and 28.7% were above 65 years. The mean age of VHA users suffering from psychosis is 56.10 years with a standard deviation of 14.40. Males constitute 86.9% of those diagnosed. Caucasians constitute 67.1% and 33% of VHA users with psychosis were married. Among three different categories of psychosis, schizophrenia accounts for 37.7%, bipolar disorder accounts for 51.9%, and other psychotic disorders constitute 10.4%.

Psychotic disorders are often comorbid with other psychiatric illnesses with a majority being depression (42.2%). Among other medical comorbidities, the majority constitute hypertension (48.2%), digestive system disease (50.4%), and arthritis (52%). 17.8% of VHA users were homeless at the time of diagnosis and 95.2% were within 40 miles of driving distance of a primary care site.

Public Health Impact and Disability in Schizophrenia

The combined costs of treatment and loss of productivity of schizophrenia (SCZ) in the general US population in 2002 were estimated to be $62.7 billion [9]. Even during periods free of active psychosis, cognitive deficits are thought to contribute to the development of functional skills deficits in patients, which are needed to maintain oneself independently in the community, in the areas of self-care, social and occupational function, and medication adherence as well as other aspects of management of the illness [10, 11].

Recognizing the major impact of SCZ on the psychosocial function of the more than 100,000 veterans with the disorder in the Veterans Affairs (VA) system, the VA funded, and recently completed, the collection and genotyping of 4000 veterans with SCZ and another 5000 with bipolar disorder (BPD) in the study "Genetics of Disability in Schizophrenia and Bipolar Illness (CSP#572)" [12], all of whom were extensively assessed for neurocognitive function and disability.

Prodromal Symptoms

Early presentation of a psychotic disorder such as schizophrenia does not always start with psychotic symptoms. Military members in Singapore were studied for prodromal symptoms before the first psychotic break compared with non-psychotic members treated in mental health, and analysis found that psychotic members were more likely to experience social withdrawal, deterioration in school, and concentration problems. Common problems that were not distinguished between the psychotic and non-psychotic groups were sleep disturbance, anxiety, depressed mood, and anger [2].

In the case of service members with exposure to combat or psychological trauma, evaluations aim to untangle psychosis from symptoms of post-traumatic stress disorder (PTSD). Common symptoms of PTSD and schizophrenia may include: distrust of others, discomfort in crowded places, poor concentration, disruption of mood, social isolation, dissociative episodes, memory impairment, negative beliefs about the world, decreased activities or interests, irritability, verbal and physical aggression, and sleep disturbance. Furthermore, there may exist both conditions of PTSD and schizophrenia, thus complicating the focus of treatment and recovery.

Minimization of Symptoms

Prevalence was discussed previously in this chapter with noting a delay of 1.6 years from first noticing psychiatric symptoms to eventual referral to a medical separation process [4]. Service members experiencing early or mild psychiatric symptoms of any disorder may experience fear of stigma, shame, or separation.

Military training promotes the unity of all members, and diversion from the norm is discouraged. A young military member is encouraged to develop teamwork, leadership, physical stamina, and military proficiency. Training involves long hours of physical fitness, classroom work, drills, and on-the-job training. Service members may experience hesitation to request to be removed from their peers and training for medical appointments, including behavioral health. Stigma is further discussed later in this chapter.

Three pathways usually exist that bring members with psychosis to behavioral health. The first is voluntary self-referral. Direct, open physician-patient communication of a schizophrenia diagnosis has been shown to improve medication adherence with odds ratio of 5.82 in community studies [13].

The second pathway of referral occurs when a member with psychotic symptoms and impaired insight into their illness may be noticed by peers or supervisors to be having behavioral disturbances concerning to their health and the mission. These individuals are referred to behavioral health evaluation via a command directed evaluation [14]. A behavioral health provider seeing a member that was command directed will need to use keen evaluation skills, collateral information from peers, supervisors, and family members, and review of the consistency of the story to determine the presence or absence of a psychiatric problem, including psychotic symptoms.

The third pathway of referral occurs when a member having a severe psychotic break with life-threatening concerns will require an emergency room visit or direct admission to inpatient treatment. Discussing the diagnosis with the patient is best done in a multidisciplinary approach. Team-based treatment teams are more effective and successful [15].

Mortality in Psychotic Disorders in Veterans Compared with Civilian Population

Between the years 1997 and 2000, patients treated for serious mental illness at eight state public mental health systems died on average 25 years earlier than the general population in USA [16]. However, this disparity is less severe with patients treated at VHA. Cardiovascular disease is the leading cause for mortality in individuals with SMI [17]. In the year 2015, about 9.8 million adults in USA were suffering from SMI [18] and 3% of VHA users with psychosis died in the year 2015 [5].

Medication Treatment and Metabolic Syndrome

Veterans receiving antipsychotic medications on an outpatient basis are at risk of developing metabolic syndrome, which basically refers to disturbances in lipid and glucose metabolism associated with excess weight gain. Affected individuals may have co-existing hypertension, abdominal obesity, hyperglycemia, and lipid abnormalities resulting in higher risk for cardiovascular disease, stroke, diabetes, and accelerated atherosclerosis.

For a person to be given the diagnosis of metabolic syndrome, at least three of the following five criterion must be met (1). A waist circumference of 40 inches or more in men and 35 inches or more in women (2). Serum triglycerides of 150 mg/dl or more (3). High-density lipoprotein (HDL) cholesterol of 40 mg/dl or less in men and 50 mg/dl or less in women (4). Blood pressure of 130/85 or more (5). Fasting blood glucose of 100 mg/dl or more.

In addition to the use of antipsychotic medications, multiple other factors contribute to the development of metabolic syndrome. Obesity combined with lifestyle risk factors like physical inactivity, high-fat diet, psychosocial stress, smoking, and heavy alcohol consumption play a major role. Advanced age, the relative deficiency of type-1 muscle fibers and genetic predisposition are also implicated in its causation [19].

While veterans may benefit from antipsychotics in terms of improvement from psychosis, the risk of metabolic syndrome can be increased. Critical decisions have to be made by healthcare providers in switching the antipsychotic medication with a balance maintained between metabolic syndrome risk and psychotic symptom control. There has been a greater concern after the introduction of second-generation antipsychotics that can potentially increase the risk of metabolic derangements like hyperglycemia, dyslipidemia, diabetes, weight gain, and serious complications like diabetic ketoacidosis.

Among different antipsychotics of choice, clozapine and olanzapine have a greater tendency to cause elevation of triglycerides [20], whereas ziprasidone and aripiprazole are associated with the lowest risk for weight gain. Central obesity and weight gain play a major role in the pathophysiology of metabolic syndrome induced by antipsychotics, predisposing the individuals for a greater risk of diabetes, insulin resistance, and dyslipidemias [21].

If left untreated, patients eventually develop various cardiovascular changes often resulting in premature death due to myocardial infarction. Further, individuals with genetically aberrant folate metabolism and hyperhomocysteinemia have a greater risk for metabolic syndrome with the use of antipsychotic medications [22]. Sedentary lifestyle and poor dietary habits are often prevalent in individuals with a serious mental illness that makes them vulnerable to metabolic abnormalities. Use of antipsychotic medications in this vulnerable group can further potentiate the risk of metabolic syndrome.

Monitoring a Veteran Started on Antipsychotic Medication

Health care providers should consider the assessment of family history, weight, body mass index (BMI), blood pressure, fasting lipid profile, and fasting glucose levels when a service member or veteran is started on antipsychotic medication. American Psychiatric Association and American Diabetes Association (APA-ADA)

Consensus Guidelines require periodic assessment of weight at 4, 8, and 12 weeks after initiation or change of an antipsychotic medication and should be continued quarterly. Fasting plasma glucose levels, blood pressure, and lipid profile should be assessed every 3 months upon the initiation of antipsychotic medication and more frequently in patients with increased baseline risk. An increase in the weight of 5% or more should warrant lifestyle modifications like exercises and dietary changes with consideration of change in medication [21].

Guideline-concordant management for hyperglycemia include administration of metformin or thiazolidinedione class of medications, participation in weight reduction and exercise programs, change in dietary habits, and switching over to antipsychotic medication with a lower tendency to cause weight gain [21, 22]. Upon clinical indication, 3-hydroxy-3-methyl-glutaryl-coenzyme A (HMG-CoA) reductase inhibitors, nicotinic acid, bile acid sequestrants, and fibric acid agents can be used to correct lipid abnormalities. Low-dose aspirin can be considered to address the prothrombotic state induced by metabolic syndrome [21]. Thus, following the recommended guidelines when a patient is started on antipsychotic medication can minimize the risk of developing metabolic syndrome.

Frequency of Metabolic Syndrome in Patients with SMI

Caroff et al. [23] examined 10,132 veterans with serious mental illness and found the presence of metabolic syndrome in 48.8% of the patients. Increased prevalence is seen in elderly, men, African-American, and those receiving disability pension benefits. Those who received antipsychotic medications, antidepressants, and anticonvulsants experienced greater prevalence of metabolic syndrome. Also, these patients had higher rates of coronary artery disease, cerebrovascular disease, and mortality [23]. Khatana, Kane, Taveira, Bauer, and Wu [24] retrospectively examined 1401 veterans with serious mental illness suffering either from schizophrenia or schizoaffective disorder or bipolar disorder. 21.4% of these veterans were not monitored for the presence of metabolic syndrome and 48.4% of monitored patients with serious mental illness had metabolic syndrome [24]. This highlights the importance of metabolic monitoring in individuals with serious mental illness, making critical decisions as warranted.

Genetics and the Boundaries of Psychosis

One of the oldest and most influential nosological schemas in psychiatry is Emil Kraepelin's distinction between *Dementia Praecox* and Manic-Depressive Illness on the basis of having a chronic deteriorating vs relapsing-remitting course, respectively [62]. These of course went on to be called schizophrenia and bipolar disorder. While earlier family studies did not find significant evidence for familial coaggregation of the two disorders, at least two suggested that psychotic BPD overlaps genetically with schizophrenia [63, 64]. This was supported by linkage studies reporting increased evidence of linkage when psychotic BPD was included in the definition of affection of schizophrenia [65]. However, a very large registry-based family study in Sweden reported significantly increased risk of BPD in biological relatives of schizophrenia probands and vice versa [26]. The first convincing molecular evidence of genetic overlap was reported by the International Schizophrenia Consortium, which showed that polygenic risk scores (PRSs) based on the results of a genome-wide association study (GWAS) of schizophrenia significantly predicted case-control status in independent BPD data sets but did not do so in non-psychiatric disorders [32]. This was further confirmed by a more powerful analysis of several disorders using the genome-wide complex trait analysis (GCTA) methodology. This showed that the genetic correlations (r_g) of schizophrenia were 0.68, 0.43, and 0.16 to BPD, major depressive disorder (MDD), and autism, respectively [66].

While schizophrenia and BPD clearly have clinical and biological overlap, they also comprise different clusters of symptoms at different times in their clinical course, which respond to different treatments. Their diagnostic distinction is therefore therapeutically pragmatic. More recently, a study tested for variants *distinguishing* the two [67] by conducting GWAS of schizophrenia vs BPD as opposed to cases vs controls. No individual loci reached genome-wide significance. However, several were moderately significant ($P < 10^{-5}$), and more importantly, a polygenic score of schizophrenia vs BPD was seen to significantly predict the schizophrenia vs BPD status in independent samples. This was the first time that any two psychiatric disorders could be distinguished genetically, which suggests that genetics could potentially play a role in diagnostic refinement.

Genetics and the Clinical Heterogeneity of Schizophrenia

SCZ has long been noted to be heterogeneous with respect to symptoms, course, and age of onset, among other features. Indeed, Kraepelin subsumed under the rubric of Dementia Praecox the previously described conditions catatonia, paranoia, and hebephrenia. He himself described ten subtypes of Dementia Praecox [62]. Bleuler, working simultaneously with Kraepelin, posited that psychotic disorders were a "Group of Schizophrenias" [68]. Furthermore, he distinguished accessory from fundamental symptoms. The latter comprise what we think of today as negative symptoms, to which he clearly accorded primacy.

DSM-3 was the first classification system to include subtypes, namely, the paranoid, catatonic, disorganized, and residual. Several decades of work have resulted in little empirical support for the validity, reliability, or longitudinal stability of these constructs, and there has been decreased usage of them in the research literature [69]. This has led to their elimination in diagnostic and statistical manual of mental disorders, fifth edition (DSM-5) [70]. Nevertheless, there have been a number of genetic studies of SCZ that attempted to identify loci influencing either clinical subtypes or symptomatic dimensions of the illness. In a GWAS of the latter in the Multicenter Genetic Studies of Schizophrenia (MGS) sample, 19 independent loci were moderately associated with positive, negative/disorganized, or affective symptoms [71]. More interestingly, the schizophrenia PRS correlated with the negative/disorganized dimension, but not the positive or affective dimensions.

The use of subtypes, either a priori determined or statistically constructed based on latent variable modeling, as phenotypes of interest have yielded a number of interesting findings. However, this approach, because of its inherently reducing sample size by dividing cases into distinct groups, is bound to risk reducing statistical power, even if it increases the signal-to-noise ratio by using more biologically homogeneous phenotypes. Deficit syndrome–like subtypes were significantly linked to 1q [72] and suggestively linked to 20p [73], while a cognitive deficit subtype was linked to 6p [74]. At the time of writing, no GWAS has been published using such phenotypes, although a number of efforts are ongoing in the Psychiatric Genomics Consortium (PGC) using latent class and cluster analysis.

Heritability of Psychotic Illness

Family [25, 26], twin [27], adoption [28], linkage [29], and association [30, 31] studies together strongly suggest that SCZ is highly heritable (~80%) [27]. Data from a variety of sources suggest genetic complexity, as the illness does not follow patterns consistent with Mendelian inheritance, demonstrating evidence of incomplete penetrance, polygenicity, genetic heterogeneity (locus and allelic), and phenocopies. A polygenic model was first hypothesized in the etiology of schizophrenia by Gottesman and Shields. This was thought to be more consistent with inheritance patterns seen in the disorder than were simpler, earlier models postulating one or a few genes.

Common Genetic Variants

GWASs of SCZ began in 2006, but the first ones with the power to detect significant, and subsequently replicated effects, were conducted in three consortia [32–34], which later merged to form the Psychiatric Genomics Consortium (PGC) Schizophrenia Workgroup (PGC SCZ) for the purpose of conducting a single, systematic analysis ("mega-analysis") [35]. PGC-SCZ now contains most of the world's extant SCZ GWAS samples, currently comprising about 37,000 cases and 45,000 controls from 49 case-control samples of European and Asian ancestry [36].

The most recent PGC-SCZ report provides the most complete and accurate picture of common variation in SCZ to date [36]. A total of 108 independent genomic loci were identified, 75% of which include at least one protein-coding gene. Interestingly, only 10 of these were the association signal attributable to a protein-coding variant, suggesting that most common variations influencing SCZ risk by altering the expression levels of proteins rather than their structure. The association signals were enriched at enhancers in brain tissue as well as immunity-related tissues such as B-lymphocyte lineages, which are encoded by genes in the major histocompatibility complex (MHC) region of 6p. Among the genes implicated, many had not been previously nominated and in some cases suggested novel etiopathogenic mechanisms.

The most significant locus in this study was in the MHC region. A breakthrough study reported that the MHC signal was driven in part by SCZ-associated haplotypes in Complement C4, which was also shown to have decreased cortical expression in SCZ, as well as play a role in synaptic pruning [36]. This study demonstrated the power of GWAS to tightly focus the search for specific risk haplotypes, when jointly analyzed with sequence data. It also demonstrated for the first time that such analyses could not only identify specific genetic risk factors, such as haplotypes, but when creatively used to inform gene expression and animal models, they could elucidate previously unsuspected etiopathogenic processes.

Rare Copy Number Variants

Copy number variant (CNV) studies have reported deletions in 1q21.1, 15q13.3, 22q11.21 [37–39]. The latter is further supported by a recent study demonstrating that duplications of this region are actually protective. Deletions were later shown to be found in 3q29, 7q36.3, 7q11.23 (reciprocal deletion), 11q11.12, and 16p12.2. Several genes have been shown to have deletions associated with SCZ, including *NXN1* [39, 40] and *VIPR2* [39]. Duplications associated with SCZ include 1p36.3, 16p11.2 [41, 42], and overall increase in CNV burden genome-wide [37, 43]. The penetrance of CNVs is variable and has been calculated to range from 2% to 100%. CNVs associated with SCZ can be inherited as well as de novo. De novo CNVs have been demonstrated to be enriched in the N-methyl-D-aspartate (NMDA) receptor and several dihydrolipoamide dehydrogenase (DLG) genes. The latter make up the membrane-associated guanylate kinase (MAGUK) complex, a component of the post-synaptic density (PSD). The third major group was the voltage-gated ion channel genes, including *CACNA1C*, which has been significantly associated with both SCZ [44] and BPD [45, 46] in GWAS. The most recent meta-analysis of the majority of the world's microarray data showed a significant excess of CNV burden genome-wide in cases, which was driven by CNVs within genes [47]. A further analysis of the data, which excluded previously implicated genes, suggested that a considerable portion of risk CNVs were ultra-rare (i.e., with a minor allele frequency of 0.1%). A few CNVs were found to have a protective role, although this did not survive genome-wide correction. However, with a larger sample size, one or more of these could be confirmed. These include duplications of 22q11.2 and *MAGEA11* along with deletions and duplications of *ZNF92*. The implicated CNVs strongly suggested enrichment in genes encoding synaptic proteins, which was consistent with previous lines of evidence [48–51]. Such gene sets included synaptic cell adhesion and scaffolding proteins, glutamatergic ionotropic receptors, and protein complexes such as the activity-regulated cytoskeleton-associated protein (ARC) complex and dystrophin-glycoprotein complex (DGC).

Rare Single Nucleotide Variants

While the heritability of SCZ has been estimated to be 80% [27], reflecting both common and rare variation, common alleles only account for a portion of that. Furthermore, CNVs as a class, on the whole, are too rare to comprise a substantial portion of heritability by themselves. This suggests that a substantial portion of the "missing heritability" is due to rare single nucleotide variants (SNVs) or point mutations, defined as having a minor allele frequency (MAF) of <1%. While exome sequencing (ES) studies had been conducted in SCZ before, it was only this year that adequately powered studies demonstrating significant effects in specific gene groups have been published [46, 47]. These provide the most complete picture to date of rare variation at the single nucleotide level in schizophrenia.

The broadest finding, in a sample of 2500 cases and 2500 controls from Sweden, was that individuals with SCZ had a higher rate of rare disruptive mutations (defined as nonsense, essential splice site, and frameshift) than controls [46]. This analysis was limited to about 2500 genes previously implicated in GWAS, CNV, and de novo SNV studies. Gene sets found to be particularly enriched for disruptive SNVs in cases included ARC and NMDA receptor (*NMDAR*) genes, which in part comprise PSD genes, which were also enriched. The third major gene group found to be enriched was the voltage-gated calcium channel group. This includes *CACNA1C*, which has been significantly associated with both SCZ and BPD.

In a parallel study of over 600 Bulgarian trios, enrichment for de novo mutations in ARC, NMDAR, and PSD genes was also found, as was enrichment in genes previously implicated in SCZ [47]. Furthermore, genes repressed by the fragile X mental retardation protein (FMRP) were also enriched. One of the more interesting findings in this study was that genes with de novo mutations in SCZ overlapped those affected by de novo mutations in both autism and intellectual disability. This highlights the importance of cognitive dysfunction as an underlying phenotype of the presentation of SCZ, which is perhaps more proximal to the effects of genes than is disease risk overall.

Whole-Genome Sequencing: Rationale and Recent Successes

In recent years, it has become increasingly clear that whole-genome sequencing (WGS) is the most powerful platform for genomic studies of complex disease. GWAS studies are only able to reliably provide information about common variants. Exome sequencing (ES), which has been successfully used to assay the impact of rare variants in SCZ [48, 49], is limited in scope to the 1% of the human genome comprised of coding deoxyribonucleic acid (DNA), or a total of about 30 MB. Each individual, on average, has about 3.5 million genetic variants, of which only about 20,000 are exonic. The non-coding genome is replete with elements of potential impact on somatic and behavioral phenotypes, including promoters, enhancers, non-coding ribonucleic acid (RNA), etc. One of the most significant results of the largest GWAS of SCZ to date is that only 10% of genome-wide significant loci were attributable to a protein-coding variant [30]. The association signal was enriched at brain-expressed enhancers, which are important elements of non-coding regulatory machinery.

The cost of WGS has decreased by more than a million-fold since it was first introduced, and it currently stands as 2–2.5 times more expensive than exome sequencing. Even in studying the exome, WGS has distinct advantages over ES, in part because the latter is dependent on the performance of capture kits. A recent study showed that WGS covered 10.8% more coding exons than ES did [52]. In another study, 74.8% of coding regions were covered by WGS at 40X, compared to only 48% coverage in ES [53]. In detecting rare CNVs, WGS is vastly superior to microarrays. It was recently demonstrated that 95.6% of small CNVs detected by WGS were not detected by high-resolution microarrays [53].

In the last 3 years, a number of WGS studies have successfully identified rare variants contributing to common, complex disease, in both case-control [55–57] and family samples [52–54]. In psychiatric illness, this has been most notable in autism [52, 53], which has been shown to have overlapping genetic risk factors with SCZ, including CNVs [58, 59] and overall single nucleotide polymorphism (SNP)-coheritability [60] due to common alleles. In a study of 32 families segregating autistic disorders, Jiang et al. identified variants that were either de novo or inherited autosomal dominant or X-linked, in 22 genes. Of these variants, 1 was a splice site, 3 were frameshift, 3 were nonsense, and the remainder missense [52]. Interestingly, four of the genes were not previously known autism spectrum disorder (ASD) risk genes and suggested potentially new pathways for drug targets.

A study of 85 ASD families identified such variants in 34 genes, 14 of which were known in neurodevelopmental disorders, but not ASD [53]. In both studies, although the focus was coding regions, several of the identified variants would not have been discovered had exome sequencing been performed. These studies highlight the power of WGS to discover etiologically relevant variation that is essentially invisible to GWAS and exome sequencing, even in the exome itself. Another significant development has been the ability to impute rare variants discovered in WGS studies into much larger GWAS datasets with the power to detect association. In a study of type 2 diabetes, this resulted in the discovery of two rare and two low-frequency risk variants [56]. WGS studies of SCZ have yet to be reported, although a number are being conducted at the time of writing, some of which are included in the Whole-Genome Sequencing Consortium [61].

Differential Diagnosis and Additional Considerations

Military members and veterans may come from anywhere in the country and could have deployed anywhere in the world. Behavioral health providers must expand diagnostic considerations for members presenting with psychosis. A new onset of symptoms requires a medical and laboratory review for other conditions, and in certain situations imaging and additional studies are indicated. Psychosis that is combined with delirium, unstable vital signs, or visual hallucinations are suspect of an internal biological problem that may require hospitalization and further investigation.

Magnetic resonance imaging may reveal infection, white matter disease, or gross anatomic changes. Leukoencephalopathies are white matter diseases caused by autoimmune diseases, toxins, or cancers, which may cause delusions, hallucinations, and neurologic abnormalities. New onset psychosis with suspicion of drug abuse warrants testing for the presence of synthetic cannabinoids and bath salts in urine or blood samples. Tumors can precipitate anti-N-methyl-D-aspartate-receptor antibodies that can be found in cerebrospinal fluid, with a presentation of seizures, catatonia, aggression, and paranoia. Pentraxin-related protein 3 (PTX3), an immune and inflammation protein, was low in schizophrenia military members vs healthy controls by 3.0 odds ratio [75]. This decrease in PTX3 in schizophrenia was not found in bipolar patients.

Stigma of Serious Mental Illness

Despite all that is known about veterans and SMI, an often ignored social and clinical variable has the potential to disrupt or even prevent otherwise high-quality treatment from occurring. This variable is the stigma of mental illness. Specifically, veterans with serious mental illnesses like schizophrenia, bipolar disorder, and major depressive disorder experience negative effects of discrimination, prejudices, and stereotypes from the public frequently preventing them from receiving the services they need. Unfortunately, veterans with SMI are exposed to even more stigma than other groups, often resulting in a lack of help for those who need it most. Concerned researchers have studied stigma of mental illness attempting to understand and counteract the harm caused by stigma.

Self-Stigma, Public-Stigma and Provider Stigma

Researchers examining stigma of mental illness in veterans have discovered that it takes many forms and is active in many environments. Critically, researchers have delineated stigma into three common types; self-stigma, public-stigma, and provider-stigma. Self-stigma occurs when veterans with mental illness internalize the public attitudes of discrimination and prejudice and suffer from resultant negative consequences like low levels of hope, self-esteem, and decreased help-seeking behavior [76, 77]. Public stigma refers to the negative impact created by members of the general population when they endorse negative stereotypes about individuals with mental illness [78], thereby making them undesirable or socially unacceptable [79].

Provider stigma is a part of public stigma where health care providers display discriminatory attitudes and behaviors toward veterans with the serious mental illness [80]. Each of these three types of stigma interact to reduce treatment engagement and efficacy, suggesting counter-stigma efforts may need to address the entire spectrum of stigma to be effective. However, research has shown that even with social and clinical counter-stigma programs, stigma is difficult to improve due to other messages veterans receive about SMI and accompanying treatments.

In addition to society at large, the advertising and film industry often regard mental illness as a socially unacceptable, negatively stereotyped, and a fear-inducing condition which is frequently associated with the usage of derogatory terminology. With the reinforcement of existing social stigma from stigma depicted within the advertising and film industry, effective available treatments are often not utilized and social integration is frequently prevented [81]. The public often characterizes mentally ill veterans as unpredictable, incompetent, and dangerous. The combination of prejudices, stereotypes, and discriminatory behaviors explain public stigma. "Fear" and "danger" play a large role in the public perception of veterans with mental illnesses often resulting in a strong desire for social distance [82].

In addition to the danger posed by self and public stigma, health care provider stigma significantly reduces treatment engagement and treatment efficacy, a troubling and perhaps unexpected process, given the ostensible role of health care providers to help, not harm, veterans under their care [83]. This can be explained on the basis of physician bias such as attributing poor prognosis to the patient based on mental illness diagnosis and misattribution of signs and symptoms of physical illness to existing mental illness [84]. The experience of working with severely, mentally ill veterans on a routine basis may result in attributing the serious course of the disease to all patients with the same diagnosis, a phenomenon described as "clinical illusion" [80]. Also, providers' stereotype unconsciously depends on patient categories such as race/ethnicity, gender, age, sexual orientation, and socioeconomic status [85]. A finding illustrates that even with a high degree of professional training, providers are not immune to the social and psychological processes driving stigma.

Consequences of Public Stigma of Mental Illness

Given what is known about the structure and process of stigma in veterans, researchers have still asked why patients, the public, and providers develop and maintain stigma. As has been discussed, individuals likely to benefit from receiving psychiatric services often do not seek treatment or poorly adhere to the treatment because of fear of being stigmatized by the public. This occurs more commonly with serious mental illnesses.

Researchers have identified the Health Belief Model as a potential explanation of WHY stigma occurs. According to the Health Belief Model, individuals choose treatments with greater perceived benefits than threats. Since pursuing treatment for psychiatric illness is associated with being labeled as "mentally ill" by the public, and a consequent lower self-esteem, these individuals avoid that perceived threat. Older age, less education, and poverty are also associated with stigma for receiving treatment. In contrast to expectations, people with more knowledge of mental illnesses, like medical students, often refuse to seek help because of the fear of being stigmatized [86]. These findings shed light on the traditionally perplexing nature of stigma.

Research further suggests that veterans with stigmatizing mental illness tend to react in three different ways. If the individual with mental illness does not identify himself with stigmatizing behaviors of the public, he will likely remain unresponsive. On the other hand, if the individual identifies himself with stigmatizing attitudes of the public, he will likely suffer low self-esteem and self-efficacy. And some people regard public stigma to be totally unfair and seek right health services [86]. This reiterates the fact that the complex nature of stigma can result in diversified effects on persons experiencing it.

While there are numerous negative consequences, the most pertinent one is discrimination. The veteran with mental illness may not be given equal opportunity for employment. Right for self-determination may be taken away, and the person might suffer segregation in the society [87]. Comparatively, stigmatized individuals are more likely to experience homelessness, discrimination in housing, and unemployment [88]. Relative to individuals having minor mental health issues, those with serious mental illnesses like schizophrenia, bipolar, and schizoaffective disorder experience greater stigma because of perceived danger by the public. Of particular note is the discrimination in health care settings toward individuals with substance abuse problems that can further hamper help-seeking behavior [89].

In conclusion, addressing the public stigma of mental illness can improve the help-seeking behavior of service users, also increasing the compliance with mental health care facilities. People living in countries with better knowledge about tackling mental health issues experienced less internalized and perceived stigma [89], which further strengthens the idea of implementing effective anti-stigma interventions.

Improving Transition of Care

Service members preparing for change are susceptible to increased stress on their support systems, finances, and coping strategies. Strengthening a transition of care from the military treatment facility (MTF) to the next location of care is critical. Some members who receive a medical retirement may not transition their care and continue treatment at the MTF. However, since most military members are more likely to move back to their home of origin, they will require assistance to receive ongoing care. Gaining consent to include family discussion is essential. A direct provider-to-provider discussion (i.e., a warm handoff) is ideal, and the clinical team should even emphasize setting an appointment date before the member physically departs for home.

A change in care may increase risk for a lapse in treatment adherence, which would cause a relapse in symptoms. Successful transitions that reduce morbidity and crisis events have huge reduction in morbidity and social costs. Hospital costs associated with schizophrenia patients with suicide attempts were $46,024, for recurrent hospitalizations $37,329, arrests $31,081, and violent behaviors $18,778 [90] (Fig. 8.2).

Innovations in Treatments

VA has developed specialized programs for veterans with serious mental illness including those with psychotic disorders to foster recovery, rehabilitation, and integration in the community. Psychosocial Rehabilitation and Recovery Centers (PRRC) are outpatient specialty mental health transitional learning centers designed for veterans with serious mental illness and severe functional impairment to promote recovery and reintegration into meaningful community roles based on their personal goals and preferences. Programming is curriculum based and focuses on building up veteran skills and talents to achieve one's chosen goals in all domains of life. PRRC services are part of the mental health continuum of care and are coordinated with

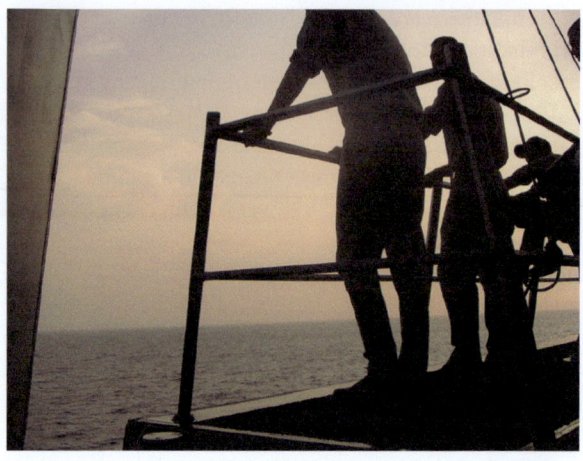

Fig. 8.2 Sunset on naval warship. (Photograph by Philip Yam, MD)

other services in the Veterans Health Administration (VHA) and in the community. To instill hope in veterans suffering from serious mental illness, efforts must focus on building up the skills and strengths necessary for successful re-integration into community-based on their own values, preferences, and goals [92].

Core services being offered by PRRC include:

1. Services that promote hope and self-respect by enhancing skills based on individual preferences and strengths.
2. Facilitating enhanced life quality in various domains of life.
3. Providing services to address the unique needs based on cultural norms.
4. Recovery planning and coaching to meet the clinical needs of individual. This is done more frequently during the initial period and less frequently after the clinical goals are achieved.
5. Individual psychotherapy.
6. Social skills training classes.
7. Psychoeducational classes.
8. Illness Management and Recovery classes using substance abuse and mental health services administration (SAMHSA) illness management and recover (IMR) Tool-Kit Material.
9. Wellness programming to promote healthy and active lifestyle using SAMHSA Action Planning for Wellness and Prevention.
10. Family psychoeducational and family educational programs.
11. Peer support services.
12. PRRC bridge groups (psychoeducational groups provided by PRRC staff members on acute and non-acute inpatient mental health units to educate about PRRC programs and other recovery-oriented programs also assisting them with transition).
13. Treatment of co-occurring substance use disorders.

Therapeutic and Supported Employment Services

The therapeutic and supported employment services (TSES) program is designed to provide vocational rehabilitation for veterans recovering from chronic mental illness, substance abuse, and homelessness to enhance overall well-being as they reintegrate back into community [91]. Components of the program include Compensated Work Therapy (CWT) programs (supported employment, transitional work, sheltered workshops, and veterans construction team), incentive therapy (IT), and vocational assistance.

All veterans in VHA mental health treatment programs who are interested in developing work-related skills can participate in the TSES program regardless of their psychiatric diagnosis, symptoms, work history, or cognitive impairment.

Services offered by TSES include:

1. *Sheltered Workshops:* Veterans participate in workshops under close clinical supervision by CWT staff. Monetary benefit would be provided on a piece rate basis.
2. *Transitional Work Experience (TWE):* Intended to provide supportive services for veterans to successfully transition into competitive employment. Veterans participate in actual work settings and get paid on hourly basis during this period.
3. *Supported Employment (SE):* Meant for veterans with serious mental illness having employment barriers. An employment specialist helps in finding the jobs that match their interests, also considering the barriers.
4. *Veterans Construction Team (VCT):* A form of transitional work for veterans interested in the construction industry. Employment is in VA or other Federal organizations that are supervised by experienced tradespersons.

Conclusion

Military members and veterans face a multitude of challenges from intensive training, time separation from family, deployments, combat trauma, and health problems. However, schizophrenia and other psychotic disorders instill tremendous impacts on a service member's career and ability to function after the military. The stigma of serious military illness, including schizophrenia, imposes a large barrier to seeking and receiving treatments that are available.

Research efforts in the genetics of schizophrenia have achieved large gains through genome-wide association studies. The large impacts of psychotic disorders in the veteran population requires collaboration of Veterans Affairs, public health efforts, and military treatment facilities. Innovative treatment modalities and expansion of outreach efforts are needed to facilitate recovery and reintegration in the community.

References

1. Tan HY, Ang YG. First-episode psychosis in the military: a comparative study of prodromal symptoms. Aust N Z J Psychiatry. 2001;35(4):512–9.
2. Kazis LE, Miller DR, Clark J, Skinner K, Lee A, Rogers W, Spiro A 3rd, Payne S, Fincke G, Selim A, Linzer M. Health-related quality of life in patients served by the Department of Veterans Affairs: results from the Veterans Health Study. Arch Intern Med. 1998; 158(6):626–32.
3. Herrell R, Henter ID, Mojtabai R, Bartko JJ, Venable D, Susser E, Merikangas KR, Wyatt RJ. First psychiatric hospitalizations in the US military: the National Collaborative Study of Early Psychosis and Suicide (NCSEPS). Psychol Med. 2006;36(10):1405–15. Epub 2006 Jul 31.
4. Millikan AM, Weber NS, Niebuhr DW, Torrey EF, Cowan DN, Li Y, Kaminski B. Evaluation of data obtained from military disability medical administrative databases for service members with schizophrenia or bipolar disorder. Mil Med. 2007;172(10):1032–8.
5. Care for veterans health administration clients with psychosis, FY2015. 17th Annual Report, VHA National Psychosis Registry: Serious Mental Illness Treatment Resource and Evaluation Center. Retrieved from http://vaww.smitrec.va.gov/National_Psychosis_Registry.asp.
6. Molinari V, Hobday JV, Roker R, Kunik ME, Kane R, Kaas MJ, et al. Impact of serious mental illness online training for certified nursing assistants in long term care. Gerontol Geriatr Educ. 2017;38(4):359–74.
7. Kessler RC, Berglund PA, Bruce ML, Koch JR, Laska EM, Leaf PJ, et al. The prevalence and correlates of untreated serious mental illness. Health Serv Res. 2001;36(6 Pt 1):987.
8. Gold KJ, Kilbourne AM, Valenstein M. Primary care of patients with serious mental illness: your chance to make a difference: a primary care visit may lead to regular care of side effects and comorbidities, especially if you coordinate care. J Fam Pract. 2008;57(8):515–26.
9. McEvoy JP. The costs of schizophrenia. J Clin Psychiatry. 2007;68(Suppl 14):4–7.
10. Bowie CR, et al. Predicting schizophrenia patients' real-world behavior with specific neuropsychological and functional capacity measures. Biol Psychiatry. 2008;63:505–11.
11. Harvey PD, et al. Validating the measurement of real-world functional outcomes: phase I results of the VALERO study. Am J Psychiatry. 2011;168:1195–201.
12. Harvey PD, et al. The genetics of functional disability in schizophrenia and bipolar illness: methods and initial results for VA cooperative study #572. Am J Med Genet B Neuropsychiatr Genet. 2014;165B:381–9.
13. McCabe R, Healey PG, Priebe S, Lavelle M, Dodwell D, Lauharne R, Snell A, Bremner S. Shared understanding in psychiatrist-patient communication: association with treatment adherence in schizophrenia. Patient Educ Couns. 2013;93(1):73–9.
14. Mental Health Evaluations of Members of the Military Services. Department of Defense Instruction 6490.04. Mar 4, 2013.
15. Outram S, Harris G, Kelly B, Cohen M, Bylund CL, Landa Y, Levin TT, Sandhu H, Vamos M, Loughland C. Contextual barriers to discussing a schizophrenia diagnosis with patients and families: need for leadership and teamwork training in psychiatry. Acad Psychiatry. 2015;39(2):174–80.
16. Centers for Disease Control and Prevention, National Center for Health Statistics. Underlying Cause of Death 1999–2016 on CDC WONDER Online Database, released December, 2017. Data are from the Multiple Cause of Death Files, 1999–2016, as compiled from data provided by the 57 vital statistics jurisdictions through the Vital Statistics Cooperative Program. Accessed at http://wonder.cdc.gov/ucd-icd10.html on 12 Feb 2018.
17. Kilbourne AM, Ignacio RV, Kim HM, Blow FC. Datapoints: are VA patients with serious mental illness dying younger? Psychiatr Serv. 2009;60(5):589.
18. Bose J, Hedden SL, Lipari RN, Park-Lee E, Porter JD, Pemberton MR. Key substance use and mental health indicators in the United States: results from the 2015 National Survey on Drug Use and Health. Substance Abuse and Mental Health Services Administration website. 2016.

https://www.samhsa.gov/data/sites/default/files/NSDUH-FFR1-2015/NSDUH-FFR1-2015/NSDUH-FFR1-2015.pdf. Published September.
19. Han TS, Lean ME. Metabolic syndrome. Medicine. 2015;43(2):80–7.
20. Li C, Mittal D, Owen RR. Impact of patients' preexisting metabolic risk factors on the choice of antipsychotics by office-based physicians. Psychiatr Serv. 2011;62(12):1477–84.
21. Narasimhan M, Raynor JD. Evidence-based perspective on metabolic syndrome and use of antipsychotics. Drug Benefit Trends. 2010;22:77–88.
22. Viverito K, Owen R, Mittal D, Li C, Williams JS. Management of new hyperglycemia in patients prescribed antipsychotics. Psychiatr Serv. 2014;65(12):1502–5.
23. Caroff SN, Leong SH, Ng-Mak D, Campbell EC, Berkowitz RM, Rajagopalan K, et al. Socioeconomic disparities and metabolic risk in veterans with serious mental illness. Community Ment Health J. 2018;54:725.
24. Khatana SAM, Kane J, Taveira TH, Bauer MS, Wu WC. Monitoring and prevalence rates of metabolic syndrome in military veterans with serious mental illness. PLoS One. 2011;6(4):e19298.
25. Kendler KS, et al. The Roscommon Family Study. I. Methods, diagnosis of probands, and risk of schizophrenia in relatives. Arch Gen Psychiatry. 1993;50:527–40.
26. Lichtenstein P, et al. Common genetic determinants of schizophrenia and bipolar disorder in Swedish families: a population-based study. Lancet. 2009;373:234–9.
27. Sullivan PF, Kendler KS, Neale MC. Schizophrenia as a complex trait: evidence from a meta-analysis of twin studies. Arch Gen Psychiatry. 2003;60:1187–92.
28. Kendler KS, Gruenberg AM, Kinney DK. Independent diagnoses of adoptees and relatives as defined by DSM-III in the provincial and national samples of the Danish Adoption Study of Schizophrenia. Arch Gen Psychiatry. 1994;51:456–68.
29. Ng MY, et al. Meta-analysis of 32 genome-wide linkage studies of schizophrenia. Mol Psychiatry. 2009;14:774–85.
30. Schizophrenia Working Group of the Psychiatric Genomics Consortium. Biological insights from 108 schizophrenia-associated genetic loci. Nature. 2014;511:421–7.
31. Aberg KA, et al. A comprehensive family-based replication study of schizophrenia genes. JAMA Psychiat. 2013;70:1–9.
32. Purcell SM, et al. Common polygenic variation contributes to risk of schizophrenia and bipolar disorder. Nature. 2009;460:748–52.
33. Shi J, et al. Common variants on chromosome 6p22.1 are associated with schizophrenia. Nature. 2009;460:753–7.
34. Stefansson H, et al. Common variants conferring risk of schizophrenia. Nature. 2009;460:744–7.
35. Cichon S, et al. Genomewide association studies: history, rationale, and prospects for psychiatric disorders. Am J Psychiatry. 2009;166:540–56.
36. Sekar A, et al. Schizophrenia risk from complex variation of complement component 4. Nature. 2016;530:177–83. https://doi.org/10.1038/nature16549.
37. International Schizophrenia Consortium. Rare chromosomal deletions and duplications increase risk of schizophrenia. Nature. 2008;455:237–41.
38. Stefansson H, et al. Large recurrent microdeletions associated with schizophrenia. Nature. 2008;455:232–6.
39. Levinson DF, et al. Copy number variants in schizophrenia: confirmation of five previous findings and new evidence for 3q29 microdeletions and VIPR2 duplications. Am J Psychiatry. 2011;168:302–16.
40. Rujescu D, et al. Disruption of the neurexin 1 gene is associated with schizophrenia. Hum Mol Genet. 2009;18:988–96.
41. McCarthy SE, et al. Microduplications of 16p11.2 are associated with schizophrenia. Nat Genet. 2009;41:1223–7.
42. Bergen SE, et al. Genome-wide association study in a Swedish population yields support for greater CNV and MHC involvement in schizophrenia compared with bipolar disorder. Mol Psychiatry. 2012;17:880–6. https://doi.org/10.1038/mp.2012.73.
43. Grozeva D, et al. Rare copy number variants: a point of rarity in genetic risk for bipolar disorder and schizophrenia. Arch Gen Psychiatry. 2010;67:318–27.

44. Ripke S, et al. Genome-wide association study identifies five new schizophrenia loci. Nat Genet. 2011;43:969–76.
45. Sklar P, et al. Large-scale genome-wide association analysis of bipolar disorder identifies a new susceptibility locus near ODZ4. Nat Genet. 2011;43:977–83.
46. Sklar P, et al. Whole-genome association study of bipolar disorder. Mol Psychiatry. 2008;13:558–69.
47. Marshall CR, et al. Contribution of copy number variants to schizophrenia from a genome-wide study of 41,321 subjects. Nat Genet. 2017;49:27–35. https://doi.org/10.1038/ng.3725.
48. Purcell SM, et al. A polygenic burden of rare disruptive mutations in schizophrenia. Nature. 2014;506:185–90.
49. Fromer M, et al. De novo mutations in schizophrenia implicate synaptic networks. Nature. 2014;506:179–84.
50. Walsh T, et al. Rare structural variants disrupt multiple genes in neurodevelopmental pathways in schizophrenia. Science. 2008;320:539–43.
51. Xu B, et al. Strong association of de novo copy number mutations with sporadic schizophrenia. Nat Genet. 2008;40:880–5.
52. Jiang YH, et al. Detection of clinically relevant genetic variants in autism spectrum disorder by whole-genome sequencing. Am J Hum Genet. 2013;93:249–63.
53. Yuen RK, et al. Whole-genome sequencing of quartet families with autism spectrum disorder. Nat Med. 2015;21:185–91.
54. Iossifov I, et al. The contribution of de novo coding mutations to autism spectrum disorder. Nature. 2014;515:216–21.
55. Helgason H, et al. A rare nonsynonymous sequence variant in C3 is associated with high risk of age-related macular degeneration. Nat Genet. 2013;45:1371–4.
56. Steinthorsdottir V, et al. Identification of low-frequency and rare sequence variants associated with elevated or reduced risk of type 2 diabetes. Nat Genet. 2014;46:294–8.
57. Morrison AC, et al. Whole-genome sequence-based analysis of high-density lipoprotein cholesterol. Nat Genet. 2013;45:899–901.
58. Guilmatre A, et al. Recurrent rearrangements in synaptic and neurodevelopmental genes and shared biologic pathways in schizophrenia, autism, and mental retardation. Arch Gen Psychiatry. 2009;66:947–56.
59. Stefansson H, et al. CNVs conferring risk of autism or schizophrenia affect cognition in controls. Nature. 2014;505:361–6.
60. Lee SH, et al. Genetic relationship between five psychiatric disorders estimated from genome-wide SNPs. Nat Genet. 2013;45:984–94.
61. Sanders SJ, et al. Whole genome sequencing in psychiatric disorders: the WGSPD consortium. Nat Neurosci. 2017;20:1661–8. https://doi.org/10.1038/s41593-017-0017-9.
62. Kraepelin, E. Manic-depressive insanity and paranoia. Edinburgh, Scotland: E & S Livingstone; 1921.
63. Erlenmeyer-Kimling L, et al. The New York High-Risk Project. Prevalence and comorbidity of axis I disorders in offspring of schizophrenic parents at 25-year follow-up. Arch Gen Psychiatry. 1997;54:1096–102.
64. Kendler KS, et al. The Roscommon Family Study. II. The risk of nonschizophrenic nonaffective psychoses in relatives. Arch Gen Psychiatry. 1993;50:645–52.
65. Fanous AH, et al. Genetic overlap of schizophrenia and bipolar disorder in a high-density linkage survey in the Portuguese Island population. Am J Med Genet B Neuropsychiatr Genet. 2012;159B:383–91.
66. Yang J, Lee SH, Goddard ME, Visscher PM. GCTA: a tool for genome-wide complex trait analysis. Am J Hum Genet. 2011;88:76–82.
67. Ruderfer DM, et al. Polygenic dissection of diagnosis and clinical dimensions of bipolar disorder and schizophrenia. Mol Psychiatry. 2014;19(9):1017–24.
68. Bleuler E. Dementia praecox, or The group of schizophrenias. New York: International Universities Press; 1950.
69. Braff DL, Ryan J, Rissling AJ, Carpenter WT. Lack of use in the literature from the last 20 years supports dropping traditional schizophrenia subtypes from DSM-5 and ICD-11. Schizophr Bull. 2013;39:751–3.

70. Tandon R, et al. Definition and description of schizophrenia in the DSM-5. Schizophr Res. 2013;150:3–10.
71. Fanous AH, et al. A genome-wide scan for modifier loci in schizophrenia. Am J Med Genet B Neuropsychiatr Genet. 2007;144:589–95.
72. Holliday EG, McLean DE, Nyholt DR, Mowry BJ. Susceptibility locus on chromosome 1q23-25 for a schizophrenia subtype resembling deficit schizophrenia identified by latent class analysis. Arch Gen Psychiatry. 2009;66:1058–67.
73. Fanous AH, et al. Novel linkage to chromosome 20p using latent classes of psychotic illness in 270 Irish high-density families. Biol Psychiatry. 2008;64:121–7.
74. Hallmayer JF, et al. Genetic evidence for a distinct subtype of schizophrenia characterized by pervasive cognitive deficit. Am J Hum Genet. 2005;77:468–76.
75. Weber NS, Larsen RA, Yolken RH, Cowan DN, Boivin MR, Niebuhr DW. Predictors of the onset of schizophrenia in US military personnel. J Nerv Ment Dis. 2015;203(5):319–24.
76. Corrigan PW, Rao D. On the self-stigma of mental illness: stages, disclosure, and strategies for change. Can J Psychiatry. 2012;57(8):464–9.
77. Mittal D, Sullivan G, Chekuri L, Allee E, Corrigan PW. Empirical studies of self-stigma reduction strategies: a critical review of the literature. Psychiatr Serv. 2012;63(10):974–81.
78. Corrigan PW, Kuwabara SA, O'Shaughnessy J. The public stigma of mental illness and drug addiction: findings from a stratified random sample. J Soc Work. 2009;9(2):139–47.
79. Mullen PR, Crowe A. Self-stigma of mental illness and help seeking among school counselors. J Couns Dev. 2017;95(4):401–11.
80. Mittal D, Corrigan P, Drummond KL, Porchia S, Sullivan G. Provider opinions regarding the development of a stigma-reduction intervention tailored for providers. Health Educ Behav. 2016;43(5):577–83.
81. Schulze B, Richter-Werling M, Matschinger H, Angermeyer M. Crazy? So what! Effects of a school project on students' attitudes towards people with schizophrenia. Acta Psychiatr Scand. 2003;107(2):142–50.
82. Link BG, Phelan JC, Bresnahan M, Stueve A, Pescosolido BA. Public conceptions of mental illness: labels, causes, dangerousness, and social distance. Am J Public Health. 1999;89(9):1328–33.
83. Charles JL, Bentley KJ. Measuring mental health provider-based stigma: development and initial psychometric testing of a self-assessment instrument. Community Ment Health J. 2018;54(1):33–48.
84. Thornicroft G, Rose D, Kassam A. Discrimination in health care against people with mental illness. Int Rev Psychiatry. 2007;19(2):113–22.
85. Burgess DJ, Fu SS, Van Ryn M. Why do providers contribute to disparities and what can be done about it? J Gen Intern Med. 2004;19(11):1154–9.
86. Rüsch N, Angermeyer MC, Corrigan PW. Mental illness stigma: concepts, consequences, and initiatives to reduce stigma. Eur Psychiatry. 2005;20(8):529–39.
87. Corrigan PW, Shapiro JR. Measuring the impact of programs that challenge the public stigma of mental illness. Clin Psychol Rev. 2010;30(8):907–22.
88. Parcesepe AM, Cabassa LJ. Public stigma of mental illness in the United States: a systematic literature review. Adm Policy Ment Health Ment Health Serv Res. 2013;40(5):384–99.
89. Henderson C, Evans-Lacko S, Thornicroft G. Mental illness stigma, help seeking, and public health programs. Am J Public Health. 2013;103(5):777–80.
90. Zhu B, Ascher-Svanum H, Faries DE, Peng X, Salkever D, Slade EP. Costs of treating patients with schizophrenia who have illness-related crisis events. BMC Psychiatry. 2008;8:72.
91. Department of Veterans Affairs. Psychosocial rehabilitation and recovery centers. VHA Handbook, 1163.03. 2016.
92. Department of Veterans Affairs. Therapeutic and supported employment services program. VHA Handbook, 1163.02. 2011.

Alcohol and Alcohol Use Disorder

Thomas W. Meeks, Nicole M. Bekman,
Nicole M. Lanouette, Kathryn A. Yung, and Ryan P. Vienna

Clinical Care: Part I

Sergeant X is a 25yo male Marine with 6 years of active duty service. He had no formal psychiatric history prior to being diagnosed with alcohol use disorder in the context of an alcohol-related incident in the military. Sgt X's development history is significant for some school truancy and a history of physical abuse by his father. He graduated high school on time with average grades. His father and uncle use alcohol heavily. His mother is treated for anxiety and depression. He first began using alcohol at 16 years of age, initially having 1–2 drinks once a month, but his use increased to about 6 drinks on Friday and Saturday nights at 18 years of age. He attended a junior college briefly, where his use increased to 3–4 nights weekly, but he dropped out after a few months due to poor academic performance.

T. W. Meeks (✉)
University of California, Davis, Davis, CA, USA

Sacramento VA Medical Center, Department of Psychiatry, Mather, CA, USA
e-mail: Thomas.Meeks@va.gov

N. M. Bekman · R. P. Vienna
Naval Medical Center San Diego, Substance Abuse Rehabilitation Program,
San Diego, CA, USA

N. M. Lanouette · K. A. Yung
Uniformed Services University of the Health Sciences, Naval Medical Center San Diego,
Substance Abuse Rehabilitation Program, Point Loma, San Diego, CA, USA

© Springer Nature Switzerland AG 2019
E. C. Ritchie, M. D. Llorente (eds.), *Veteran Psychiatry in the US*,
https://doi.org/10.1007/978-3-030-05384-0_9

Sgt X enlisted in the Marines when he was 19 years old. He successfully completed basic training and had no notable disciplinary issues. Afterward, he progressively spent more free time drinking and partying with fellow Marines, often to the point of blacking out, but the alcohol use did not overtly interfere with his performance at work. He deployed twice while on active duty, one time to Korea and then later to Afghanistan, where he was exposed to combat. Two members of his unit were killed in combat operations. When Sgt X returned from his second deployment, he began to find that he had lost interest in some of his typical activities, isolated from friends and family, had more trouble sleeping, and felt frequently anxious and irritable. His alcohol use also increased in frequency and quantity, ultimately drinking eight or more standard drinks daily. His work performance suffered, and one morning he arrived late to work and his supervisor suspected that he was "hung over." When confronted about concerns regarding his alcohol use, he minimized his drinking but did endorse some suicidal ideation.

Historical Perspectives

> Anchors aweigh, my boys,
> Anchors aweigh.
> Farewell to foreign shores,
> We sail at break of day-ay-ay-ay.
> Through our last night ashore,
> Drink to the foam,
> Until we meet once more.
> Here's wishing you a happy voyage home.
> -----
> MCPON John Hagen, USN (Ret)

Members of the US military seem uniquely poised to develop problems with alcohol use disorders (AUDs). They are steeped in their own traditional culture and history and one such unofficial tradition is heavy alcohol consumption. Nearly every quasi-permanent military installation, large or small, stateside or overseas, has a bar or club where liquor is available and that has typically been the center of socialization during nonduty hours. The United States Marine Corps (USMC) was founded in a brewery in Philadelphia in 1775 [82].

During the American Revolution, Dr. Benjamin Rush, one of the founding fathers of the United States and Surgeon General of the Continental Army, expressed concern about the deleterious effect of heavy alcohol use in military members [73]. The US Navy had inherited the British Navy's tradition of a daily ration of rum prior to the order. The US Navy stopped this tradition during the American Civil War; however, the Confederate Navy continued the daily ration in the hope that this would assist recruitment from other countries' navies. The US Navy became officially "dry" in 1914 when the Secretary of the Navy Josephus Daniels, a supporter of the temperance movement, gave the official order. This "dry" status ultimately met its demise along with the whole of the Prohibition era, and alcohol again enjoyed a long reign as the king of military social life for decades.

On 26 May 1981, 14 military members were killed and 48 injured in an aircraft crash aboard the aircraft carrier USS Nimitz. Six of those killed had cannabis detected in their bodies and this was considered a contributing factor in the incident. In December 1981, the Department of Defense (DoD) established the "zero tolerance" policy for illicit drug use, which authorized punitive actions for illicit drug use. The rate of use of illicit drugs in the military has dropped dramatically as a result; use of illicit drug rates are much higher in the civilian population compared to the military population at present. Recent estimates place rates of prior-month illicit substance use at 2.7% among military members, compared to 22.3% among civilians age 18–25 years [63]. With such strong policies regarding illicit drugs, alcohol became even more entrenched as the substance of choice for recreation and revelry, but also for respite, among service members.

Military members face significant stressors as part of their routine jobs. They give up many of their traditional rights (absolute freedom of speech, freedom of movement, freedom to dress as they wish, freedom to refuse direction without severe penalty, etc.) in order to protect the rights of their fellow citizens. They face separation from loved ones and experience long working hours, boredom, and frequent sleep deprivation. Service members often face significant injury and death not only in active combat zones but also in daily training exercises and routine operations. Their relative youth may leave them with fewer adaptive or mature coping skills to deal with emotional stressors and peer pressure. The use of alcohol for many is a way to quickly and reliably change internal feeling states and thus relieve emotional distress in the short term, as well as create a sense of belongingness through shared experiences with peers.

As discussed above, military culture has historically accepted, if not implicitly fostered, heavy drinking with practices such as widespread reduced-price-alcohol on military installations. Aside from the official pro-alcohol practices and historical events already discussed, a culture tolerant of alcohol use emerged in less direct ways. Stigmatization of mental illness in military culture, albeit lessening over time, has left many service members and veterans with untreated psychological symptoms that they attempted to suppress with alcohol.

For many years, alcohol use has been celebrated and ritualized in military culture, whereas mental health treatment has been taboo, even career-ending. For example, after the Vietnam conflict, there was relatively little acknowledgment in military and broader American culture about the profound traumatic effect of this experience on service members. Veterans, often left to their own devices to cope, sometimes turned to alcohol and drugs when other means failed. Other times, addiction developed as a continuation of behaviors that had taken root while deployed, as substances were often used in theater to relieve fear, guilt, disenchantment, anger, and boredom [80].

Epidemiology

Alcohol use, unhealthy use (variably labelled as risky, hazardous, harmful, heavy, and binge use), and use disorder are prevalent among US military service members and veterans, often at rates higher than their civilian counterparts. Bray and colleagues

[11] reviewed data from the 2008 Health Related Behaviors (HRB) survey of military service members regarding heavy drinking and binge drinking (defined by frequency of use and quantity used per occasion).

For nearly two decades, the rate of heavy drinking had been declining, until 1998. That declining trend likely originated in part from military policy changes in the 1980s such as raising the minimum drinking age to 21 years on military bases. In support of this explanation, another study noted rates of treatment for AUD fell more substantially for veterans (60%) compared to civilians (20%) aged 25–34 during a span of 12 years that closely followed this policy change [89]. However, from 1998 to 2008 there was a 5% increase in heavy drinking, reversing the decades-long trend of decline. Binge drinking followed a similar pattern, increasing from 35% in 1998 to 47% in 2008.

Overall, the prevalence of heavy drinking among service members (active duty and reserve) was 20%. Significantly higher rates occurred among those serving in the Marine Corps and Army, males, non-Hispanic whites or Hispanics, those without a college degree, those single or separated from their spouse, and those of lower ranks [11, 41]. In comparison with civilian rates from the 2007 National Survey on Drug Use and Health, service members age 18–35 were more likely to drink heavily, while those aged 46 and above were less likely to do so [11, 12, 41].

There are a variety of definitions of "unhealthy drinking." For example, using Alcohol Use Disorders Identification Tests (AUDIT) scores in the same 2008 HRB survey, approximately one-third of military service members exhibited either hazardous (24.6%, AUDIT 8–15), harmful (4.2%, AUDIT 16–19), or probable dependent (4.5%, AUDIT ≥20) use [3, 11]. Alternatively, using clinical health records to identify diagnostic codes indicative of AUD, rates from 2000 to 2009 ranged from a low of 1.25% in the Air Force to a high of 4.1% in the Army [22, 41]. Important caveats in interpreting all these data include clinical under-identification of AUD (pertinent for studies reviewing medical records) and a social desirability response tendency in self-report assessments of alcohol use. Both factors increase the risk of underestimating unhealthy drinking. This is true among civilians, but potentially even more relevant when the confidentiality of medical records that could impact one's career is in doubt by some military service members.

Using Veterans Affairs (VA) administrative data in retrospective cross-sectional analyses on nearly a half-million Iraq and Afghanistan (OEF/OIF) veterans entering VA healthcare from 2001 to 2009, Seal and colleagues [77] noted 10% received AUD diagnoses (10.5% of men and 4.5% of women), 5% drug use disorder diagnoses (DUD), and 3% both. A systematic literature review on alcohol misuse and use disorders in women veterans noted that rates in the reviewed studies were 4–37% for misuse, 7–25% for binge drinking, and 3–10% for AUDs. There was no clear difference in rates of binge or heavy drinking between females civilians and veterans, and rates were again lower for female than male veterans (as is true in the general population) [37].

Since veterans seeking care at the VA are not necessarily representative of all veterans, data from national surveys are also important. Surveying a national sample of OEF/OIF veterans within 1 year of returning from deployment, Eisen and colleagues [29] found that 39.2% (41.4% of men and 17.0% of women) screened positive for possible AUD (≥ 5 on the AUDIT-C). The National Health and Resilience in Veterans Study (NHRVS) was a web-based survey of a nationally representative sample of over 3000 US military veterans aged 21 and older, and it reported the prevalence of lifetime AUDs (assessed by DSM-IV diagnostic criteria) was 42.2%. Past-year positive screens for AUD (using AUDIT-C) were reported among 14.8% of veterans [32].

Comorbidity

Numerous variables have been examined as potential risk factors for AUD and its associated comorbidities among service members and veterans. Such studies often lacked the prospective design needed to establish a direction of causality between these variables and alcohol use outcomes, but they are nonetheless clinically informative. Compared to those without AUD, veterans with life-time AUD had significantly higher rates of life-time and current mood disorders, anxiety disorders, and drug use disorders, as well as life-time suicide attempt and current suicidal ideation [32]. Other examples of factors associated in more than one study with unhealthy alcohol use among service members and veterans include male sex, younger age, unmarried status, depressive and PTSD symptoms, premorbid substance abuse, premorbid low resilience, traumatic brain injury (TBI), and psychological trauma history, including combat exposure and sexual assault [13, 19, 21, 32–34, 37, 56, 77, 92].

Any association of adverse health outcomes, including alcohol-related problems, with combat and military sexual trauma is of heightened interest for many policymakers and veteran advocates. Among OEF/OIF veterans diagnosed with substance use disorders (SUDs), 55–75% also received PTSD or depression diagnoses, and SUDs were 3–4.5 times more likely among veterans with PTSD and depression [77]. The same study noted the prevalence of AUD diagnoses was similar to that reported in previous surveys of Vietnam Veterans, which reported that 11.2–14% of males and 2.4% of females met criteria for current alcohol dependence [15, 50].

Specific aspects of combat may increase risk for problematic alcohol use, including reported exposure to threat of death/injury or to atrocities of war [92]. It is commonly assumed that alcohol use among combat veterans relates to attempts to self-medicate PTSD symptoms. This is likely one important causal explanation. Service members and veterans with PTSD may experience a biphasic quality to their affective states [47]. Periods of emotional flooding and overwhelmingly painful affect (re-experiencing and hyperarousal symptoms) may alternate with extreme affective numbing and difficulty with interpersonal attachment. Alcohol can play a role in alleviating (albeit temporarily) distress in both extremes, settling powerful affects while heightening positive emotions and perceived social connection; ultimately, unhealthy alcohol use only worsens affective symptoms and increases social isolation.

The Millennium Cohort Study compared pre-deployment and post-deployment alcohol use patterns among nearly 50,000 OEF/OIF combat veterans. Baseline prevalence of heavy weekly drinking, binge drinking, and alcohol-related problems was 9.0%, 53.6%, and 15.2%, respectively. Post-deployment prevalence of each changed in variable ways, reported as 12.5%, 53%, and 11.9%. Although the overall pre- vs post- deployment rates were similar, new-onset heavy use, binge use, and alcohol-related problems prevalence was 8.8%, 25.6%, and 7.1%, respectively. Reserve and National Guard personnel and younger service members were at highest risk for developing new-onset unhealthy patterns of alcohol use [42].

Another study demonstrated that childhood trauma increased the risk of problematic alcohol use among Reserve and National Guard members, but that combat trauma worsened alcohol outcomes primarily among those with low childhood adversity [87]. These and other studies underscore that combat exposure does not have a simple linear relationship with post-deployment alcohol use; other factors such as premorbid alcohol use patterns, psychiatric comorbidity, non-combat trauma history, and various psychosocial variables also play a role in post-deployment risk for unhealthy alcohol use.

Tragically, each day approximately 20 US veterans die by suicide, a rate over 20% higher than the general US population [23]. Please see Chap. 5 for a full review of suicide risk factors and prevention strategies among military members/veterans. Alcohol has long been identified as a risk factor for suicide among veterans [43, 84] and merits specific attention because it has additive risk-amplifying effects when combined with other risk factors, such as depression or impulsivity.

When faced with a veteran at risk for suicide, as part of a comprehensive exam, clinicians should thoroughly assess substance use, and if an alcohol or other SUD is identified, keep in mind that veterans with SUDs have higher suicide mortality rates that those without [9, 39]. Risk is substantially magnified when veterans have comorbid mental health and SUDs [93]. Of note, the more days a veteran has had problems with alcohol use, the greater their suicide risk [39].

Two-thirds of veteran suicides are by firearm, a particularly lethal method [9]. Alcohol use has been found to increase the likelihood of firearm suicide and self-injury [10], highlighting the importance of addressing both alcohol use and firearm access/safety among veterans.

While US men have long been known to complete suicide at higher rates than women, among veterans that suicide "gender gap" is much smaller [23, 91], and the rates of suicide from 2001 to 2014 increased most substantially (by 85.2%) in female veterans. SUDs further close the gap and may even elevate women veterans' risk beyond that of male veterans with SUDs [16]. While SUDs should always be considered an important suicide risk factor, they may be an especially concerning signal of suicide risk among women veterans [9, 40]. Please see Chap. 18 for a detailed review of special issues for women service members and veterans.

When caring for a veteran with AUD, it is critical for clinicians to screen for suicidality and other suicide risk factors, particularly comorbid mental illness, access to firearms, and other psychosocial factors. Engagement with care, including substance abuse treatment, reduces veteran's suicide risk [23, 39] but only 30% of veterans who died by suicide in 2014 were engaged with care [23]. In another report, among OEF/OIF veterans with unhealthy alcohol use, only 31% reported having received mental health treatment and only 2.5% specific SUD treatment in the prior year [13]. This highlights the importance of interventions discussed elsewhere in this book (Chap. 4) to increase veteran involvement with mental health and substance use treatment, as well as the importance of providing integrated mental health and SUD care.

Psychosocial Treatments

Until the First World War, the standing/regular army of the United States was relatively small compared to modern levels [85]. If substance abuse was identified in a military member (especially in the officer corps), he would typically be referred to a local temperance society to take the "pledge of allegiance" to the society and to abstain from all intoxicating beverages. For example, Ulysses S. Grant took such steps to try to save his Army career [79]. The options for military SUD treatment, or lack thereof, mirrored the dearth of options for the civilian population. As the military grew during the Second World War, the military itself began to recognize the negative potential of addiction on mission readiness.

Treatment for SUDs in the military began at a grass roots level in the 1940s, via active duty service members who had achieved abstinence from alcohol via the traditional 12-step mutual support model of Alcoholics Anonymous (AA). These members began sharing their personal experiences with others in their commands in the AA tradition of carrying the message to other alcoholics [83].

In 1970, the Government Accounting Office (GAO) was tasked by Senator Harold E. Hughes, who identified as a recovering alcoholic, with reporting on the extent of alcoholism in the US military. There was little data available from the Department of Defense due to the stigma associated with the problem. The typical attitude toward the military member who suffered from alcohol addiction was punitive, which resulted in the problem being ignored or going underground. The GAO report stated:

> Military regulations and certain statutes deal punitively with those intemperate in the use of alcohol…The official stated policy of DoD and the military services on alcoholic consumption by military personnel is "to encourage abstinence, enforce moderation, and punish overindulgence." [86]

The GAO Report revealed that commanders had many options to approach the military member in question: ignore the problem, transfer the member to a different command, refer the member for counseling, or punish the member (which could include reprimand, loss of security clearance, reduction in rank, and/or administrative separation). These options appeared to be chosen somewhat arbitrarily at times [86].

In 1969 there were three specific alcohol treatment programs available to military members: Long Beach Naval Station, Fort Benning (Army), and Wright Patterson

Air Force Base. The program at the Long Beach Naval Station was the most well-known. In 1965, a retired Navy commander, who shared his story of recovery using AA, convinced the medical director to allow an AA meeting on base. This led to a formal outpatient treatment program and ultimately an inpatient residential program based on the Minnesota Model.

Such an approach allowed military members to be relieved of their usual duties temporarily in order to focus on treatment. Most patients were referred by their commands, but about 10% self-referred. The program also focused on education about alcoholism and its impact on the family, as well as the development of better psychological coping skills. The program gained some fame as a result of treating the brother of a US president, a former First Lady, and an astronaut who had walked on the moon. Due to such pioneering programs and the advocacy of Senator Hughes and his committee, all branches of the military now have prevention and screening programs, as well as all levels of care based on the American Society of Addiction Medicine (ASAM) criteria.

The cornerstone of substance abuse treatment in the military, as in the civilian population, remains an abstinence-based model of treatment that has incorporated the principles of Alcoholics Anonymous (AA) and other 12-step mutual support groups. Founded in 1935, AA and other 12-step peer support organizations are currently the most commonly sought source for help with substance abuse, and are free and widely available worldwide [36]. As the field of substance use treatment began to place increased emphasis on the provision of evidence-based treatment, researchers have attempted to evaluate the effectiveness of 12-step support in improving outcomes.

Though challenged by the strict anonymity and the uncontrolled, unstandardized nature of 12-step involvement, research has been able to demonstrate that more frequent and more active participation in 12-step meetings (e.g., obtaining a sponsor, "working the steps," and identifying with other group members) reduces risk for relapse [59] by facilitating changes in social networks, boosting coping skills to manage cravings and distressing emotions, and increasing motivation for and self-efficacy to maintain abstinence [45]. Twelve-Step Facilitation Therapy was developed as an evidence-based treatment designed to encourage active engagement in 12-step peer support.

Research has demonstrated comparable outcomes between this and other addictions treatment modalities [60]. Notably, younger active duty service members and veterans may benefit from initially attending 12-step meetings with similar-aged peers early in the recovery process while becoming comfortable with the program. Later, attending meetings with more experienced members may become more important [6].

Addiction treatment in the military and VA systems has become increasingly informed by evidence-based strategies with foundations in behavioral and cognitive theories, such as motivational interviewing, cognitive behavioral therapy, contingency management, and relapse prevention. Such interventions are not based on 12-step philosophy though not necessarily incompatible with its simultaneous use. These alternative treatment models may more easily accommodate patients who are not motivated to fully abstain from alcohol, who adamantly oppose the use of spirituality in recovery, or who reject a disease model of addiction and/or self-identification as "alcoholic."

While many such persons may ultimately develop a positive opinion of AA over time, many others do not, so a broad toolbox of treatment approaches is helpful. In addition to the professional treatments outlined below, there are secular and religion-based alternatives to AA in the form of community mutual support groups (e.g., Celebrate Recovery, SMART Recovery, Life Ring), albeit with more limited geographical distribution. Although abstinence is the safest recommendation for patients with AUD, for those unwilling to consider this as a goal, a harm reduction treatment approach may be appropriate. Harm reduction is officially not an acceptable treatment recommendation for active duty members with moderate-to-severe AUD. Administrative regulations aside, however, it may be a starting point to keep patients engaged in treatment while helping them work through the stages of change.

Motivational interviewing (MI) has become a critical element to the treatment of SUDs, although research evidence has been mixed. Developed by Rollnick and Miller [72], MI makes use of strategic open-ended questions, affirmation, reflective listening, and summary statements to assist patients in challenging their ambivalence regarding making behavioral changes. These techniques have been shown to be more effective for patients with less severe AUDs and for those who are more treatment-resistant [1]. This is particularly useful for service members who are referred to treatment via command intervention or veterans referred to treatment by the legal system and who do not personally believe that their current pattern of use is problematic (e.g., in precontemplation or contemplation stage of change) [69].

Cognitive-behavioral therapy (CBT) focuses on assisting patients in identifying dysfunctional thoughts and maladaptive behaviors that encourage substance use, as well as recognizing potential internal (emotional or cognitive) and external (situational) cues or triggers that precede substance use [48]. Cognitive strategies target patients' beliefs regarding their self-efficacy or ability to effectively change their current pattern of use. It also entails working to identify and implement healthier coping skills for managing cravings and stressors. Relapse prevention uses CBT to specifically improve the above-described skills, as well as to help patients analyze the chain of events, thoughts, and behaviors that led to past decisions to use a substance/relapse. This enables the identification of steps in the decision-making process that can be challenged or modified in the future to reduce relapse risk [55].

CBT has also been adapted for use in treating comorbid PTSD and SUD via a manualized treatment called Seeking Safety [8]. This emphasizes the concurrent treatment of both disorders, which runs contrary to historical beliefs that treatment for co-occurring conditions (or "dual diagnosis") should be sequential; typically, this meant substance treatment first followed by mental health treatment after some specified period of abstinence.

Increasingly, the standard of care has shifted to integrated, simultaneous treatment of both SUDs and mental illness (PTSD or otherwise) [49]. Seeking Safety uses several stand-alone modules addressing cognitive, behavioral, and interpersonal topics that can affect recovery from PTSD and SUD. The treatment focuses on coping skills, present-life issues (i.e., not delving into trauma history), and basic elements of clinical safety (e.g., self-harm behaviors, violent relationships, hazardous substance use, and prolonged dissociation) [61].

Other valuable additions to SUD treatment were developed based upon behavioral theory, including contingency management (CM) and community reinforcement (CR). While SUD introduces a number of natural negative consequences, these are not typically sufficient to combat addictive behavior, and the failure of these to impact substance use is in fact one diagnostic criterion. CM involves reducing the positive associations to substance use while increasing the reward associated with abstinence [67].

Target behaviors may include sustained abstinence evidenced by negative biological tests (e.g., breathalyzer or urine ethyl glucuronide in the case of alcohol), regular medication usage (e.g., observed disulfiram dosing), and increased attendance of treatment activities or peer support meetings. Examples of rewards are monetary payments, lottery entries, vouchers, and prizes. Frequently, CM rewards a patient achieving the target goal consecutively over time with progressively larger payout, thus incentivizing continuous behavior changes.

To be effective, rewards must be practical, valued by the participant, and provided as quickly as possible after the target behavior is achieved [31]. CM has demonstrated effectiveness in the treatment of patients dependent on multiple substances, including alcohol [68]. Notably, in 2011 the VA began a nationwide implementation of CM for the treatment of SUDs, resulting in the effective dissemination of CM; this led to increased treatment attendance and resulted in over 90% of urine samples collected testing negative for the target substance [24].

A community reinforcement approach (CRA) combines elements of MI and CM to assist patients in increasing personal motivation, as well as analyzing what specific positive reinforcements substance use provides to patients [58]. In this model, therapists assist patients by initiating a trial of sobriety, identifying the triggers and payouts for substance use, and helping patients modify their environment to increase positive reinforcement of sobriety and decrease positive reinforcement of substance use. CRA includes role-play and practice of effective coping skills (e.g., assertive communication, drink refusal) and enlists significant others in the treatment to further reinforce sobriety and improve communication.

Both CRA and Community Reinforcement and Family Training (CRAFT, a CRA that specifically assists family members of individuals who are abusing substances and refusing treatment) have been tested among active duty service members and veterans [64, 76]. Family involvement is frequently limited for active duty patients engaged in substance use treatment due to geographical barriers. As such, Osilla and colleagues specifically designed a web-based intervention to reach military families impacted by this barrier.

Military and VA settings often present unique challenges in substance use treatment. Substance use treatment among active duty populations is complicated by the need to balance the confidentiality of the patient with the needs of the organization. As such, patients frequently hesitate to divulge their substance use patterns and mental health symptoms due to legitimate concern that honest reporting may endanger their careers.

Due to the nature of military treatment referrals, many patients arrive to treatment with the firm belief that their substance use is not problematic and does not warrant the level of treatment recommended. Although service members cannot be mandated to treatment, they are also aware that failure to comply with treatment recommendations may result in separation from the military and loss of certain veteran benefits. Conversely, such potential looming negative consequences frequently encourage treatment engagement by individuals who otherwise would not receive such early intervention for SUD.

The nature of military service, including close scrutiny of members' behaviors, also enables treatment referral earlier in the course of AUD than is typical of civilian populations. Early treatment may reduce patient morbidity, mortality, and functional impairments. The choices facing service members identified with an SUD have similarities with civilians facing legal charges who are offered SUD treatment (or "drug court") in lieu of incarceration, as well as professionals such as pilots and physicians who are offered SUD treatment to avoid licensure revocation. Notably, evidence suggests coerced or mandated treatment among veterans as well as civilian professionals can lead to equally or more positive outcomes than among self-referring individuals [28, 46], although ethical issues related to individual autonomy are cited by opponents to such approaches.

For veterans, who are more frequently struggling with multiple complex physical, mental, and psychosocial treatment needs than active duty members, chronic SUDs may be better treated in longer-term programs that provide housing, vocational training, and long-term structured support. Additionally, while veterans may be further along in their addiction and less resistant to believing their pattern of substance use is problematic, they may require additional support to enhance motivation to regularly attend treatment, as well as to challenge cognitions that they will not be able to effectively modify their behavior after potentially multiple treatment courses and/or relapses.

Medical Aspects

Ethanol is a simple two-carbon alcohol with anything but simple effects on the human body. Aside from its central nervous system intoxicant effects, alcohol directly and indirectly interacts with multiple body systems, creating a plethora of unintended medical morbidity and mortality. Approximately 3.8% of all worldwide deaths are attributable to alcohol use [71]. Its deleterious effects on health and physical functioning likewise have been documented among military service members and veterans [54, 90]. Clinicians working with active duty and veteran patients should conduct adequate medical evaluation of individuals with known AUD, as well as monitor for medical signs of harmful alcohol use among persons who may underreport their use. In the latter case, the medical consequences may be the only clue that provides an opportunity to intervene and refer patients for substance use treatment.

Heavy alcohol use is particularly toxic to the neurological system. Neurological consequences of chronic heavy alcohol use include peripheral neuropathy, cognitive impairment (including Wernicke-Korsakoff syndrome and dementia), psychiatric symptoms (e.g., insomnia, anxiety, and depression), and cerebellar atrophy.

During alcohol withdrawal, tremors, seizures, hallucinations, and delirium tremens may occur [26, 74]. Alcohol withdrawal itself is also neurotoxic, creating a kindling effect such that subsequent withdrawal episodes are more easily triggered and progressively more severe [5]. Wernicke's syndrome is classically characterized by ataxia, ophthalmoplegia, and disorientation, while Korsakoff's syndrome is characterized by retrograde and anterograde amnesia prototypically compensated by the patient via confabulation. Wernicke's and Korsakoff's syndromes may or may not co-occur.

Aging, and increased cumulative exposure to alcohol, increases susceptibility to these neurological sequelae, making these more common among veterans than active duty service members, with the probable exception of alcohol-induced psychiatric symptoms that may occur earlier in the course of AUD. Nonetheless, even subtle neurocognitive impairments can significantly reduce mission readiness and contribute to workplace accidents among service members [88].

Alcohol-related neurological symptoms may result from direct neuronal toxicity, nutritional deficiencies (e.g., thiamine), increased risk of cerebrovascular disease, accumulation of toxins from hepatic impairment, and increased risk of head trauma [20]. In addition to combat-related traumatic brain injury (TBI), alcohol is another common etiological factor in head injuries in the military and elsewhere; the cause-and-effect directionality of the association between substance use and TBI is an area of active research [4, 7].

Probably the most well-known medical morbidity of AUD is liver disease. Hepatic steatosis is an early finding that progresses to cirrhosis in 10–20% of those with moderate-to-severe AUD [81]. End-stage cirrhosis results in a widespread chain of physiological events, including portal hypertension, decreased production of vital hepatic proteins (e.g., clotting factors), inefficient elimination of toxic compounds (e.g., urea), and alterations of biochemical pathways (e.g., sex hormone metabolism).

Veterans in VA health care, especially those with SUDs, are also at increased risk of hepatitis C [27], which further compounds alcoholic liver disease and cirrhosis risk. While cirrhosis is rare among younger active duty service members who drink heavily, they are still susceptible to bouts of acute alcoholic hepatitis. This usually resolves without medical treatment and without chronic sequelae among healthy young adults, but severe cases may progress to liver failure and death.

With the increasing numbers of women enlisting in the military and then transitioning to VA healthcare, it is important to consider the unique health effects of alcohol among women. Women have a significantly higher blood alcohol level than men after consuming equivalent amounts, and they incur adverse health outcomes faster than men with similar lifetime alcohol exposure. Women with AUD have increased risk of breast cancer, infertility, miscarriage, and sexual assault [14].

During pregnancy, alcohol can have serious adverse effects on the developing fetus [25]. Classic fetal alcohol syndrome includes characteristic facial dysmorphisms, growth retardation, and abnormal neurobehavioral development. The concept of fetal alcohol syndrome has been expanded to fetal alcohol spectrum disorders

(FASD), as research has demonstrated that even relatively small amounts of intrauterine alcohol exposure can create a variable range of adverse effects on fetal and childhood development.

With this expanded definition, the prevalence of FASD has recently been estimated as high as 1–5% among US school-age children [57]. Children with FASD are more likely to experience attention deficit-hyperactivity disorder (ADHD), intellectual disability, sensorimotor impairments, learning disorders, and deficits in emotional regulation [38]. Because treating AUD in pregnancy can present ethical dilemmas, the American College of Obstetrics and Gynecology issued a statement for clinicians, emphasizing respect for the pregnant woman abusing substances, confidentiality to the extent allowed by local laws, and advocacy against separating the mother from her child(ren) based solely on an SUD diagnosis [2].

A wide array of other medical conditions, among men and women, are associated with heavy alcohol use and are summarized in Table 9.1. Many of these conditions can occur through multiple intersecting physiological effects of alcohol. For instance, alcohol-related anemia can result from nutritional malabsorption, direct bone marrow suppression, and/or gastrointestinal bleeding. Alcohol-related hyperglycemia can result from pancreatitis, elevated cortisol, and/or insulin resistance. Subdural hematomas may occur with the convergence of alcohol-related effects such as cerebral atrophy, coagulopathy due to liver disease, and falls related to ataxia from cerebellar toxicity. These are just a few examples of how the widespread bodily effects of alcohol interact to cause over a 7-year reduction in life expectancy among those with moderate-severe AUD [75].

For all these reasons, it is important to conduct a thorough medical assessment of persons in treatment for AUD. Physical exam can reveal some classic indications of chronic AUD, alcohol intoxication, and alcohol withdrawal, as indicated in Fig. 9.1. History obtained from the patient or collateral sources should include time of last alcohol use, typical amount consumed (in *standard* drinks), known alcohol-related medical comorbidities, basic review of systems, history of withdrawal episodes (e.g., past seizures or delirium tremens), and history of other substances being used.

Concurrent use of opioids or sedative-hypnotics both increases the risk of accidental overdose during intoxication and the risk of complicated withdrawal upon cessation. Prescription opioids may contain acetaminophen that, often unwittingly to the user, compounds the risk of alcohol-related hepatic injury. Concurrent use of cocaine and alcohol results in the metabolite cocaethylene, which is particularly cardiotoxic [30].

Comprehensive drug screens should accompany self-report histories. Drug screens in the military are complicated by the potential to be used for administrative rather than therapeutic purposes. This potential therapeutic dilemma should be openly discussed with the service member, and disciplinary actions by military commands should be restricted to drug screens obtained through a proper chain of custody procedure. For clinicians, this dual agency at times requires a delicate balance between advocating for patient treatment, and adhering to regulations ensuring a service member does not endanger mission readiness or the safety of fellow service members [51].

Table 9.1 Medical complications of heavy alcohol use and relevant diagnostic procedures or findings

Bodily System	Medical complication	Pertinent diagnostics/findings
Cardiovascular [78]	Atrial fibrillation	Electrocardiogram
	Cardiomyopathy	Echocardiogram
	Hypertension	Elevated systolic and diastolic blood pressure
Endocrine [70]	Acute and chronic pancreatitis	Serum amylase/lipase ($\uparrow$); electrolytes; glucose Abdominal ultrasound/CT scan
	Erectile dysfunction/menstrual irregularities/infertility	Estrogen-to-testosterone ratio ($\uparrow$); prolactin ($\uparrow$); sperm count ($\downarrow$)
	Hyper- and hypo-glycemia	Glucose; hemoglobin A1c
	Pseudo-Cushing's syndrome	Cortisol; blood pressure; glucose
Gastrointestinal [78]	Alcoholic hepatitis	Liver functions; renal function; CBC; INR; hepatic ultrasound
	Ascites[a]	Paracentesis; abdominal ultrasound
	Cancer[b]	Endoscopy; fecal occult blood
	Esophageal varices[a]	Upper GI endoscopy; CBC
	Gastritis/esophagitis	Upper GI endoscopy; CBC
	Gastroesophageal reflux	Upper GI endoscopy
	Hemorrhoids[a]	Fecal occult blood
	Hepatic steatosis, cirrhosis	Liver functions; INR; hepatic ultrasound; liver biopsy
	Nutrient malabsorption	Thiamine ($\downarrow$); folate ($\downarrow$); B12 ($\downarrow$)
Hematological [52]	Anemia	CBC; iron panel; folate; B12
	Coagulopathy[a]	INR; liver functions
	Immune suppression	PPD skin test; chest X-ray
	Macrocytosis	Mean corpuscular volume of red blood cells ($\uparrow$)
	Pancytopenia	CBC; bone marrow biopsy
	Thrombocytopenia[a]	CBC; liver functions
Musculoskeletal [17, 65, 70]	Gout	Uric acid ($\uparrow$); synovial fluid analysis
	Myopathy	Creatine phosphokinase ($\uparrow$); electromyography; muscle biopsy
	Osteopenia	Vitamin D ($\downarrow$); calcium; parathyroid hormone; Bone density scan
Neurological [26, 74]	Cerebellar degeneration	Brain MRI/head CT scan
	Delirium tremens	Vital signs; head CT scan
	Dementia/cerebral atrophy	Brain MRI/head CT scan; neuropsychological testing
	Peripheral neuropathy	Nerve conduction studies
	Stroke (hemorrhagic > ischemic)	Brain MRI/head CT scan
	Traumatic brain injury	Brain MRI/head CT scan; neuropsychological testing
	Wernicke-Korsakoff syndrome	Thiamine; brain MRI (e.g., mammillary body petechial hemorrhages)
	Withdrawal seizures	EEG; vital signs; head CT scan

Table 9.1 (continued)

Bodily System	Medical complication	Pertinent diagnostics/findings
Renal [66]	Beer potomania	Sodium (↓)
	Electrolyte disturbances/renal tubular dysfunction	Magnesium (↓); calcium (↓); potassium (↓); phosphate (↓)
	Hepatorenal syndrome[a]	Glomerular filtration rate (↓); serum creatinine (↑)
	Metabolic ketoacidosis	Bicarbonate (↓); arterial blood gas (PCO_2 ↓, pH ↓)

Abbreviations: CBC complete blood count, *CT* computerized tomography, *GI* gastrointestinal, *INR* international normalized ratio, *MRI* magnetic resonance imaging, *PPD* purified protein derivative
(↑) Value is typically increased; (↓) value is typically decreased
[a]Complications secondary to portal hypertension/cirrhosis
[b]Includes oral, pharyngeal-laryngeal, esophageal, liver, and colon cancer

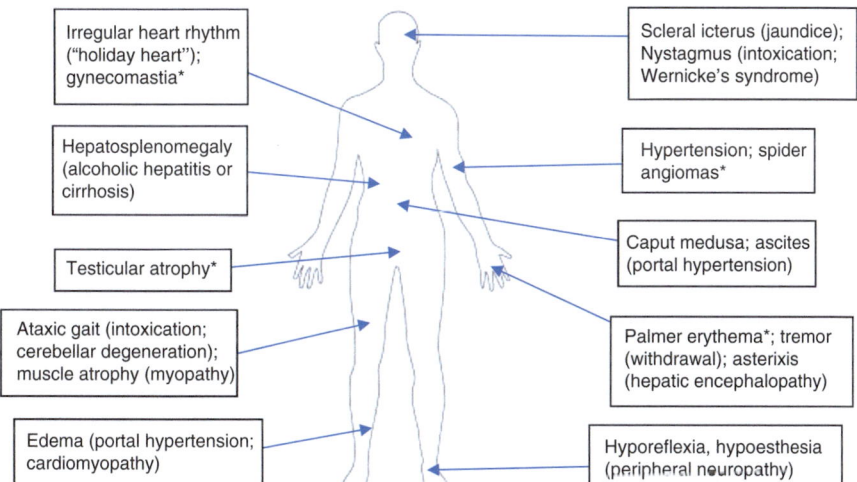

Fig. 9.1 Possible physical exam findings with chronic heavy alcohol use. Items with (*) are related to effects of alcohol on sex hormones, including an increase in estrogen-to-testosterone ratio

Other basic laboratory screenings should include complete blood count, renal function panel with electrolytes including phosphorus and magnesium, and liver function tests. Females with childbearing potential should be screened for pregnancy. Optional additional diagnostic tests, depending on the medical history of the individual, include international normalized ratio (INR) to assess for cirrhosis-induced coagulopathy, vitamin levels (vitamin B12, folate, thiamine, vitamin D), amylase and lipase (if abdominal pain is present), and screening for sexually transmitted diseases.

Persons with SUDs have elevated rates of risky sexual behaviors and sexual trauma. Hepatitis serology among those with elevated liver functions can evaluate for comorbid viral hepatitis as well as identify those who may benefit from initial or repeat hepatitis A and B immunizations. In cases of questionable reliability of patient self-report of alcohol use, several laboratory tests can suggest alcohol use indirectly (e.g., certain liver function tests) or directly (i.e., biomarkers specific to ethanol ingestion). The advantages and disadvantages of such tests are summarized in Table 9.2.

The treatment of most medical complications of AUD is beyond the scope of this chapter. A few illustrative examples are discussed instead. Clinicians should have some working familiarity with the management of alcohol withdrawal. The standard of care is benzodiazepines, which can be ordered as fixed tapers or via symptom-triggered dosing regimens. In the latter case, rating scales for withdrawal severity, such as Clinical Institute Withdrawal Assessment (CIWA), determine the amount and frequency of benzodiazepine dosing. Such an approach allows uniform order sets, lowers total benzodiazepine doses, and shortens detoxification duration.

However, patients with past complicated withdrawal or fragile medical status may fare better by staying ahead of withdrawal symptoms using fixed tapers or with one or more loading doses followed by transition to symptom-triggered protocols. Chlordiazepoxide and diazepam are the most commonly used benzodiazepines due to their long half-lives. In cases of severe liver dysfunction or elderly patients, shorter-acting agents less reliant on hepatic metabolism, such as lorazepam or oxazepam, are preferred. Anticonvulsants such as gabapentin and carbamazepine may have some utility for managing mild alcohol withdrawal or in the rare instance that benzodiazepines are contraindicated [44]. Please see Chap. 10 for a review of pharmacotherapy for the treatment of AUD itself.

For acute alcoholic hepatitis, tools such as Maddrey's discriminant function, calculated via specific lab values, can help determine the severity and suggest when corticosteroids are indicated for treatment [53]. Other laboratory-based calculations, MELD (Model for End-stage Liver Disease) and Child-Pugh scores, are predictive of mortality rates of alcoholic hepatitis and cirrhosis. They can be used to guide referral for liver transplantation.

Liver transplants for alcoholic liver disease often require 6 months of sobriety, except in emergent cases. The stigma of SUDs has at times created public controversy about prioritization of alcoholic liver disease versus other etiologies on transplant lists. Although longer sobriety may improve post-transplant outcomes, there are several studies that call this into question, and overall post-transplant mortality rates are similar for alcoholic liver disease and other liver disorders [18, 81].

Clinical Case: Part II

Sergeant X was referred by his command's substance use liaison for additional evaluation. When assessed by an addiction specialist, he reported that his command "overreacted" to him "just having a few beers" and denied any symptoms of anxiety, depression, or suicidal ideation. His labs were significant for a gamma glutamyltransferase level of 99 IU/L (reference range <40 IU/L) and a phosphatidylethanol level of 553 ng/mL. When the implications of these results were discussed, Sgt X

Table 9.2 Laboratory indicators of alcohol use [35, 62]

Marker	Window of detection	Level of drinking detected	Comments
Gamma-glutamyltransferase (GGT)	2–6 weeks	Moderate-to-heavy	Also elevated by viral hepatitis, obesity, biliary disease, hypertriglyceridemia, and certain medications (e.g., statins); sensitivity ~30–60%, even lower in young adults
Aspartate aminotransferase (AST)	1–2 weeks (highly variable)	Heavy	Also elevated by viral hepatitis, obesity, certain medications, autoimmune disease, and hemochromatosis; less sensitive than GGT; AST:ALT[a] ratio >2 is suggestive of heavy alcohol use but not definitive
Red blood cell mean corpuscular volume (MCV)	Can take months to return to normal (RBC $t_{1/2}$ c. 40 days)	Heavy	Also elevated by hypothyroidism, hyperglycemia, certain medications, non-alcoholic liver disease and B12 or folate deficiency; more sensitive combined with GGT
Carbohydrate-deficient transferrin (CDT)	2–4 weeks	~4 or more drinks[a]/day for 2–3 weeks or more	%CDT (≥1.7%) more accurate than total CDT, especially for females; sensitivity similar to GGT but better specificity; a calculation using GGT and CDT had sensitivity and specificity >90% in one study
Ethyl glucuronide (EtG)	48–80 h (urine)	Light drinking, even incidental exposure	Minor ethanol metabolite; can be detected in very small amounts from alcohol in food, medication, mouthwash, hand sanitizer, etc. Values ≥500 ng/mL are unlikely to be related to incidental exposure
Phosphatidylethanol (PEth)	2–3 weeks (up to 6 weeks for heavy drinkers) Mean $t_{1/2}$ 4 days (range 3–10 days)	≥25 ng/mL: not abstinent[b] ≥70 ng/mL: ≥7 drinks/week[b] ≥140 ng/mL: ≥14 drinks/week[b] ≥300 ng/mL: highly suggestive of hazardous or dependent use[b]	Phospholipid in red blood cell membrane formed only in the presence of ethanol; probably the most specific laboratory measure of heavy alcohol use and the most linearly correlated with amount of alcohol use; Interpretation of exact cut-off values requires additional research; PEth continues to form in vitro after sample collection if blood alcohol level is elevated at time of collection, invalidating results

Abbreviations: ALT alanine aminotransferase, $t_{1/2}$ half-life

[a]A standard drink in the United States is defined as 14 grams of ethanol, which is equivalent to 12 ounces of beer (5% alcohol), 5 ounces of wine (12% alcohol), and 1.5 ounces (a "shot") of 80-proof (40% alcohol) liquor

[b]Values are for the PEth isoform 16:0/18:1 (c.40% of total PEth) are suggested as conservative estimates (sacrificing sensitivity for very high specificity) and should be interpreted in the context of accompanying clinical information. Cut-off values are generally derived from individuals with chronic ethanol ingestion; they may be less useful in interpreting binge alcohol use because values are disproportionately elevated immediately after acute use and thus may not reflect an accurate average alcohol use pattern

ultimately revealed, "Well, maybe I am overdoing it." He was referred to an intensive outpatient program (IOP) for AUD, where he had an intake with a psychiatrist. He had previously denied symptoms related to his deployment because he felt "weak" and worried it could sabotage his career. After discussing his nightmares, hypervigilance, and other related symptoms, he was diagnosed with PTSD as well as alcohol use disorder. He was referred to the Seeking Safety group therapy in addition to mutual help meetings for alcohol. He was started on sertraline for PTSD, prazosin for sleep, and naltrexone for alcohol use disorder. After completing the IOP, Sgt X was referred to weekly aftercare groups to support sobriety and individual cognitive processing therapy for PTSD; at 6-month follow-up he remained sober, had moderate improvement of PTSD symptoms, and was being considered for a rank promotion at work.

Conclusion

In conclusion, the myriad of medical effects of chronic alcohol use requires that clinicians from a wide variety of disciplines remain vigilant for detecting alcohol-related medical illness. Veterans and active duty service members with SUDs often neglect their physical and emotional health, and clinicians should take advantage of any encounter to promote better health outcomes for such individuals. Physical exam, labs, radiological imaging, and other diagnostic tests can assist providers in the assessment and treatment of individuals with AUD.

For some, news of a serious medical illness due to alcohol use is a key turning point in their decision to access life-saving substance use treatment. Of course, as with most disorders, the medical assessment of AUD still starts and stops with the conversation and personal relationship between provider and patient, which should remain professional, respectful, and adherent to the ethical standards of the medical profession.

References

1. Allen JP, Mattson ME, Miller WR, Tonigan JS, Connors GJ, Rychtarik RG, et al. Matching alcoholism treatments to client heterogeneity. J Stud Alcohol. 1997;58(1):7–29.
2. American College of Obstetrics and Gynecology. Committee opinion no. 633: alcohol abuse and other substance use disorders: ethical issues in obstetric and gynecologic practice. Obstet Gynceol. 2015;125(6):1529–37.
3. Babor TF, Higgins-Biddle JC, Saunders JB, Monteiro MG. Alcohol Use Disorders Identification Test: guidelines for use in primary care. 2nd ed. Geneva: World Health Organization; 2001.
4. Beaulieu-Bonneau S, St-Onge F, Blackburn MC, Banville A, Paradis-Giroux AA, Ouellet MC. Alcohol and drug use before and during the first year after traumatic brain injury. J Head Trauma Rehabil. 2017;33(3):E51–60
5. Becker HC. Kindling in alcohol withdrawal. Alcohol Health Res World. 1998;22(1):25–33.
6. Bergman BG, Kelly JF, Nargiso JE, McKowen JW. The age of feeling in-between: addressing challenges in the treatment of emerging adults with substance use disorders. Cogn Behav Pract. 2016;23(3):270–88.

7. Bjork JM, Grant SJ. Does traumatic brain injury increase risk for substance abuse? J Neurotrauma. 2009;26(7):1077–82.
8. Boden MT, Kimerling R, Jacobs-Lentz J, Bowman D, Weaver C, Carney D, Walser R, Trafton JA. Seeking Safety treatment for male veterans with a substance use disorder and post-traumatic stress disorder symptomatology. Addiction. 2012;107(3):578–86.
9. Bohnert KM, Ilgen MA, Louzon S, McCarthy JF, Katz IR. Substance use disorders and the risk of suicide mortality among men and women in the US Veterans Health Administration. Addiction. 2017;112(7):1193–201.
10. Branas CC, Han S, Wiebe DJ. Alcohol use and firearm violence. Epidemiol Rev. 2016;38(1):32–45.
11. Bray RM, Pemberton MR, Hourani LL, Witt M, Olmsted KL, Brown JM, Weimer B, Lance ME, Marsden ME, Scheffler S. Department of Defense survey of health related behaviors among active duty military personnel. RESEARCH TRIANGLE INST (RTI) RESEARCH TRIANGLE PARK NC; 2009.
12. Bray RM, Pemberton MR, Lane ME, Hourani LL, Mattiko MJ, Babeu LA. Substance use and mental health trends among U.S. military active duty personnel: key findings from the 2008 DoD Health Behavior Survey. Mil Med. 2010;175(6):390–9.
13. Burnett-Zeigler I, Ilgen M, Valenstein M, Zivin K, Gorman L, Blow A, et al. Prevalence and correlates of alcohol misuse among returning Afghanistan and Iraq veterans. Addict Behav. 2011;36(8):801–6.
14. Center for Disease Control and Prevention [Internet]. Fact sheets—excessive alcohol use and risks to women's health. c2016 [cited 2018 Feb 26]. Available from: https:www.cdc.gov/alcohol/fact-sheets/womens-health.htm.
15. Centers for Disease Control. Vietnam Experience Study: Health status of Vietnam veterans: I. Psychosocial characteristics. JAMA. 1988;259(18):2701–7.
16. Chapman SL, Wu LT. Suicide and substance use among female veterans: a need for research. Drug Alcohol Depend. 2014;136:1–10.
17. Choi HK, Atkinson K, Karlson EW, Willett W, Curhan G. Alcohol intake and risk of incident gout in men: a prospective study. Lancet. 2004;363(9417):1277–81.
18. Choudhary NS, Kumar N, Saigal S, Rai R, Saraf N, Soin AS. Liver transplantation for alcohol-related liver disease. J Clin Exp Hepatol. 2016;6(1):47–53.
19. Clarke-Walper K, Riviere LA, Wilk JE. Alcohol misuse, alcohol-related risky behaviors, and childhood adversity among soldiers who returned from Iraq or Afghanistan. Addict Behav. 2014;39(2):414–9.
20. Costin BN, Miles MF. Molecular and neurologic responses to chronic alcohol use. Handb Clin Neurol. 2014;125:157–71.
21. Cucciare MA, Darrow M, Weingardt KR. Characterizing binge drinking among U.S. military Veterans receiving a brief alcohol intervention. Addict Behav. 2011;36(4):362–7.
22. Department of Defense. Comprehensive plan on prevention, diagnosis, and treatment of substance use disorders and disposition of substance use offenders in the armed forces. Washington, DC: Office of the Under Secretary of Defense; 2011.
23. Department of Veterans Affairs. Suicide among Veterans and other Americans 2001–2014. Washington, DC: Office of Suicide Prevention; 2016.
24. DePhilippis D, Petry NM, Bonn-Miller MO, Rosenbach SB, McKay JR. The national implementation of Contingency Management (CM) in the Department of Veterans Affairs: attendance at CM sessions and substance use outcomes. Drug Alcohol Depend. 2018;185:367–73.
25. DeVido J, Bogunovic O, Weiss RD. Alcohol use disorders in pregnancy. Harv Rev Psychiatry. 2015;23(2):112–21.
26. Diamond I, Messing RO. Neurologic effects of alcoholism. West J Med. 1994;161(3):279–87.
27. Dominitz JA, Boyko EJ, Koepsell TD, Heagerty PJ, Maynard C, Sporleder JL, et al. Elevated prevalence of hepatitis C infection in users of United States veterans medical centers. Hepatology. 2005;41(1):88–96.

28. DuPont RL, McLellan AT, White WL, Merlo LJ, Gold MS. Setting the standard for recovery: Physicians' Health Programs. J Subst Abus Treat. 2009;36(2):159–71.
29. Eisen SV, Schultz MR, Vogt D, Glickman ME, Elwy AR, Drainoni ML, et al. Mental and physical health status and alcohol and drug use following return from deployment to Iraq or Afghanistan. Am J Public Health. 2012;102(Suppl 1):S66–73.
30. Farooq MU, Bhatt A, Patel MB. Neurotoxic and cardiotoxic effects of cocaine and ethanol. J Med Toxicol. 2009;5(3):134–8.
31. Fletcher JB, Dierst-Davies R, Reback CJ. Contingency management voucher redemption as an indicator of delayed gratification. J Subst Abus Treat. 2014;47(1):73–7.
32. Fuehrlein BS, Mota N, Arias AJ, Trevisan LA, Kachadourian LK, Krystal JH, et al. The burden of alcohol use disorders in US military veterans: results from the National Health and Resilience in Veterans Study. Addiction. 2016;111(10):1786–94.
33. Green KT, Beckham JC, Youssef N, Elbogen EB. Alcohol misuse and psychological resilience among U.S. Iraq and Afghanistan era veterans. Addict Behav. 2014;39(2):406–13.
34. Grossbard J, Malte CA, Lapham G, Pagulayan K, Turner AP, Rubinsky AD, et al. Prevalence of alcohol misuse and follow-up care in a national sample of OEF/OIF VA patients with and without TBI. Psychiatr Serv. 2017;68(1):48–55.
35. Hahn JA, Anton RF, Javors MA. The formation, elimination, interpretations and future research needs of phosphatidylethanol (PEth) for research studies and clinical practice. Alcohol Clin Exp Res. 2016;40(11):2292–5.
36. Hedden SL. Behavioral health trends in the United States: results from the 2014 National Survey on Drug Use and Health. Washington DC: Substance Abuse and Mental Health Services Administration, Department of Health & Human Services; 2015.
37. Hoggatt KJ, Jamison AL, Lehavot K, Cucciare MA, Timko C, Simpson TL. Alcohol and drug misuse, abuse, and dependence in women veterans. Epidemiol Rev. 2015;37:23–37.
38. Hoyme HE, Kalberg WO, Elliott AJ, Blankenship J, Buckley D, Marais AS, et al. Updated clinical guidelines for diagnosing fetal alcohol spectrum disorders. Pediatrics. 2016;138(2):e20154256.
39. Ilgen MA, Harris AHS, Moos RH, Tiet QQ. Predictors of a suicide attempt one year after entry into substance use disorder treatment. Alcohol Clin Exp Res. 2007;31(4):1–8.
40. Ilgen MA, Bohnert AS, Ignacio RV, McCarthy JF, Valenstein MM, Kim HM, Blow FC. Psychiatric diagnoses and risk of suicide in veterans. Arch Gen Psychiatry. 2010;67(11):1152–8.
41. Institute of Medicine. Substance use disorders in the U.S. armed forces. Washington, DC: The National Academies Press; 2013. https://doi.org/10.17226/1344.
42. Jacobson UG, Ryam MA, Hooper TI, Smith TC, Amoroso PJ, Boyko EJ, et al. Alcohol use and alcohol-related problems before and after military combat deployment. JAMA. 2008;300(6):663–75.
43. Kang HK, Bullman TA. Risk of suicide among US veterans after returning from the Iraq or Afghanistan war zones. JAMA. 2008;300(6):652–3.
44. Kattimmani S, Bharadwaj B. Clinical management of alcohol withdrawal: a systematic review. Ind Psychiatry. 2013;22(2):100–8.
45. Kelly JF. Is Alcoholics Anonymous religious, spiritual, neither? Findings from 25 years of mechanisms of behavior change research. Addiction. 2017;112(6):929–36.
46. Kelly JF, Finney JW, Moos R. Substance use disorder patients who are mandated to treatment: characteristics, treatment process, and 1-and 5-year outcomes. J Subst Abus Treat. 2005;28(3):213–23.
47. Khantzian EJ. The self-medication hypothesis revisited: the dually diagnosed patient. Prim Psychiatry. 2003;10(9):47–54.
48. Kleber HD, Anton Jr RF, George TP, Greenfield SF, Kosten TR, O'Brien CP, et al. Treatment of patients with substance use disorders. American Psychiatric Association Practice Guidelines for the Treatment of Psychiatric Disorders: Compendium 2006. 2006;291.
49. Kuehn BM. Integrated care key for patients with both addiction and mental illness. JAMA. 2010;303(19):1905–7.

50. Kulka RA, Schlenger WE, Fairbank JA, Hough RL, Jordan BK, Marmar CR, et al. Trauma and the Vietnam war generation: report of findings from the National Vietnam Veterans Readjustment Study. New York: Brunner/Mazel Publishers; 1990.
51. Larson MJ, Wooten NR, Adams RS, Merrick E. Military combat deployments and substance use: review and future directions. J Soc Work Pract Addict. 2012;12(1):6–27.
52. Latvala J, Parkkila S, Niemelä O. Excess alcohol consumption is common in patients with cytopenia: studies in blood and bone marrow cells. Alcohol Clin Exp Res. 2004;28(4):619–24.
53. Lucey MR, Mathurin P, Morgan TR. Alcoholic hepatitis. N Engl J Med. 2009;360(26):2758–69.
54. Mansell D, Penk W, Hankin CS, Lee A, Spiro A 3rd, Skinner KM, et al. The illness burden of alcohol-related disorders among VA patients: the veterans health study. J Ambul Care Manage. 2006;29(1):61–70.
55. Marlatt GA, Donovan DM, editors. Relapse prevention: maintenance strategies in the treatment of addictive behaviors. New York: Guilford Press; 2005.
56. Marshall BD, Prescott MR, Liberzon I, Tamburrino MB, Calabrese JR, Galea S. Coincident posttraumatic stress disorder and depression predict alcohol abuse during and after deployment among Army National Guard soldiers. Drug Alcohol Depend. 2012;124(3):193–9.
57. May PA, Chambers CD, Kalberg WO, Zellner J, Feldman H, Buckley D, et al. Prevalence of fetal alcohol spectrum disorders in 4 US communities. JAMA. 2018;319(5):474–82.
58. Miller WR, Meyers RJ, Hiller-Sturmhöfel S. The community-reinforcement approach. Alcohol Res Health.1999;23(2):116–21.
59. Montgomery HA, Miller WR, Tonigan JS. Does Alcoholics Anonymous involvement predict treatment outcome? J Subst Abus Treat. 1995;12(4):241–6.
60. Morgenstern J, McKay JR. Rethinking the paradigms that inform behavioral treatment research for substance use disorders. Addiction. 2007;102(9):1377–89.
61. Najavits L. Seeking safety: a treatment manual for PTSD and substance abuse. New York: Guilford Publications; 2002.
62. Nanau RM, Neuman MG. Biomolecules and biomarkers used in diagnosis of alcohol drinking and in monitoring therapeutic interventions. Biomol Ther. 2015;5(3):1339–85.
63. National Institutes of Health [Internet]. National survey of drug use and health. c2015–6 [cited 2018 Apr 20]. Available from: https://www.drugabuse.gov/national-survey-drug-use-health.
64. Osilla KC, Pedersen ER, Tolpadi A, Howard SS, Phillips JL, Gore KL. The feasibility of a web intervention for military and veteran spouses concerned about their partner's alcohol misuse. J Behav Health Serv Res. 2018;45(1):57–73.
65. Owczarek J, Jasińska M, Orszulak-Michalak D. Drug-induced myopathies: an overview of the possible mechanisms. Pharmacol Rep. 2005;57(1):23–34.
66. Palmer BF, Clegg DJ. Electrolyte disturbances in patients with chronic alcohol-use disorder. N Engl J Med. 2017;377(14):1368–77.
67. Petry NM. Contingency management for substance abuse treatment: a guide to implementing this evidence-based practice. New York: Routledge; 2013.
68. Petry NM, Martin B, Cooney JL, Kranzler HR. Give them prizes and they will come: contingency management for treatment of alcohol dependence. J Consult Clin Psychol. 2000;68(2):250.
69. Prochaska JO, DiClemente CC. The transtheoretical approach: crossing traditional boundaries of therapy. Homewood: Dow Jones-Irwin; 1984.
70. Rachdaui N, Sarkar DK. Effects of alcohol on the endocrine system. Endocrinol Metab Clin N Am. 2013;42(3):593–615.
71. Rehm J, Mathers C, Popova S, Thavorncharoensap M, Teerawattananon Y, Patra J. Global burden of disease and injury and economic cost attributable to alcohol use and alcohol-use disorders. Lancet. 2009;373(9682):2223–33.
72. Rollnick S, Miller WR. What is motivational interviewing? Behav Cogn Psychother. 1995;23(4):325–34.
73. Rush B. Medical inquiries and observations upon the diseases of the mind. Philadelphia: Kimber & Richardson; 1812.
74. Sachdeva A, Chandra M, Choudhary M, Dayal P, Anand KS. Alcohol-related dementia and neurocognitive impairment: a review study. Int J High Risk Behav Addict. 2016;5(3):e27976.

75. Schoepf D, Heun R. Alcohol dependence and physical comorbidity: increased prevalence but reduced relevance of individual comorbidities for hospital-based mortality during a 12.5-year observation period in general hospital admissions in urban North-West England. Eur Psychiatry. 2015;30(4):459–68.
76. Scruggs SM, Meyers RJ, Kayo R. Community reinforcement and family training, support and prevention (CRAFT-SP). Oklahoma City: Veterans Administration Medical Center; 2005.
77. Seal KH, Cohen G, Waldrop A, Cohen BE, Maguen S, Ren L. Substance use disorders in Iraq and Afghanistan veterans in VA healthcare, 2001–2010: implications for screening, diagnosis and treatment. Drug Alcohol Depend. 2011;116(1–3):93–101.
78. Shield KD, Parry C, Rehm J. Chronic diseases and conditions related to alcohol use. Alcohol Res. 2013;35(2):155–71.
79. Smith G. Lee and Grant: a dual biography. New York: McGraw Hill; 1984.
80. Stanton MD. Drugs, Vietnam, and the Vietnam veteran: an overview. Am J Drug Alcohol Abuse. 1976;3(4):557–70.
81. Stickel F, Datz C, Hampe J, Bataller R. Pathophysiology and management of alcoholic liver disease: update 2016. Gut Liver. 2017;11(2):173–88.. Erratum in: Gut Liver. 2017;11(3):447.
82. Sturkey MF. Warrior culture of the US Marines. 3rd ed. Plum Branch: Heritage Press International; 2009.
83. Swegan WE, Chestnut GF. The psychology of alcoholism. Bloomington: iUniverse; 2011.
84. US Army Reports [Internet]. Army health promotion, risk reduction, suicide prevention. Washington, DC: Department of the US Army; c2010 [cited 2018 Apr 20]. Available from: http://www.army.mil/article/42934/.
85. US House of Representatives[Internet]. The establishment of the Department of War [cited 2018 Jan 28]. Available from: http://history.house.gov/HistoricalHighlight/Detail/35480?ret=True.
86. US Senate Comptroller General's report [Internet]. Alcoholism among military personnel c1971 [cited 2018 Apr 20]. Available from: https://www.gao.gov/assets/210/201628.pdf.
87. Vest BM, Hoopsick RA, Hornish DL, Daws RC, Hornish GG. Childhood trauma, combat trauma, and substance use in National Guard and Reserve soldiers. Subst Abus. 2018:1–31.. (epub ahead of print).
88. Vrijkotte S, Roelands B, Meeusen R, Pattyn N. Sustained military operations and cognitive performance. Aerosp Med Hum Perform. 2016;87(8):718–27.
89. Wallace AE, Wallace A, Weeks WB. The U.S. military as a natural experiment: changes in drinking age, military environment, and later alcohol treatment episodes among veterans. Mil Med. 2008;173(7):619–25.
90. Waller M, McGuire AC, Dobson AJ. Alcohol use in the military: associations with health and wellbeing. Subst Abuse Treat Prev Policy. 2015;10:27.
91. Weiner J, Richmond TS, Conigliaro J, Wiebe DJ. Military veteran mortality following a survived suicide attempt. BMC Public Health. 2011;11:374–83.
92. Wilk JE, Bliese PD, Kim PY, Thomas JL, McGurk D, Hoge CW. Relationship of combat experiences to alcohol misuse among U.S. soldiers returning from the Iraq war. Drug Alcohol Depend. 2010;108(1–2):115–21.
93. Zivin K, Kim HM, McCarthy JF, Austin KL, Hoggatt KJ, Walters H, et al. Suicide mortality among individuals receiving treatment for depression in the Veterans Affairs health system: associations with patient and treatment setting characteristics. Am J Public Health. 2007;97(12):2193–8.

Alcohol Pharmacotherapy

Jasmine Carpenter and Shannon Tulk

Pharmacotherapy has been proven effective in assisting with the treatment of alcohol use disorder (AUD). These agents have been shown to decrease heavy drinking and increase days of abstinence [1]. Currently there are three FDA approved medications for the treatment of AUD, which include naltrexone, acamprosate, and disulfiram (outlined in Table 10.1). Furthermore, there are a number of other off-labeled medications that have also been found effective for AUD (outlined in Table 10.2). This chapter will provide a detailed review of these agents and how they can be used for the treatment of AUD.

Labeled Medications for the Treatment of AUD

Naltrexone

Naltrexone was FDA approved in 1994 for the treatment of AUD and is considered a first line agent for the treatment of AUD by the VA/DOD Treatment Guidelines [2]. Alcohol consumption is known to enhance endogenous opioid activity, therefore by blocking the mu-opioid receptors naltrexone can decrease the reinforcing effects of alcohol consumption [3, 4]. A number of studies have shown that naltrexone is effective in reducing heavy drinking and increasing days of abstinence. The Combined Pharmacotherapies and Behavioral Interventions (COMBINE) trial found that naltrexone, in addition to medical management, reduced the risk of a heavy drinking day by 28% [5]. This same study found that naltrexone plus

J. Carpenter (✉)
Veterans Affairs Medical Center, Washington DC, Pharmacy Service/Mental Health Service, Washington, DC, USA

S. Tulk
Minneapolis VA Health Care System, Pharmacy Service,
Minneapolis, MN, USA

Table 10.1 Summary of labeled medications for alcohol use disorder: naltrexone, acamprosate, disulfiram [3, 4, 8, 13, 20]

	Dose	Dose adjustments	Contra-indications (CI)/precautions	Adverse reactions	Drug interactions	Monitoring
Naltrexone	*Initial (Oral):* 25–50 mg daily *Maintenance:* 50–150 mg daily *Long-acting injectable* 380 mg every 4 weeks	*Renal:* Not studied in <50 ml/min *Hepatic:* Not studied in Child-Pugh class C	*Contraindicated:* Concomitant use of opioids Acute Hepatitis *Precautions* Hepatitis/liver dysfunction Suicidal thinking/behavior Eosinophilic pneumonia	GI upset (nausea, vomiting, diarrhea) Headache Anxiety Dizziness Syncope Injection site reactions	Opioids	Liver Function Tests (ALT, AST) Serum creatinine (SCr)
Acamprosate	666 mg three times daily	*Renal:* CrCl 30–50 ml/min: 333 mg three times daily CrCl <30 ml/min: Not recommended	*Precautions* CNS depression Suicidal thinking/behavior May contain sulfites	Diarrhea, flatulence, nausea Pruritus Anxiety, depression		Serum creatinine (SCr)
Disulfiram	*Initial:* 500 mg po daily *Maintenance:* 125–250 mg po daily		*Contraindicated:* Alcohol intoxication or without consent Psychoses Severe myocardial disease or coronary occlusion Hepatic toxicity	Hepatitis Optic neuritis Allergic dermatitis Drowsiness Headache Peripheral neuropathy Altered taste	Metronidazole Dronabinol Amprenavir Paraldehyde Tinidazole Diazepam Fosphenytoin Omeprazole Phenytoin Theophylline Warfarin	BMP LFTs CBC

Table 10.2 Summary of off-label medications for alcohol use disorder: topiramate, gabapentin, baclofen, ondansetron [24, 27, 32, 34, 35, 38, 39, 42, 45, 46]

	Dose	Dose adjustments	Contra-indications (CI)/ precautions	Adverse reactions	Drug interactions	Monitoring
Topiramate	*Initial:* 25 mg daily *Maintenance:* max: 300 mg daily in 2 divided doses	*Renal:* CrCl <70 ml/min reduce dose by 50% *Hepatic:* use caution	Caution in elderly Metabolic acidosis Hepatic impairment Nephrolithiasis Visual field defects/acute myopia Suicidal thinking/behavior CNS depression	Dizziness Confusion Impaired cognition, memory, concentration Mood disturbances Fatigue Weight loss	Contraception CNS depressants Anticholinergics Carbonic anhydrase inhibitors Diuretics Metformin	BMP SCr Ammonia Weight
Gabapentin	*Initial:* 300 mg daily *Maintenance:* Up to 1800 mg daily in three divided doses	*Renal:* CrCl 30–59 ml/min 200–700 mg BID 15–29 ml/min 200–700 mg day <15 ml/min Use with caution	Caution in elderly Anaphylaxis, angioedema, and eosinophilia and systemic symptoms (DRESS) CNS depression Suicidal thinking/behavior	Ataxia Fatigue Dizziness Nystagmus Nausea/vomiting Peripheral edema	Orlistat CNS depressants	SCr
Baclofen	*Initial:* 5 mg three times a day *Maintenance:* 10 mg three times a day	*Renal:* CrCl 50–80 ml/min 5 mg po BID; 30–49 ml/min: 2.5 mg po TID; <30 ml/min 2.5 mg po BID	Avoid abrupt withdrawal Seizures Psychiatric disorders Renal impairment	Hypotonia Drowsiness Confusion Headache Nausea/vomiting Hypotension Urinary retention Constipation	CNS depressants	SCr
Ondansetron	2–16 mg BID or Weight-based: 16 mcb/kg	*Hepatic:* Child-Pugh class C: Do not exceed 8 mg daily	QTc prolongation Phenylketonurics Serotonin syndrome	Headache Fatigue Constipation Diarrhea Hypoxia Anxiety	QTc prolonging agents CYP3A4 inducers Serotonin modulators P-glycoprotein inhibitors	BMP ECG

medical management had a higher percent of days abstinent when compared to those receiving only the placebo and medical management [5]. Additionally, a meta-analysis comparing the efficacy of naltrexone with acamprosate found that naltrexone significantly reduced the return to heavy drinking more than acamprosate [6].

Dosing and Precautions

Naltrexone is available as an oral tablet and as a long-acting injectable. The usual dose of the oral formulation is 50 mg daily. Doses as high as 150 mg daily have been found safe and effective, however the risk of hepatotoxicity increases as the dose of naltrexone increases [4, 6, 7].

The long-acting injectable formulation of naltrexone is a great option for patients who have difficulty with adherence to the oral formulation of naltrexone. The dose of the long-acting injectable formulation is 380 mg monthly and it is administered as a gluteal intramuscular injection [8]. Treatment with this formulation has been associated with longer treatment participation and it was also found to decrease inpatient and emergency healthcare costs [9].

Naltrexone has a black box warning for hepatocellular toxicity, therefore it is contraindicated in patients with acute hepatitis or hepatic failure [3]. Additionally, since naltrexone is a mu-opioid antagonist it should be avoided in patients actively taking opioids. In order to prevent precipitated withdrawal, patients should be abstinent from opioids for approximately 7–10 days prior to initiating naltrexone. Additional precautions can be found in Fig. 10.1.

Naltrexone should be **avoided** in patients who:	Are currently taking opioids or those with anticipated opioid use within the next 7 days/ Positive opioid UA	
	Have active hepatitis or liver failure	
Naltrexone should be used with **caution** in patients with:	Liver impairment	Should still be avoided in patients with LFTs > 5 times the upper limited of normal
	Patients with severe renal impairment	
	Pregnant women/women of childbearing age	

Fig. 10.1 Naltrexone: warnings and precautions [3]

Side Effects and Monitoring Parameters

The side effects of naltrexone are usually mild and resolve over time. The most common side effect reported is nausea and other less common side effects include headache, fatigue, and appetite suppression. For patients who experience bothersome side effects, providers may consider initiating a patient on 25 mg daily for 7 days, and then titrate to 50 mg [3]. For the long-acting formulation of naltrexone, patients may experience injection site reactions. Lastly, naltrexone has also been associated with causing depression and suicidal ideation and therefore patients should be monitored for changes in mood during treatment.

Due to naltrexone's potential to lead to hepatotoxicity providers should monitor liver function test (LFTs) at baseline and periodically throughout therapy, generally 1 month after initiation, followed by 6 months after initiation, and annually thereafter. It is recommended to avoid or discontinue treatment with naltrexone if the LFTs are or become 5× greater than the upper limit of normal [4]. Providers can also perform toxicology screening prior to initiation to ensure that the patient is clear of opioids.

Acamprosate

Acamprosate was FDA approved in the United States for the treatment of AUD in 2004 and is also considered a first-line agent for the treatment of AUD by the VA/DOD SUD guidelines [2]. The FDA approval was largely based on three randomized, double-blind, placebo-controlled European trials which found that acamprosate, in combination with psychosocial interventions, had higher abstinence rates when compared to placebo [10–12]. Acamprosate's mechanism of action for the treatment of AUD is not clearly understood; however, it has been hypothesized that acamprosate restores the balance between excitatory glutamate and inhibitory γ-aminobutyric acid (GABA), which is normally altered during chronic alcohol consumption [13–16].

Unlike naltrexone, acamprosate is not as effective for decreasing heavy drinking but multiple studies have found that it significantly assists with prolonging abstinence from alcohol. A Cochrane review of 24 randomized controlled trials found that acamprosate reduced the risk of returning to any drinking after detoxification by 86% [17]. This review also found that patients who received acamprosate had an increase in the total days of abstinence. Similarly, a meta-analysis of 17 trials conducted by Mann and Lehert also found that acamprosate increased six-month abstinence rates when compared to the placebo [18].

Dosing and Precautions

Acamprosate is only available as a delayed release tablet and the usual dose is 666 mg three times daily. The dose should be decreased to 333 mg three times daily in patients with mild to moderate renal impairment [13]. It can be initiated in patients still consuming alcohol but studies show that acamprosate is more effective at maintaining abstinence in patients who have been abstinent prior to the initiation, thus it is typically recommended that acamprosate be initiated 5 days following abstinence from alcohol [19].

Acamprosate is contraindicated in patients with severe renal impairment and should be avoided in patients with a CrCl <30 ml/min. Because it does not undergo hepatic metabolism, it can be used in patients with hepatic impairment. Therefore, it can be used as an alternative for naltrexone in patients with hepatic impairment.

Side Effects and Monitoring Parameters

The most common side effect seen with acamprosate includes diarrhea and other less common side effects include insomnia, nausea, and headache [13]. As with naltrexone, acamprosate is also associated with the possibility of an increased risk for suicidal ideation.

It is recommended for providers to monitor renal function at baseline and periodically throughout treatment. Providers should also monitor for changes in mood following initiation.

Disulfiram

Disulfiram was FDA approved in 1951 and was the first medication indicated for alcohol dependence. Unlike naltrexone and acamprosate, disulfiram does not influence the cravings or the reinforcing effects of alcohol. It is utilized as an aversive medication that causes an unpleasant reaction when combined with alcohol, which is intended to discourage the consumption of alcohol [20].

Pharmacologically, disulfiram disrupts the metabolism of alcohol by inhibiting aldehyde dehydrogenase, thus leading to a rapid accumulation of acetaldehyde when alcohol is consumed [21]. This rise in acetaldehyde leads to a disulfiram-reaction that is characterized by severe nausea, vomiting, flushing, palpitations, and headache. This reaction typically begins within 10–30 min after alcohol ingestion and can last for several hours [4].

The findings reviewing the efficacy of disulfiram for the treatment of AUD are mixed. A study evaluating the efficacy of disulfiram in veterans found that disulfiram was not effective in delaying time to relapse or in enhancing continuous abstinence more than counseling alone [22]. However, a meta-analysis found that in opened label studies disulfiram was more beneficial in preventing alcohol consumption when compared to naltrexone, acamprosate, and placebo [23]. Disulfiram has been found to be more effective when the administration is supervised or when treatment is court-ordered [24–26]. However, there remains to be limited studies supporting its use.

Dosing and Precautions

Disulfiram is available as an oral tablet and its dose can range from 125 to 500 mg, with 250 mg as the usual maintenance dose [20]. It should only be initiated in patients who have been abstinent from alcohol for at least 12 h or patients who have a blood alcohol concentration of zero. It should be avoided in patients who are taking metronidazole or any alcohol-containing preparations. Patients should also be counseled to avoid using or ingesting any kind of alcohol including mouthwash.

Hepatotoxicity has been associated with disulfiram and it should be used with caution in patients with hepatic impairment. It should also be avoided in patients with severe myocardial disease and/or coronary occlusion. Additional contraindications, precautions, and adverse reactions have been outlined in Table 10.1.

Side Effects and Monitoring Parameters

Disulfiram has a number of side effects that include mild drowsiness, fatigue, metallic aftertaste, and allergic dermatitis [20].

Due to disulfiram's potential to lead the hepatotoxicity, providers should monitor LFT at baseline, 2 weeks after initiation, monthly for the first 6 months of therapy, and then every 3 months thereafter [20]. Patients should be educated on the alcohol-disulfiram effects and the importance of avoiding alcohol-containing products in disguised forms such as mouthwash and cough mixtures.

Off-Label Medications for the Treatment of AUD

Topiramate

Topiramate is an antiepileptic agent that has been found to be effective for the treatment of a number of neurological and psychological conditions, including AUD (off-label). Pharmacologically, topiramate is involved in enhancing GABAergic transmission and inhibiting glutamatergic transmission, via antagonism of the alpha-amino-3-hydroxy-5-methylisoxazole-4-propionic acid receptors (AMPA)/kainate glutamate receptors. It has been hypothesized that this effect reduces cortico-mesolimbic dopamine release, which may lead to a decrease in alcohol reinforcement (Fig. 10.2) [27].

A number of randomized controlled trial (RCT) have found topiramate to be more effective than placebo in improving alcohol outcomes [28, 29]. A 14-week multisite RCT found that topiramate significantly reduced the percentage of heavy drinking days and drinks per drinking day by more than 8.5% when compared to placebo [28].

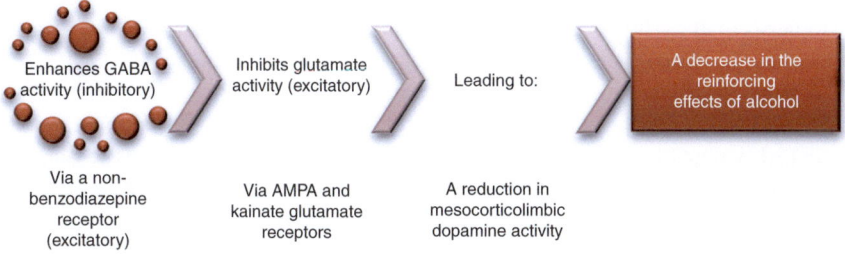

Fig. 10.2 Topiramate: mechanism of action for alcohol use disorder [27]

Similar to naltrexone, topiramate has also been found to be effective in reducing alcohol consumption. More specifically, one study found that 300 mg of topiramate reduced heavy drinking days by more than 8.5% more than the placebo. It has also been found to decrease alcohol cravings compared to placebo. Another RCT performed by Baltieri and colleagues found that topiramate was significantly superior to placebo on a number of measured outcomes, which included heavy drinking weeks (3.4 vs 5.9 weeks), time to first relapse (7.8 vs 5.0 weeks), and abstinence duration (8.2 vs 5.6 weeks) [30].

Lastly, topiramate may provide a unique benefit to the veteran patient population with AUD. An RCT evaluating the use of topiramate for the treatment of AUD in veterans with a comorbidity of PTSD found that topiramate reduced the frequency of alcohol use and alcohol cravings along with also reducing PTSD symptom severity [31]. More specifically, topiramate was found to reduce PTSD-related hyperarousal symptoms compared to placebo.

Dosing and Side Effects

Topiramate is available as a number of formulations, however the immediate release tablet is recommended for the treatment of AUD. The extended release tablets are contraindicated after recent alcohol use; therefore, this formulation should be avoided when being used for the treatment of AUD [32].

When used for the treatment of AUD, topiramate can be initiated at 50 mg daily and increased weekly to a maximum of 300 mg/day in divided doses [24, 27]. In order to decrease the number of adverse effects, a slower titration schedule is recommended over at least an 8-week period.

A 50% dose reduction when initiating treatment and a slower titration schedule is recommended for those with a CrCl <70% as well [32].

Common side effects include paresthesia, taste perversion, cognitive impairment, difficulty concentration, and anorexia. There is also an increased risk of nephrolithiasis thus topiramate is not recommended in those with a history of kidney stones. Adequate hydration is strongly encouraged during therapy [32].

Gabapentin

Originally used as an antiepileptic, gabapentin has also been found effective as an off-label medication for the treatment of AUD. Its exact mechanism in alcohol use disorder is unclear, however it is likely it is the modulation of GABA activity in the amygdala that leads to decreased cravings and increased abstinence [33].

Several trials have found gabapentin superior to placebo for AUD. One trial in particular was a 12-week, double blinded, randomized controlled trial that randomized 150 patients to either gabapentin 900 mg, gabapentin 1800 mg, or placebo. Both gabapentin groups were found to improve rates of abstinence, decrease heavy drinking, and reduce alcohol cravings. The higher 1800 mg dose of gabapentin had slightly better results, thus it is recommended to titrate up to 1800 mg if tolerated for this indication [34]. Another trial found that the combination of gabapentin and naltrexone significantly reduced heavy drinking in comparison to naltrexone monotherapy. Gabapentin may be particularly useful for those patients who have a history of insomnia and/or alcohol withdrawal syndrome [35].

Dosing

Gabapentin should be initiated at a dose of 300 mg po daily and titrated by 300 mg/day until a dose of 900–1800 mg/day in three divided doses is achieved as tolerated [34, 35]. Slower titration and lower doses are indicated in patients with renal impairment. Slower titration can also be completed for those at risk or sensitive to the adverse effects, which include drowsiness, dizziness, and fatigue. As gabapentin is renally cleared and dosed, serum creatinine should be monitored at baseline and periodically during therapy [33].

Baclofen

Baclofen, which is FDA approved for muscle spasticity, has also been found to be beneficial for the treatment of AUD. Its hypothesized mechanism for this indication is believed to be through the modulation of GABA activity and inhibition of dopaminergic neurons. It may be of particular use in patients with liver cirrhosis as it is renally cleared [36]. In March 2014, France issued a temporary recommendation for the use of baclofen in AUD due to the increasing amount of evidence in case studies and trials [37].

Dosing

A variety of doses have been studied for baclofen's use for the treatment of AUD. One study in particular started with a dose of 5 mg three time daily and increased to a dose 10 mg po three time daily [38]. This early low dose demonstrated the safety and efficacy of baclofen over placebo in increasing abstinence (62.8 vs 30.8 cumulative abstinent days, respectively) [39]. However, more recently doses up to 275 mg daily have been used for some patients [40].

Dose adjustments should be made in renal impairment. Caution should also be exercised in the elderly due to its anticholinergic and CNS depressant side effects such as drowsiness, confusion, nausea, vomiting, urinary retention, and constipation. Baclofen can also cause withdrawal symptoms when abruptly discontinued [41].

Ondansetron

Ondansetron is FDA approved for prophylaxis and the treatment of chemotherapy, radiation, and post-operative nausea and vomiting [42]. Its antagonism of the 5-HT3 receptor is theorized to reduce the serotonin-mediated dopaminergic effects in AUD. This reduction of dopamine is believed to reduce the reinforcing effects of alcohol consumption [43, 44]. Interestingly, ondansetron's positive effects on AUD has primarily been demonstrated in those with an early-onset to the disorder (defined as AUD prior to age 25) rather than those with late-onset. It is theorized those with early-onset AUD may share a genetic predisposition for serotonin dysfunction that can lead to the disease [45].

Dosing

A variety of doses have also been studied with ondansetron. One RCT found 16 mcg/kg and 4 mcg/kg twice daily to be superior in reducing the amount of drinks per drinking day. [45] These low doses of ondansetron require the use of ondansetron liquid formulation. Thus, other studies have used the commercially available 4 and 8 mg tablets. Another study found 16 mg of ondansetron to be superior over placebo in reducing the proportion of heavy drinking days [46].

Caution should be used in anyone with a significant cardiovascular history as ondansetron can prolong the QTc interval. Thus, baseline and periodic monitoring of potassium, magnesium, and an electrocardiogram (ECG) is recommended for those patients. Other common side effects of ondansetron include fatigue, dizziness, headache, and serotonin syndrome. The sign and symptoms of serotonin syndrome include agitation, fever, restlessness, and tachycardia and can lead to seizures, extrapyramidal reactions, and QTc prolongation [42].

Conclusion

The use of alcohol pharmacotherapy has been proven effective in the treatment of AUD. With the disparity in the prevalence of AUD in the military and veteran patient population, the utilization of these agents may provide a significant benefit and improve veteran alcohol consumption outcomes [47].

References

1. Jonas DE, Amick HR, Feltner C, et al. Pharmacotherapy for adults with alcohol use disorders in outpatient settings: a systematic review and meta-analysis. JAMA. 2014;311(18):1889–900.
2. Management of substance use disorder in the primary care setting. Washington, DC: VA/DoD Evidence-Based Clinical Practice Guideline Working Group, Veterans Health Administration, Department of Veterans Affairs, and Health Affairs, Department of Defense; 2009. Office of Quality and Performance publication 10Q-CPG/SUD-09.
3. ReVia® [package insert]. Pomona: Duramed Pharmaceuticals; 2013.
4. Center for Substance Abuse Treatment. Incorporating alcohol pharmacotherapies into medical practice. Treatment Improvement Protocol (TIP) Series 49. HHS Publication No. (SMA) 09-4380. Rockville: Substance Abuse and Mental Health Services Administration; 2009.
5. Anton RF, O'Malley SS, Ciraulo DA, et al. Combined pharmacotherapies and behavioral interventions for alcohol dependence: the COMBINE study: a randomized controlled trial. JAMA. 2006;295:2003–17.
6. Anton RF. Naltrexone for the management of alcohol dependence. N Engl J Med. 2008;359(7):715–21.
7. Oslin DW, Pettinati HM, Volpicelli JR, Wolf AL, et al. The effects of naltrexone on alcohol and cocaine use in dually addicted patients. J Subst Abus Treat. 1999;16(2):163–7.
8. Vivitrol® [package insert]. Waltham: Alkermes, Inc.; 2010.

9. Bryson WC, Mcconnell J, Korthuis PT, Mccarty D. Extended-release naltrexone for alcohol dependence: persistence and healthcare costs and utilization. Am J Manag Care. 2011;17(Suppl 8):S222–34.
10. Paille F, Guelfi J. Double-blind randomized multicentre trial of acamprosate in maintaining abstinence from alcohol. Alcohol Alcohol. 1995;30(2):239–47.
11. Pelc I, Verbanck P, Le Bon O, Gavrilovic M, Lion K, Lehert P. Efficacy and safety of acamprosate in the treatment of detoxified alcohol-dependent patients. A 90-day placebo-controlled dose-finding study. Br J Psychiatry. 1997;171(1):73–7.
12. Sass H, Soyka M, Mann K, Zieglgänsberger W. Relapse prevention by acamprosate: results from a placebo-controlled study on alcohol dependence. Arch Gen Psychiatry. 1996;53:673–80.
13. Campral® [package insert]. St. Louis: Forest Laboratories Inc; 2012.
14. Lhuintre J, Moore N, Saligaut C. Ability of calcium bis acetyl homotaurine, a GABA agonist, to prevent relapse in weaned alcoholics. Lancet. 1985;325:1014–6.
15. Kiefer F, Mann K. Acamprosate: how, where, and for whom does it work? Mechanism of action, treatment targets, and individualized therapy. Curr Pharm Des. 2010;16(19):2098–102.
16. Olive MF, Cleva RM, Kalivas PW, Malcolm RJ. Glutamatergic medications for the treatment of drug and behavioral addictions. Pharmacol Biochem Behav. 2012;100(4):801–10.
17. Rösner S, Hackl-Herrwerth A, Leucht S, Lehert P, et al. Acamprosate for alcohol dependence. Cochrane Database Syst Rev. 2010;9:1–118.
18. Mann K, Lehert P, Morgan MY. The efficacy of acamprosate in the maintenance of abstinence in alcohol-dependent individuals: results of a meta-analysis. Alcohol Clin Exp Res. 2004;28(1):51–63.
19. Maisel NC, Blodgett JC, Wilbourne PL, et al. Meta-analysis of naltrexone and acamprosate for treating alcohol use disorders: when are these medications most helpful? Addiction. 2013;108(2):275–93.
20. Antabuse [package insert]. North Wales: Teva Pharmaceuticals; 2015.
21. Ait-Daoud N, Johnson BA. Medications for the treatment of alcoholism. In: Johnson BA, Ruiz P, Galanter M, editors. Handbook of clinical alcoholism treatment. Baltimore: Lippincott Williams & Wilkins; 2003. p. 119.
22. Fuller RK, Branchey L, Brightwell DR, et al. Disulfiram treatment of alcoholism. A Veterans Administration cooperative study. JAMA. 1986;256(11):1449.
23. Skinner MD, Lahmek P, Pham H, Aubin HJ. Disulfiram efficacy in the treatment of alcohol dependence: a meta-analysis. PLoS One. 2014;9(2):e87366.
24. Jørgensen CH, Pedersen B, Tønnesen H. The efficacy of disulfiram for the treatment of alcohol use disorder. Alcohol Clin Exp Res. 2011;35(10):1749–58.
25. Martin BK, Clapp L, Alfers J, Beresford TP. Adherence to court-ordered disulfiram at fifteen months: a naturalistic study. J Subst Abuse Treat. 2004;26(3):233–6.
26. Martin B, Mangum L, Beresford TP. Use of court-ordered supervised disulfiram therapy at DVA medical centers in the United States. Am J Addict. 2005;14(3):208–12.
27. Johnson BA. Recent advances in the development of treatments for alcohol and cocaine dependence: focus on topiramate and other modulators of GABA or glutamate function. CNS Drugs. 2005;19(10):873–96.
28. Johnson BA, Rosenthal N, Capece JA, Wiegand F, Mao L, Beyers K, et al. Topiramate for treating alcohol dependence: a randomized controlled trial. JAMA. 2007;298(14):1641–51.
29. Johnson BA, Ait-Daoud N, Akhtar FZ, et al. Oral topiramate reduces the consequences of drinking and improves the quality of life of alcohol-dependent individuals: a randomized controlled trial. Arch Gen Psychiatry. 2004;61(9):905–12.
30. Baltieri DA, Daro FR, Ribeiro PL, de Andrade AG. Comparing topiramate with naltrexone in the treatment of alcohol dependence. Addiction. 2008;103(12):2035–44.
31. Batki S, Pennington D, Lasher B, et al. Topiramate treatment of alcohol use disorder in veterans with posttraumatic stress disorder: a randomized controlled pilot trial. Alcohol Clin Exp Res. 2014;38(8):2169–77.
32. Topamax [package insert]. Titusville: Janssen Pharmaceuticals Inc; 2017.
33. Neurontin [package insert]. New York: Pfizer; 2015.

34. Mason J, Quello S, Goodell V, Shandan F, Kyle M, Begovic A. Gabapentin treatment for alcohol dependence: a randomized clinical trial. JAMA Intern Med. 2014;174(1):70–7.
35. Anton RF, Myrick H, Wright TM, et al. Gabapentin combined with naltrexone for the treatment of alcohol dependence. Am J Psychiatry. 2011;168(7):709–17.
36. Addolorato G, Leggio L. Safety and efficacy of baclofen in the treatment of alcohol-dependent patients. Curr Pharm Des. 2010;16(19):2113–7.
37. Baraha E, Salemink E, Goudriaan A, et al. Efficacy and safety of high-dose baclofen: for the treatment of alcohol dependence: a multicentre, randomised, double-blind controlled trial. Eur Neuropsychopharmacol. 2016;26:1950–9.
38. O'Shea R, Dasarathy S, McCullough A, the Practice Guideline Committee of the American Association for the Study of Liver Diseases and the Practice Parameters Committee of the American College of Gastroenterology. Alcoholic liver disease. Hepatology. 2010;51(1):307–28.
39. Addolorato G, Leggio L, Ferrulli A, et al. Effectiveness and safety of baclofen for maintenance of alcohol abstinence in alcohol-dependent patients with liver cirrhosis: a randomized, double-blind, controlled study. Lancet. 2007;370(9603):1915–22.
40. Dore GM, Lo K, Juckes L, et al. Clinical experience with baclofen in the management of alcohol-dependent patients with psychiatric comorbidity: a selected cases series. Alcohol Alcohol. 2011;46:714–20.
41. Baclofen tablet [package insert]. Pulaski: AvKare Inc; 2014.
42. Zofran [package insert]. East Hanover: Norvartis Pharmaceuticals; 2017.
43. Barnes N, Sharp T. A review of central 5-HT receptors and their function. Neuropharmacology. 1999;38(8):1083–152.
44. Johnson B, Campling G, Griffiths P, Cowen P. Attenuation of some alcohol-induced mood changes and the desire to drink by 5-HT3 receptor blockade: a preliminary study in health male volunteers. Psychopharmacology. 1993;112:142–4.
45. Johnson B, Roache J, Javors M, et al. Ondansetron for reduction of drinking among biologically predisposed alcoholic patients: a randomized controlled trial. JAMA. 2000;284:963–71.
46. Filho J, Baltieri D. A pilot study of full-dose ondansetron to treat heavy-drinking men withdrawing from alcohol in Brazil. Addict Behav. 2013;38:2044–51.
47. Jones E, Fear NT. Alcohol use and misuse within the military: a review. Int Rev Psychiatry. 2011;23:166–72.

Opiate Use in the Military Context

11

Mike Colston

Introduction

Opiates include a number of compounds that are natural (e.g., morphine processed from the dried latex of the opium poppy), semi-synthetic (e.g., hydrocodone, hydromorphone), or synthetic (e.g., methadone, oxycodone, oxymorphone, and fentanyl). Opiates have been used in the treatment of pain for millennia. Assyrian, Egyptian, Greek, and Roman empires used opium widely [1], and military surgeons used the compound to complete surgical procedures. Unprocessed opium was used as a military analgesic through the American Civil War, before being replaced by morphine and its successor compounds, which allowed better titration of dosage and analgesic effect.

Today, opiates are widely used for pain control and, unfortunately, as drugs of abuse. A scourge of addiction and overdose death has overcome the nation. Opioids—both prescription and illicit— comprise the large majority of all drug overdose deaths. Opioids were involved in over 42,000 deaths in 2016. The states with the highest rates of death due to drug overdose were West Virginia, at 52.0 per 100,000, Ohio at 39.1 per 100,000, and New Hampshire at 39.0 per 100,000 [2].

Five times more Americans died of opioid overdose deaths in 2016 than 1999 [2]. The trend started with a precipitous rise in overdoses of prescription opioids, followed by a steep rise in heroin overdose deaths (ostensibly owing to addicted persons diverting use to cheaper street drugs as the cost of pills rose in the setting of stricter prescribing practices), and now overdoses of fentanyl and its analogues that are sourced from a number of countries, including strategic adversaries and near-peers such as China.

M. Colston (✉)
Fort Belvoir Community Hospital, Mental Health Department, Fort Belvoir, VA, USA

© Springer Nature Switzerland AG 2019
E. C. Ritchie, M. D. Llorente (eds.), *Veteran Psychiatry in the US*,
https://doi.org/10.1007/978-3-030-05384-0_11

Epidemiology of Opiate Use in the Military Context

Fortunately, Service members have largely escaped the national opioid epidemic. The Department of Defense's (DoD's) rate of overdose death was 2.7 per 100,000 in 2015, compared to a national rate of 10.4 per 100,000 [3]. Many theories have been advanced to explain the discrepancy, including the deterrent effect of random drug testing, pharmacy controls, prescriber safety training and monitoring, stepped treatment of pain syndromes, and the wide availability of addiction treatment and overdose reversal capability. Further, DoD rates of opiate prescriptions decreased by 53% and positive drug tests decreased by 76% between fiscal years 2013 and 2017 [4].

Despite these trends, other trends are less sanguine. Opioid use disorder rates, which are low and decreasing among Active-Duty, National Guard, and Reserve Service members and their families [5], rise after the period of service in both Service members and beneficiaries [6]. The positive effects of military service appear to dissipate after the active duty period, despite health systems in DoD and the Veterans Health Administration (VHA) that have very similar strategies and capabilities in regard to opiate use.

One factor may be the accrual of pain syndromes as individuals age. Among DoD beneficiaries, 88% of users of long-term opiate therapy (LOT), defined as greater than 90 continuous days of use, were over 45 years of age. Fifty percent of LOT users were over 65 years of age. Most were treated outside of military treatment facilities [7]. In 2010, leaders in DoD and VHA began to strategize about national trends in opiate addiction and overdose death, and created a strategy around the sentiment that these trends stemmed from the inadequate management of opiate prescriptions and unstandardized processes to manage pain. In fact, national data from the Substance Abuse and Mental Health Services Administration, VHA, and DoD data all suggested that while some portion of opiate addiction arises from gateway drug escalation and recreational use, most addiction stemmed from pain. To that end, a Pain Task Force, chaired by the Army Surgeon General and populated with VHA, Service, and Tricare Management Agency medical leaders, developed a 5-point strategy [8] to serve as a map for the execution of strategy in DoD and VHA. Its tenets included the following:

- Implement a drug abuse assessment strategy in primary care.
- Use written opioid treatment agreements (informed consent) for chronic opioid patients.
- Mandate sole prescribers for those on chronic opioids.
- Mandate military treatment facilities (MTFs) and VA hospitals participate in state prescription drug monitoring programs (PDMPs).
- Educate providers on pain and addiction, contraindications to opioid therapy, and goals of a pain treatment plan.

By 2018, this strategy was mostly implemented across agencies, with opiate use down 50% and 15% in VHA and DoD, respectively. Drug abuse assessments were integrated into primary care workflow, and mental health and substance abuse counseling services were integrated into primary care clinics. Opioid treatment agreements, detailed in the 2017 VA/DoD Clinical Practice Guideline for Opioid Therapy for Chronic Pain, became a standard of care in the treatment of patients on LOT. Prescription monitoring programs identified patients on LOT or who otherwise were obtaining opioids from multiple providers or pharmacies, and began to restrict use to one provider, pharmacy, or emergency room as appropriate. VHA and DoD providers enrolled in state PDMPs to monitor patients' opiate use. National aggregators, such as *PMP Interconnect* and *Rx Check*, gave providers from any state (many VHA and DoD providers are licensed in states away from the facilities in which they practice) the capability to instantly query drug profiles from a number of states simultaneously. Finally, VHA and DoD collaborated to create a 12-hour Joint Pain Education Program (JPEP), which gave providers the tools to manage both pain and incipient addictive behavior in their patients.

Clinical Management of Pain-Avoiding or Minimizing Opiate Use

VHA and DoD use a stepped-care model in pain management. The model was developed and validated at VHA, and exported to DoD for implementation in 2015. It has four basic principles arrayed around a central theme—use evidence-based pain management guided by clinical practice guidelines (CPGs):

- Effectively treat acute and chronic pain.
- Promote non-pharmacologic treatment.
- Prevent acute pain from becoming chronic.
- Minimize use of opioids with appropriate prescribing only when indicated.

Starting in 2018, The Joint Commission began enforcing pain assessment and management standards at accredited hospitals, including leadership influence in regard to pain management opioid prescribing safety, provision of non-pharmacologic pain treatments (which are available at the majority of VHA and DoD treatment facilities), and monitoring of opioid use to maximize patient safety. The Stepped Care Model is a process by which the standards are implemented. Decisions regarding the escalation and de-escalation of pain care, and stratification of pain care management, are informed by the changes to the following domains [9]:

- Refractory pain: a pain condition's recalcitrance in response to treatment initiation.
- Pain severity: Patient's pain level as measured by the Defense and Veterans Pain Rating Scale (0–10 plus supplementary questions on mood, activity, sleep, and stress).

- Mood disorders: Presence of depression and anxiety as measured by the Patient Health Questionnaire (PHQ-9) and the Generalized Anxiety Disorder scale (GAD-7).
- Referrals/visits: Number of pain-related specialist referrals and visits over a given period.
- ER use: Number of pain-related Emergency Room visits over a given period.
- Dosage and duration of opiate prescription: The two most salient risk factors in the development of addiction.
- Sleep: Impact of pain on sleep duration and quality.
- Functional activity: Impact of pain on activities of daily living (ADLs) and function.
- Substance use disorder: History of substance use disorder while prescribed opioids.
- Concurrent prescription of opioids and benzodiazepines.

To these ends, the model [10] starts with pain resilience and functional continuity achieved through self-care—attention to the triad of sleep, nutrition, and exercise—all of which have been shown to have salutary effects on health across academic disciplines. The first step in the stepped care model is pain managed by a primary care physician, most likely formally trained in pain and opiate safety by mandatory Opiate Provider Safety Training (DoD) or new state licensing mandates (VHA/DoD), and trained in pain management (VHA/DoD) through the JPEP curricula.

In the event that pain treatment is unsuccessful based on the domains above, Step 2 is initiated, again managed by the primary care physician (PCP). In this case, the PCP may engage help from a local pain champion or telementoring from an extended healthcare option provider, a strategy shown to work in an academic collaboration between DoD and the University of New Mexico. An integrated behavioral health counselor arranges psychotherapeutic intervention. A care coordinator educates the patient in complementary and integrative pain modalities, two of which (chiropractic and acupuncture) are available at most MTFs and VA Medical Centers (VAMCs). Battlefield acupuncture, which focuses on five cardinal points on the ear and is easily mastered, has been taught to, and is often practiced by, over 3000 DoD and VHA providers. Other complementary and integrative modalities, including Tai Chi, Yoga, acupressure, medical massage, music therapy, biofeedback, and guided imagery, are also often available, but not in network care provided outside of either health system. A physical therapist is available to address biomechanical functional limitations from pain, and finally a clinical pharmacist scrubs the patient's chart for drug interactions and contraindicated prescriptions (such as co-administration of opiates and benzodiazepines; complementary and integrative modalities for pain are covered in more detail in another chapter in this volume).

Failure of self-care and the first two steps of the stepped care model mandates elevation of pain management to a trained pain specialist, such as an anesthesiologist, in Step 3. This approach endeavors to manage a patient's functional limitations and suffering from pain while making every effort to avoid iatrogenic harm. In the event opiates are used, they are used at the lowest dose possible among a suite of pain services (described above, with the addition of a clinical psychologist and a case manager). Low dose opiate prescriptions are paired with non-pharmacologic therapies. These include regional anesthesia and nerve space therapies, and non-opioid pharmacologic therapy, including pain adjuvants in the anti-epileptic and antidepressant classes, acetaminophen, and non-steroidal anti-inflammatory drugs.

For patients on long-term opiate therapy, effort is focused on keeping daily morphine milligram equivalents (MME) at the lowest possible dose per day. This is calculated by determining the relative potency of the drug used in relation to morphine (oxycodone has a relative potency of 1.5, hydromorphone has a relative potency of 4, and fentanyl and its analogues—sufentanil and carfentanil—have potency hundreds to thousands of times greater than morphine) times the dose used. The dosage goal is to remain under 90 MME per day, and ideally, below 50 MME per day.

Even with careful titration and monitoring of the administration of low dose opiates, there is no universal "safe" dose of opiates. Opiate naïve patients can experience respiratory depression on lower doses of opiates. Co-administration of benzodiazepines or other central nervous system (CNS) depressants lower the median lethal dose of opiates. Some opiates, such as methadone, can kill by means other than respiratory depression, such as tachycardia stemming from QT prolongation.

In addition to the disciplines above, patients in Step 3 with substance use disorders or on LOT (up to half of whom suffer from addiction) are availed to the services of an addictions specialist, as opiate use disorders carry a 20-year mortality of 40–60%. Mortality stems not only from overdose but also from infectious disease (endocarditis, HIV, Hepatitis C), accidents, violence, and more prosaic forms of death.

Three evidence-based therapies exist for opiate addiction, all of which are medication-assisted therapy (MAT), and the first two of which use opiate analgesics. Methadone has the largest body of evidence and the longest period of use for opiate use disorders. Buprenorphine, which requires a Drug Enforcement Administration waiver to administer, has a large but less robust body of evidence for its use. It has the advantage of being an antagonist-antagonist, making overdose unlikely. Further, its most common formulation adds the opiate antagonist naloxone and can be used by most patients, except for pregnant women and some others, such as individuals allergic to naloxone. This formulation of Buprenorphine prevents the drug from being snorted or intravenously injected to induce a high or stave withdrawal symptoms. Outpatient induction protocols have become a clinical norm but do require patients to first initiate withdrawal before starting buprenorphine. Its higher affinity for the mu-opiate receptor will cause immediate withdrawal symptoms if given to patients with supratherapeutic plasma levels of opioids.

Finally, naltrexone, a longer acting oral or injectable opiate antagonist used for alcohol use disorders, has proven to be effective for opiate use disorders. A recent study in Massachusetts of three modes of MAT after overdose showed increased 12-month survival of individuals with opiate use disorders in the methadone and buprenorphine groups, but was insufficiently powered to show an effect from naltrexone [11].

Overdose Reversal

Opiates are more likely to cause death from overdose than other pharmacologic agents. Pharmacokinetic and pharmacodynamics issues abound. Addicts' recent history of use, low therapeutic indices, unpredictable dose titration, unknown congeners (such as carfentanil) in illicit preparations, and a wide body of drug-drug interactions, including interaction with CNS depressants such as alcohol, all lead to morbidity and mortality in these agents.

In 2013, President Barack Obama signed an executive action mandating that DoD and VA equip first responders, such as police, firefighters, and emergency medical technicians (EMTs), with overdose reversal capability. In the ensuing period, the national standard of care evolved so that virtually all EMTs and first responders in areas where opiate addiction were endemic were equipped with naloxone, and the price of a common formulation, a nasal inhaler (Narcan ®), fell to a point where easing access to it on both the DoD and VHA regular formularies was not cost prohibitive.

Further, pilots are being introduced within the DoD and VHA to mimic the best practices of states. These include mandates that naloxone be co-prescribed to all patients with opiate doses greater than 90 MME/day, patients on LOT, and all patients with co-prescribed benzodiazepines. Pharmacists may dispense the drug based on an independent review of a patient's drug list and patients may ask for the drug at pharmacies without a doctor's prescription.

Clinical Practice Guidelines

In 2016, CDC published its CDC Guideline for Prescribing Opioids for Chronic Pain—United States, 2016, which was followed by the VA/DoD CPG for Opioid Therapy for Chronic Pain in 2017. The documents align closely, save for a slightly more expansive explanation set in the VA-DoD CPG, which includes a short section on the use of opioids for acute pain. Similarities in the recommendations abound, and are summarized as follows:

- Recommendations against the use of opioids for chronic pain, preference for non-pharmacologic therapies, and use of non-opioid pharmacologic therapies.
- Weighing benefits of opioid therapy against risks, and periodically reevaluating therapy for discontinuation or lower dosing.
- When opiates are used, prescribing the lowest effective dose of immediate-release opioids.
- Carefully considering dose titrations greater than 50 MME/day, and avoiding dose titrations greater than 90 MME/day.
- Reviewing patient's substance use histories using state PDMPs.
- Monitoring users of LOT with urine drug screens.
- Avoiding co-prescription of benzodiazepines and opiates.
- Offering evidence-based treatment, such as buprenorphine or methadone, to patients with opiate use disorders.

Conclusion

The vicissitudes of opiate use, and treatment of Service members, veterans, and their families for pain is buttressed by a comprehensive set of evidence-based principles. VHA and DoD have worked assiduously to address the suffering that stems from these issues, and the tide has turned in the effort to develop enterprise solutions to combat a national scourge of death and disability. Treatment of pain syndromes using complementary and integrative therapies, and a shift away from opiate use, is part of the solution. Comprehensive evidence-based treatments, including MAT, are necessary. Further health services research and advancements in the fields of addiction and pain may herald better outcomes for Service members, veterans, and their families in the future.

References

1. Opium. 2018, June 2. Retrieved from Wikipedia: https://en.wikipedia.org/wiki/Opium
2. Drug Overdose Death Data, 2015–2016 Increases [Internet]. 2018 [cited 2018, June 2]. Available from Centers for Disease Control: https://www.cdc.gov/drugoverdose/data/statedeaths.html
3. United States. Department of Defense. Armed Forces Medical Examiner data; 2017.
4. United States. Department of Defense. Office of Drug Demand Reduction. Report to the Department of Defense (Washington, DC): Addictive Substances Misuse Committee; 2018.
5. United States. Department of Defense. Military Health System Management Analysis and Reporting Tool Data Extraction; 2017.
6. United States. Department of Defense. Military Health System Management Analysis and Reporting Tool Data Extraction; 2018.
7. United States. Department of Defense. Military Health System Opiate Registry Data Extraction; 2017.
8. Providing a Standardized DoD and VHA Vision and Approach to Pain Management to Optimize the Care for Warriors and their Families. United States. Department of Defense. Office of the Army Surgeon General. Pain Management Task Force. Final Report; 2010.
9. Pain Campaign, Primary Care Overview. United States. Department of Defense. Defense Health Agency; Primary Care Clinical Community: 2017.
10. Defense Health Agency Procedural Instruction 6025.04 Pain Management and Opioid Safety in the Military Health System. United States. Department of Defense. Defense Health Agency; 2018.
11. Larochelle MR, Bernson D, Land T, et al. Medication for opioid use disorder after nonfatal opioid overdose and association with mortality. A cohort study. Ann Intern Med. 2018;6(19) https://doi.org/10.7326/M17-3107. American college of physicians. 2018.

Use of Stimulants for ADHD and TBI in Veterans

12

Donna L. Ticknor and Antoinette M. Valenti

Introduction

Stimulants are an important psycho-pharmacological tool to consider when treating veterans with adult attention deficit hyperactivity disorder (ADHD) and traumatic brain injury (TBI) and as a second-line agent for narcolepsy or excessive daytime sedation. Stimulants may also have a role in helping veterans with dementia-related cognitive changes such as apathy or treatment-refractory depression; however, there is less evidence supporting their role for these conditions. In use since the early 1900s, many stimulant formulations currently available can be very effective and relatively quick acting agents. However, caution must be used in veterans with significant cardiac risk factors and females of childbearing age as well as those at risk for substance use disorders, eating disorders, mania, and psychosis. In this chapter, the authors review the most common psychiatric conditions for which stimulants may be indicated in veterans as well as tips for successful prescribing practices, monitoring ongoing use as well as potential pitfalls and contraindications.

History of Stimulants

The development and subsequent clinical application of stimulants in the United States began in the early twentieth century and has grown over the years. In 1933, the base form of amphetamine was patented and marketed as Benzedrine Inhaler, to

D. L. Ticknor (✉)
Washington DC Veterans Affairs Medical Center, Department of Psychiatry, Camp Springs, MD, USA
e-mail: donnaticknormd@verizon.net

A. M. Valenti
Washington DC VA Medical Center, Department of Mental Health, Washington, DC, USA

© Springer Nature Switzerland AG 2019
E. C. Ritchie, M. D. Llorente (eds.), *Veteran Psychiatry in the US*,
https://doi.org/10.1007/978-3-030-05384-0_12

be used as needed for congestion [1]. For the next 15 years, the Benzedrine Inhaler was advertised for over-the-counter sales [2].

In 1937, the American Medical Association approved the advertisement of Benzedrine sulfate tablets for indications of minor depression, narcolepsy and post-encephalitic Parkinsonism [3]. The medication quickly gained popularity, and by World War II it had significant support to be used as a psychiatric medication, despite some reports of abuse and misuse [4]. In addition to its use within the United States, Benzedrine was supplied to soldiers of many countries during World War II, including those serving in the US military for various indications such as for use during aviation as well as other general medical conditions [5, 6].

Concurrently in 1937, Charles Bradley reported a positive effect of stimulants on children with various behavior disorders [7]. This find was purely "by chance" as he was using stimulant medication to treat severe headaches caused by pneumoencephalograms that he performed to examine structural brain abnormalities in children that were hospitalized for emotional problems and difficulty learning [8]. Although there was negligible effect on the headaches, there was a substantial improvement in the learning and behavior of these children [9, 10].

Despite the Bradley's findings and the popularity of stimulants in the 1930s, the prescription was not widely used in the treatment of children and fell out of favor until the second half of the twentieth century. For the next several years, biological and medical forms of treatment of psychological symptoms were dismissed, as psychoanalysis and behavioral-based psychotherapy became the preferred theories [10]. Bradley's reports of the benefits of stimulants had little impact on treatment and research. It was not until the 1950s, when Ritalin, a methylphenidate, was introduced [11] that stimulants began to gain wider acceptance for the treatment of "hyperkinetic children."

Now stimulant medication for the treatment of what is known as attention-deficit and hyperactivity disorder (ADHD) is the treatment of choice [12, 13]. Although Benzedrine was the first drug administered for use in the 1930s, it is no longer in use. At the time of submission of this book for publication, there are numerous FDA-approved stimulants available in a variety of formulations (see Table 12.1).

Another reason for the delay in use of stimulants for symptoms of inattention, hyperactivity, and impulsivity is that ADHD was not recognized as a psychological disorder in the first edition of the Diagnostic and Statistical Manual of Mental Disorders (DSM) that was published in 1952. The classification of these troubled children over the years was given many names, including but not limited to: brain-injured, hyperkinetic impulse disorder, clumsy child syndrome, hyperkinetic reaction of childhood, and minimal brain dysfunction [14].

The disorder was not recognized in the Diagnostic and Statistical Manual of Mental Disorders (DSM) until the 2nd edition, which was released in 1968, and was referred to as "hyperkinetic impulse disorder." In DSM III (1980), the syndrome was re-classified as "Attention Deficit Disorder" (ADD) and later "Attention Deficit and Hyperactivity Disorder" (ADHD) in the revised version of DSM III that was released in 1987, which is still how this condition is currently recognized in DSM 5 today.

Although ADHD was first recognized in the pediatric population, awareness of the disorder persisting into adulthood did not gain acceptance until the late 1990s and early 2000s. The criteria for the adult manifestation of ADHD were included in the DSM 5 that was published in 2013. The disorder as it is known today is characterized by persistent symptoms of inattention, hyperactivity, and impulsivity (Table 12.2).

Table 12.1 Commonly used stimulant medications

Drug	Stimulant classification	Formulations available	Doses recommended
Ritalin	Methylphenidate	IR, LA Tablets and Capsules	IR: 5–15 mg BID-TID LA: 20–60 QD
Metadate ER	Methylphenidate	ER Capsules and Tablets	20–60 mg divided QD-BID
Concerta	Methylphenidate	ER Tablets	18–72 mg QD
Focalin	Dexmethylphenidate	IR, XR Tablets	IR: 2.5–10 mg BID XR: 20–40 mg QD
Dexedrine	Dextroamphetamine	IR, ER capsules (spansules)	IR: 5–40 mg divided QD-BID ER: 4–40 mg QD
Adderall	Dextroamphetamine	IR, XR Tablets	IR: 5–40 mg divided QD-BID XR: 20–60 mg QD
Daytrana	Methylphenidate	Transdermal Patch	10–30 mg Patch QD × 9 h and off × 15 h
Vyvanse	Lisdexamphetamine	Capsules	30–70 mg QD
Procentra	Dextroamphetamine	Liquid	5–40 mg divided QD-TID
Quillivant XR	Methylphenidate	Liquid	20–60 mg QD
Adzenys XR-ODT	Amphetamine	Orally disintegrating tablet	12.5 mg QD
Quillichew ER (chewable)	Mehtylphenidate	Chewable	20–60 mg QD

Table 12.2 DSM 5 Criteria for ADHD

DSM 5 has specific criteria for ADHD. A persistent pattern of inattention and/or hyperactivity-impulsivity that interferes with functioning or development, as characterized by (1) and/or (2):

Inattention: Six (or more) of the following symptoms have persisted for at least 6 months to a degree that is inconsistent with the developmental level and that negatively impacts directly on social and academic/occupational activities: Note: The symptoms are not solely a manifestation of oppositional behavior, defiance, hostility, or failure to understand tasks or instructions. For older adolescents and adults (age 17 and older), at least five symptoms are required.	Often fails to give close attention to details or makes careless mistakes in schoolwork, at work, or during other activities (e.g., overlooks or misses details, work is inaccurate).
	Often has difficulty sustaining attention in tasks or play activities (e.g., has difficulty remaining focused during lectures, conversations, or lengthy reading).
	Often does not seem to listen when spoken to directly (e.g., mind seems elsewhere, even in the absence of any obvious distraction).
	Often does not follow through on instructions and fails to finish schoolwork, chores, or duties in the workplace (e.g., starts tasks but quickly loses focus and is easily sidetracked).
	Often has difficulty organizing tasks and activities (e.g., difficulty managing sequential tasks; difficulty keeping materials and belongings in order; messy, disorganized work; has poor time management; fails to meet deadlines).
	Often avoids, dislikes, or is reluctant to engage in tasks that require sustained mental effort (e.g., schoolwork or homework; for older adolescents and adults, preparing reports, completing forms, reviewing lengthy papers).
	Often loses things necessary for tasks or activities (e.g., school materials, pencils, books, tools, wallets, keys, paperwork, eyeglasses, mobile telephones).
	Is often easily distracted by extraneous stimuli (for older adolescents and adults, may include unrelated thoughts).
	Is often forgetful in daily activities (e.g., doing chores, running errands; for older adolescents and adults, returning calls, paying bills, keeping appointments).

(continued)

Table 12.2 (continued)

Hyperactivity and impulsivity: Six (or more) of the following symptoms have persisted for at least 6 months to a degree that is inconsistent with developmental level and that negatively impacts directly on social and academic/occupational activities: Note: The symptoms are not solely a manifestation of oppositional behavior, defiance, hostility, or a failure to understand tasks or instructions. For older adolescents and adults (age 17 and older), at least five symptoms are required.	Often fidgets with or taps hands or feet or squirms in seat.
	Often leaves seat in situations when remaining seated is expected (e.g., leaves his or her place in the classroom, in the office or other workplace, or in other situations that require remaining in place).
	Often runs about or climbs in situations where it is inappropriate. (Note: In adolescents or adults, may be limited to feeling restless.)
	Often unable to play or engage in leisure activities quietly.
	Is often "on the go," acting as if "driven by a motor" (e.g., is unable to be or uncomfortable being still for extended time, as in restaurants, meetings; may be experienced by others as being restless or difficult to keep up with).
	Often talks excessively.
	Often blurts out an answer before a question has been completed (e.g., completes people's sentences; cannot wait for turn in conversation).
	Often has difficulty waiting his or her turn (e.g., while waiting in line).
	Often interrupts or intrudes on others (e.g., butts into conversations, games, or activities; may start using other people's things without asking or receiving permission; for adolescents and adults, may intrude into or take over what others are doing).

B. Several inattentive or hyperactive-impulsive symptoms were present prior to age 12 years.
C. Several inattentive or hyperactive-impulsive symptoms are present in two or more settings (e.g., at home, school, or work; with friends or relatives; in other activities).
D. There is clear evidence that the symptoms interfere with, or reduce the quality of, social, academic, or occupational functioning.
E. The symptoms do not occur exclusively during the course of schizophrenia or another psychotic disorder and are not better explained by another mental disorder (e.g., mood disorder, anxiety disorder, dissociative disorder, personality disorder, substance intoxication, or withdrawal).

Clinical Indications for Stimulants

The most common clinical indication for the use of stimulants is in the treatment of childhood, adolescent, and adult ADHD. Stimulants have also been widely used as a second-line treatment for excessive daytime sleepiness in narcolepsy. Although inattention is the hallmark symptom of ADHD, poor concentration is a symptom of many psychiatric conditions, among veterans as well as the general population.

For the veteran population in particular, the increased awareness and screening for traumatic brain injury (TBI) has also driven a demand for treatment options. Stimulants have been explored as a potential treatment for the inattention and other cognitive effects of TBI. There have been several studies that have demonstrated some efficacy of methylphenidate [15–17] and some case reports supporting dextroamphetamine [18] and lisdexamfetamine [19] for improved attention after sustaining a TBI. In addition to off-label use in TBI, there has been off-label use of stimulants for treatment-refractory depression. Stimulants have been used as augmentation agents for antidepressants to target symptoms of poor concentration and energy in melancholic patients as well as apathy in elderly depressed patients.

Use of Stimulants in ADHD

When approaching the treatment of ADHD, it is advised to assess and address other comorbid psychiatric illnesses first, unless it is clear that the other psychiatric illnesses are likely secondary to untreated ADHD. For example, a patient in the midst of an episode of major depression or severe anxiety may exhibit concentration and memory problems. The recommended course of action would be to treat the anxiety and depression with customary anti-depressants or anti-anxiolytics prior to the initiation of ADHD medications. However, if the patient is exhibiting mild symptoms of anxiety or depression (e.g., anxiety before a major exam, mild depression after losing a job or failing an exam), these manifestations may be secondary to the untreated ADHD illness and more appropriately addressed with the initiation of medications targeting the ADHD symptoms.

The use of stimulants when treating comorbid ADHD and bipolar disorder is less clear as both stimulant and non-stimulant ADHD medications (atomoxetine, bupropion, tricyclic anti-depressants (TCAs)) can potentially worsen mania, mixed and psychotic symptoms. Case reports in the literature suggest ADHD medications may be helpful for some patients with comorbid bipolar disorder if they are used cautiously. In patients with bipolar disorder symptoms that are well controlled by a mood stabilizer, a slow titration of ADHD medications (stimulant or non-stimulant) with close monitoring may be considered [20].

For patients with a current or past history of substance use disorders, stimulants should be used very cautiously. Historically, it had been recommended to abstain from prescribing stimulants to any patient with a substance abuse history. However, given that up to 17–45% of patients with ADHD may experience a comorbid substance use disorder during their lifetime, [21] this would leave a large population with untreated ADHD symptoms.

For these patients, a non-stimulant, such as atomoxetine or bupropion, would be a better first choice for treatment of ADHD symptoms. After the failure of an adequate trial of a non-stimulant, stimulants may be a reasonable option in some patients. However, patients for whom stimulants are their drug-of-choice would not be good candidates for stimulant therapy, and would probably be better suited to non-stimulant alternatives or evidence-based behavioral treatments [22].

The literature suggests that treatment of ADHD with stimulants generally does not lead to new or worsening substance use and may even decrease substance use in some patients [23]. Patients who are in remission for substance use disorders or actively engaged in substance abuse treatment may be candidates for stimulants for

ADHD. To lower the risk of abuse in these patients, consider prescribing long-acting stimulants, stimulant patches, or the pro-drug lisdexamfetamine, which requires metabolism in the gastrointestinal (GI) tract to be active.

Clinicians may want to reflect on the following questions prior to initiating stimulants in patients with comorbid substance use disorders:

- Has the patient abused stimulants in the past?
- Is the patient willing to participate in random urine drug screens and how will positive results be handled?
- How is the stimulant likely to interact with the patient's drugs-of-choice should s/he relapse?
- What are the likely interference of the patient's drugs-of-choice with the ADHD therapy (i.e., cannabis's effect on concentration and memory)?
- How likely is the patient to divert his/her stimulants?
- Has the patient sold/distributed drugs in the past or traded stimulants to get his/her drug-of-choice?
- Are there members in the patient's household who are also abusing substances and able to access the patient's stimulants?

Once the decision has been made to start a trial of stimulants for ADHD, the clinician has several options from which to choose. There are two main classes of stimulants: the methylphenidate-based compounds and the amphetamine compounds. Neither class has shown superiority over the other for treating ADHD symptoms; however, some patients clearly respond or tolerate one type of agent better compared to the other. Clinicians may want to consider giving patients a trial of both stimulant types to see which medication provides the best response.

It should be noted that the only stimulants that are FDA-approved for ADHD in adults are the long-acting formulations. While short-acting formulations can be considered for off-label use, there are several reasons to consider the long-acting formulations as the first treatment choice.

Most adults need 8–12 h of coverage during the day for their ADHD symptoms. Long-acting formulations eliminate the need for multiple dosing throughout the day, which can improve compliance. It is difficult for most people to remember to take medications 2–3 times a day. It can be even more challenging for the person with ADHD who is already prone to distractibility and forgetfulness to remember to carry and take their medications.

The slower onset of the effect of the long-acting stimulants helps reduce the "rush" and jitteriness patients sometimes experience when first taking the medications in the morning. Long-acting stimulants also tend to have a gentler wearing off period rather than a "crash" of sedation that sometimes accompanies the short-acting agents. Long-acting stimulants have been reported to have less euphoria and lower "likability ratings" compared to short-acting agents and therefore possibly abused less frequently [24].

Most of the long-acting agents are now available in generic formulations and are no longer as cost-prohibitive. Sometimes, even the long-acting stimulants do not provide long enough coverage for the entire day and may stop working after 6–8 h. In this situation, a second dose of a long-acting stimulant can be given in the afternoon but usually at a lower dose to avoid insomnia at night. If the afternoon long-acting stimulant is not tolerated, a short-acting stimulant can be used.

Since both veterans and people with ADHD frequently suffer from sleep disturbances, it is important to ask about sleep behaviors at each appointment when monitoring stimulants. Dosing the stimulant too close to bedtime many delay sleep initiation and impair sleep maintenance. However, there are some patients who paradoxically sleep better with an afternoon dose of stimulants. Since many patients with ADHD tend to procrastinate and have poor time-management skills, it is important to reiterate that the stimulants are there to help with concentration, NOT to help the person stay up later to get more accomplished.

Use of Stimulants in TBI

Although not FDA-approved for this indication, stimulants are sometimes used to treat symptoms associated with Traumatic Brain Injury (TBI). Individuals with TBI may exhibit a number of neuropsychiatric symptoms including cognitive impairment, affective changes, diminished impulse control, and decreased energy, alertness, and motivation [25]. Stimulants have been used to treat similar symptoms in other psychiatric illnesses such as ADHD (inattention, impulsivity, hyperactivity, slowed cognitive processing), narcolepsy (sedation, diminished alertness), and depression or apathy associated with medical illness. Extrapolating from experience using stimulants to treat these other illnesses, stimulants have been used in TBI.

TBI-related cognitive dysfunction can include: impairments of memory, impairments of attention, impairments of executive functions, and cognitive processing speed [25]. The expected recovery from cognitive-based symptoms following TBI ranges from 1 week to 6 months. A small but significant percentage of individuals (5–15%) experience persistent cognitive symptoms beyond the acute recovery period, which can impair their ability to resume many pre-morbid activities.

It may be helpful to obtain a neuropsychological assessment for cognitive symptoms persisting after 3 months. A neuropsychological assessment may help identify impairments that are responsive to specific behavioral rehabilitation strategies such as compensatory cognitive strategies and cognitive-behavioral therapy (CBT) [26].

For cognitive symptoms failing behavioral approaches, the next step would be to assess for comorbid affective changes that are common in TBI. It is recommended that the clinician rule out and treat mood-related cognitive dysfunction prior to initiating stimulants. Affective changes include depression, apathy, irritability, and emotional lability as well as anxiety syndromes such as generalized anxiety, panic attacks, phobic disorders, and post-traumatic stress disorder (PTSD).

The Ontario Neurotrauma Foundation guidelines for treating TBI-induced cognitive dysfunction recommend selective serotonin reuptake inhibitors (SSRIs) as the first-line treatment after TBI, based upon their favorable side-effect profile and broad utility for treating both cognitive and affective impairments in TBI [27]. The

TBI literature recommends both sertraline (starting at 25 mg; targeting 50–200 mg/day) and citalopram (starting at 10 mg; targeting 20–40 mg/day) [25–28].

For patients who either fail or do not adequately respond to a trial of a SSRI or do not tolerate SSRIs, a trial of stimulants may be considered. Methylphenidate is the most commonly studied stimulant in the literature for treatment of TBI [15–17] although some studies show positive results for dextroamphetamine [18] and lisdexamfetamine [19] as well.

As TBI patients appear to be more sensitive to side effects of medications, it is wise to "start low and go slow." Small doses of immediate-release formulations with multiple daily dosing can be added as needed and tolerated. There are fewer studies in the literature using sustained-release formulations. The literature is also unclear on the benefit of long-term stimulant treatment as most of the positive stimulant trials in TBI last only weeks rather than for months or years [18].

Use of Stimulants in Depression

Treatment-refractory depression (TRD) continues to be a problem despite the development of several medications and behavioral interventions developed over the past century. Prior to the development of antidepressants, stimulants were prescribed for severe depression because of their energy and cognitive enhancing properties and rapid onset of effect. However, problems with tolerance, dependence, and usually a time-limited effect of a few weeks preclude long-term treatment for what is often a chronic illness.

After the development of antidepressants, stimulants became more commonly used as augmentation strategies to treat TRD or as a method to gain a quick antidepressant response while waiting for traditional antidepressants to start working. Some case reports and small open label studies suggested possible benefit to adding stimulants to TCAs and monoamine oxidase inhibitors (MAOIs) and later to the SSRIs. Since stimulants are known to help with fatigue, apathy, and cognitive difficulties, they can appear to be a reasonable choice for off-label antidepressant augmentation for clinicians treating refractory depression. However, side effects that include anxiety, insomnia, exacerbation of mania or psychosis, abuse potential, as well as the cardiovascular risks of hypertension and arrhythmia limit their use [29–33].

Prescribing stimulants in patients with bipolar depression is controversial. Experts recommend prescribing stimulants only in conjunction with mood stabilizers with close monitoring for manic, mixed, or psychotic symptoms [20].

Use of Stimulants for Apathy and Cognitive Changes in Dementia

As the veteran and non-veteran population ages, they become at risk for the neuropsychological changes of dementia. Stimulants have also been used for the behavioral and cognitive changes that occur with dementia. Methylphenidate has been the most commonly prescribed stimulant in these incidences. A 2010 article [34] reviewing eight studies of the use of psychostimulants in dementia showed little improvement in cognition with the use of these medications and not enough data to support its use in excess daytime sedation. The article's review of the studies did reveal some support for the use of methylphenidate in apathy. The authors of this study also warn to use careful patient selection since stimulants can increase blood pressure and heart rate as well as induce psychological changes of irritability, agitation, and psychosis in this vulnerable population.

A more recent 2018 article [35] described a 12-week, prospective, double-blind, randomized, placebo-controlled study of the use of methylphenidate 5–10 mg BID in 60 community-dwelling male veterans with mild Alzheimer's disease, which showed a significant improvement not only in apathy but also cognition, functional status, caregiver burden, clinical global impression scales (CGI) scores, and depression. While this study demonstrates a possible benefit of the use of stimulants in dementia, the limitations of the study should be noted, which includes a small sample size from only one site and the inclusion of only male veterans.

Mechanism of Action

The precise mechanism of action of stimulants is unknown but they are thought to enhance extracellular norepinephrine and dopamine [36]. It is the enhancing effect on dopamine neurotransmission that is thought to be of most significance in the treatment of symptoms seen in ADHD.

Risks of Stimulant Use

Warning labels on ADHD medications have been updated in recent years to include warnings about possible cardiovascular risks, particularly sudden death in children and adolescents with structural cardiac abnormalities or other serious heart problems as well as risks of adverse psychiatric symptoms including hallucinations, delusional thinking, or mania. Black box warnings were also issued to caution their use in alcoholism and other substance use disorders and that a marked tolerance could lead to dependence.

Given that stimulants are stimulating, caution should be used in those with underlying anxiety disorders and mania. There is also some precaution to using stimulants in PTSD as there is at least one report of stimulants being a risk factor for post-traumatic stress symptoms [37].

Risks of Psychostimulant Use in Pregnancy

There are limited studies to guide a clinician's decision to use psychostimulants in pregnant patients. However, there have been some recent articles that are worth reviewing if a veteran presents wishing to continue stimulants during pregnancy. A

2017 JAMA psychiatry study showed a small increase of cardiac malformations for the first trimester use of methylphenidate but not amphetamines [38] This study contradicts an earlier, much smaller study in the September 2016 Journal of Clinical Psychiatry, which showed no increase in prenatal major malformations. There was also an increase in hypertensive disorders of pregnancy with use of psychostimulants after the 20th week of gestation demonstrated in a study in the November 2016 Journal of Clinical Psychiatry [39]. A good review of the limited studies of psychostimulants in pregnancy and recommendations can be found on the Massachusetts General Hospital (MGH) Center for Women's Mental Health website [40].

Recommended Medical Workup Prior to Initiating Psychostimulants

Psychostimulants are known to carry some medical risks and the FDA placed black box warnings on all stimulants. There are no formally established guidelines for a medical workup prior to starting stimulants in adults. However, in 2008, the American Heart Association (AHA) established guidelines [41] for a cardiac workup in adolescents and children prior to starting stimulants. These guidelines include taking a personal and family cardiac history, performing a physical exam, and obtaining an ECG.

These guidelines have been extrapolated to adults by many medical providers. FDA labeling on Adderall and Ritalin suggest assessing cardiovascular status and risk factors in children, adolescents, or adults who are being considered for treatment with stimulant medications and warn that misuse of amphetamine may cause sudden death and serious cardiovascular adverse reactions. FDA labeling also warn that stimulants have a high potential for abuse and prolonged use may lead to dependence.

Clinicians are advised to assess for the possibility of non-therapeutic use and distribution to others. In 2011, the FDA issued a safety update on the use of stimulants [42]. The update contained two studies that evaluated frequency of myocardial infarctions and sudden deaths in a sample of adults and also assessed the frequency of strokes. Neither study showed an increased risk of serious adverse cardiovascular events in adults treated with ADHD medications. However, the FDA's recommendations remained unchanged in advising that stimulants and atomoxetine should generally not be used in patients with serious heart problems, or patients for whom an increase in blood pressure or heart rate would be problematic. The report also recommended that patients treated with stimulants should be periodically monitored for changes in heart rate or blood pressure.

In two review articles, Martinez-Raga provides a nice synopsis of the cardiovascular changes observed when prescribing ADHD medications [43] as well as an updated summary of considerations for safe prescribing practices [44]. In addition to a baseline cardiovascular workup, it is also helpful to obtain a baseline weight and sleep pattern prior to starting a stimulant since some patients may experience weight loss and insomnia after starting treatment. The risks and benefits of starting a stimulant should be carefully considered for patients with comorbid eating disorders and sleep disorders.

Ongoing Monitoring for Chronic Stimulant Use

Since ADHD is often a chronic condition, both child and adult patients are now remaining on stimulants for many years. Given the medical and abuse risks associated with these medications, it is helpful to establish ongoing monitoring protocols to evaluate the benefit versus the risk of ongoing treatment.

Symptom rating scales such as the Adult ADHD Self-Report Scale (ASRS-V1.1) for ADHD, the Patient Health Questionnaire (PHQ9) for depression, and the Epworth Sleepiness Scale (ESS) for excessive daytime sleepiness can be helpful to monitor the response to treatment. A targeted review of systems at each visit to screen for new onset of stimulant-induced cardiovascular, gastrointestinal, neurological, and psychiatric symptoms is also advised.

While most psychiatrists do not perform physical exams as a part of their routine follow-up visits, it is recommended to check blood pressure, heart rate [45], and weight periodically, especially while titrating doses. There is an average increase of 5 beats per minute in heart rate and an increase of 1–3 mm of mercury in systolic and diastolic blood pressure, although some patients may experience larger changes [46]. Referral for ECG or a more thorough physical exam by primary care or cardiology should be considered when clinically indicated, especially in older populations. For patients with an elevated risk of substance abuse or concerns about diversion, urine toxicology screens should also be considered.

For clinicians who are interested in more education on the evaluation, treatment, and monitoring of ADHD and the use of stimulants in this disorder, we recommend the following two resources. The Canadian ADHD Resource Alliance (CADDRA) is a leader in the research of ADHD and developing guidelines for the evaluation and treatment of ADHD. We suggest visiting the CADDRA website at www.caddra.ca. A free version of the Canadian ADHD Practice Guidelines is available online [47]. The American Professional Society of ADHD and Related Disorders (APSARD) is another good resource for clinicians and APSARD hosts an annual educational meeting.

Summary

Stimulants are an important psycho-pharmacological tool to consider when treating veterans with adult ADHD and TBI and as a second-line agent for narcolepsy or excessive daytime sedation. Stimulants may also have a role in helping veterans with dementia-related cognitive changes such as apathy or treatment-refractory depression, however, there is less evidence supporting their utilization for these conditions.

In use since the early 1900s, many stimulant formulations are currently available and can be very effective and relatively quick acting agents. However, caution must be used in veterans with significant cardiac risk factors and females of child bearing age as well as those at risk for substance use disorders, eating disorders, mania, and psychosis.

References

1. AMA Council on Pharmacy and Chemistry. Benzedrine. J Am Med Assoc. 1933;101:1315.
2. Jackson CO. The amphetamine inhaler: a case study of medical abuse. J Hist Med. 1971;26:187–96.
3. AMA Council on Pharmacy and Chemistry. Present status of benzedrine sulfate. J Am Med Assoc. 1937;109:2064–9.
4. Goodman L, Gilman A. The pharmalogical basis of therapeutics. New York: Macmillan; 1941.
5. Grinspoon L, Hedblom P. The speed culture: amphetamine use and abuse in America. Cambridge: Harvard University Press; 1975.
6. Green FHK, Clovell G. History of the Second World War: medical research. London: HMSO; 1953;38:p. 21–2.
7. Bradley C. The behavior of children receiving Benzedrine. Am J Psychiatry. 1937;94:577–85.
8. Rothenberger A, Neumarker KJ. Wissenschaftsgeschichte der ADHS Steinkopff, Darmstadt: Kramer-Pollnow im Spiegel der Zeit; 2005.
9. Gross MD. Origin of stimulant use for treatment of attention deficit disorder. Am J Psychiatry. 1995;152:298–9.
10. Brown WA. Charles Bradley MD, 1902–1979. Am J Psychiatry. 1998;155:968.
11. Morton WA, Stockton GG. Methylphenidate abuse and psychiatric side effects. Prim Care Companion J Clin Psychiatry. 2002;2:159–64.
12. Rosler M, Casas M, Konofal E, et al. Attention deficit hyperactivity disorder in adults. World J Biol Psychiatry. 2010;11:684–98.
13. Leonard BE, McCartan D, White J, et al. Methylphenidate: a review of its neuropharmacological, neuropsychological and adverse clinical effects. Hum Psychopharmacol Clin Exp. 2004;19:151–80.
14. Lange KW, Reichl S, Lange KM, et al. The history of attention deficit hyperactivity disorder. Atten Defic Hyperact Disord. 2010;2(4):241–55.
15. Huang CH, Huang CC, Sun CK, et al. Methylphenidate on cognitive improvement in patients with traumatic brain injury: a meta-analysis. Curr Neuropharmacol. 2016;14:272–81.
16. Johansson B, Wentzel AP, Andréll P, Rönnbäck L, Mannheimer C. Long-term treatment with methylphenidate for fatigue after traumatic brain injury. Acta Neurol Scand. 2017;135(1):100–7.
17. Zhang WT, Wang YF. Efficacy of methylphenidate for the treatment of mental sequelae after traumatic brain injury. Medicine. 2017;96:25.
18. Maksimowski MB, Tampi RR. Efficacy of stimulants for psychiatric symptoms in individuals with traumatic brain injury. Ann Clin Psychiatry. 2016;28(3):156–66.
19. Tramontana MG, Cowan RL, Zald D, Prokop JW, Guillamondegui O. Traumatic brain injury-related attention deficits: treatment outcomes with lisdexamfetamine dimesylate (Vyvanse). Brain Inj. 2014;28(11):1461–72.
20. Perugi G, Vannucchi G, Bedani F, Favaretto E. Use of stimulants in bipolar disorder. Curr Psychiatry Rep. 2017;19:7.
21. Wilens TE. The nature of the relationship between attention-deficit/hyperactivity disorder and substance use. J Clin Psychiatry. 2007;68(Suppl 11):4–8.
22. Mariani JJ, Levin FR. Treatment strategies for co-occurring ADHD and substance use disorders. Am J Addict. 2007;16(Suppl 1):45–54; quiz 55-6

23. Kollins S. Abuse liability of medications used to treat Attention-Deficit/Hyperactivity Disorder (ADHD). Am J Addict. 2007;16(Suppl 1):35–44; quiz 43-4
24. Upadhyaya H. Managing attention-deficit/hyperactivity disorder in the presence of substance use disorder. J Clin Psychiatry. 2007;68(Suppl 11):23–30.
25. Scher LM, Lomis E, RM MC. Traumatic brain injury: pharmacotherapy options for cognitive deficits. Curr Psychiatr Ther. 2011;10:10–2. 21–37.
26. Rees L. Persistent cognitive difficulties. In: Chapter 9, Guidelines for concussion/mild traumatic brain injury & persistent symptoms. 2nd ed. Toronto: Ontario Neurotrauma Foundation; 2013. p. 40–1.
27. McCullagh S, Rees L, Velikonja D. Persistent mental health disorders. In: Chapter 9, Guidelines for concussion/mild traumatic brain injury & persistent symptoms. 2nd ed. Toronto: Ontario Neurotrauma Foundation; 2013. p. 34–9.
28. Arciniegas DB, Silver JM. Psychopharmacology. In: Silver JM, Mcalister TW, Yudofsky SC, editors. Textbook of traumatic brain injury. 2nd ed. Washington, DC: American Psychiatric Publishing, Inc.; 2011. p. 553–69.
29. Barowsky J, Schwartz TL. An evidence-based approach to augmentation and combination strategies for: treatment-resistant depression. Psychiatry (Edgmont). 2006;3(7):42–61.
30. McIntyre RS, Lee Y, Zhou AJ, Rosenblat JD, Peters EM, Lam RW, Kennedy SH, Rong C, Jerrell JM. The efficacy of psychostimulants in major depressive episodes a systematic review and meta-analysis. J Clin Psychopharmacol. 2017;37:412–8.
31. Lavretsky H, Reinlieb M, St Cyr N, et al. Citalopram, methylphenidate, or their combination in geriatric depression: a randomized, double-blind, placebo-controlled trial. Am J Psychiatry. 2015;172:561–9.
32. Nelson JC. The role of stimulants in late-life depression. Am J Psychiatry. 2015;172:505–7.
33. Malhi GS, Byrow Y, Bassett D, Boyce P, Hopwood M, Lyndon W, Mulder R, Porter R, Singh A, Murray G. Stimulants for depression: on the up and up? Aust N Z J Psychiatry. 2016;50(3):203–7.
34. Dolder CR, Davis LN, McKinsey J. Use of psychostimulants in patients with dementia. Ann Pharmacother. 2010;44(10):1624–32.
35. Padala PR, Padala KP, Lensing SY, Ramirez D, Monga V, Bopp MM, Roberson PK, Dennis RA, Petty F, Sullivan DH, Burke WJ. Methylphenidate for apathy in community-dwelling older veterans with mild Alzheimer's disease: a double-blind, randomized, placebo-controlled trial. Am J Psychiatry. 2018;175(2):159–68.
36. Herbst E, McCaslin S, Kalapatapu R. Use of stimulants and performance enhancers during and after trauma exposure in a combat veteran: a possible risk factor for posttraumatic stress symptoms. Am J Psychiatry. 2017;174(2):95–9.
37. Wilens TE, Morrison NR, Prince J. An update on the pharmacotherapy of attention deficit/hyperactivity disorder in adults. Expert Rev Neurother. 2011;11:1443–65.
38. Huybrechts KF, Bröms G, Christensen LB, Einarsdóttir K, Engeland A, Furu K, Gissler M, Hernandez-Diaz S, Karlsson P, Karlstad Ø, Kieler H, Lahesmaa-Korpinen AM, Mogun H, Nørgaard M, Reutfors J, Sørensen HT, Zoega H, Bateman BT. Association between methylphenidate and amphetamine use in pregnancy and risk of congenital malformations: a cohort study from the international pregnancy safety study consortium. JAMA Psychiat. 2018;75(2):167–75.
39. Newport DJ, Hostetter AL, Juul SH, Porterfield SM, Knight BT, Stowe ZN. Prenatal psychostimulant and antidepressant exposure and risk of hypertensive disorders of pregnancy. J Clin Psychiatry. 2016;77(11):1538–45.
40. Nonacs R. Good news: more data on the use of ADHD medications during pregnancy [Internet]. 2017 Dec 22; Available from: https://womensmentalhealth.org/posts/good-news-data-use-adhd-medications-pregnancy/
41. Vetter VL, Erickson C, Berger S, et al. Cardiovascular monitoring of children and adolescents with heart disease receiving stimulant drugs: a scientific statement from the American Heart Association Council on Cardiovascular Disease in the Young Congenital Cardiac Defects Committee and the Council on Cardiovascular Nursing. Circulation. 2008;117:2407–23.

42. FDA Drug Safety Communication: Safety Review Update of Medications used to treat Attention-Deficit/Hyperactivity Disorder (ADHD) in adults. Silver Spring, MD: U.S. Food and Drug Administration (US); 2011 Dec. 12 [updated 2018 Feb 13; cited 2018 Jul 7]. Available from: https://www.fda.gov/Drugs/DrugSafety/ucm279858.htm
43. Martinez-Raga J, Knecht C, Szerman N, Martinez MI. Risk of serious cardiovascular problems with medications for attention-deficit hyperactivity disorder. CNS Drugs. 2013;27(1):15–30.
44. Martinez-Raga J, Ferreros A, Knecht C, de Alvaro R, Carabal E. Attention-deficit hyperactivity disorder medication use: factors involved in prescribing, safety aspects and outcomes. Ther Adv Drug Saf. 2017;8(3):87–99.
45. Wilens TE, Hammerness PG, Biederman J, Kwon A, Spencer TJ, Clark S, Scott M, Podolski A, Ditterline JW, Morris MC, Moore H. Blood pressure changes associated with medication treatment of adults with attention-deficit/hyperactivity disorder. J Clin Psychiatry. 2005;66(2):253–9.
46. Adler LA. Pharmacotherapy for adult ADHD. J Clin Psychiatry. 2009;70(5):e12.
47. Canadian Attention Deficit Hyperactivity Disorder Resource Alliance (CADDRA): Canadian ADHD Practice Guidelines, 3rd ed. Toronto ON; CADDRA, 2011. Available from: http://www.caddra.ca.

Use of Complementary and Integrative Health for Chronic Pain Management

13

Marina A. Khusid, Elissa L. Stern, and Kathleen Reed

Introduction

Chronic pain is one of the most common health concerns in Veterans. Several recent studies show that 44–47% of Operation Enduring Freedom (OEF)/Operation Iraqi Freedom (OIF) Veterans complain of pain and about half of them report daily or constant pain of moderate to severe intensity that lasts longer than a year [1–3]. Pain commonly co-occurs with psychiatric disorders [4], such as major depressive disorder (30–47%), posttraumatic stress disorder (30–43%), substance use disorder (28%), and sleep disturbance (48%) [5]. It increases depression risk three- to five-fold, raises risk of posttraumatic stress disorder (PTSD) and insomnia [6], and is associated with increased recurrence of depression and anxiety [7].

Inversely, adults with mental health conditions are statistically more likely to be prescribed opioids. They receive 51.4% of the total opioid prescriptions in the United States each year, even though opioids generally exacerbate psychiatric and sleep disorders [8]. This complex relationship between chronic pain, opioid use, and psychological health suggests that addressing pain should be a vital component of any mental health treatment plan.

The growing costs of pain-related morbidity, mortality, and disability and increasing evidence that conventional treatment does not adequately address pain

M. A. Khusid (✉)
Jesse Brown Veterans Affairs Medical Center, University of Illinois at Chicago, Department of Family Medicine, Chicago, IL, USA
e-mail: marina.khusid@va.gov

E. L. Stern
Jesse Brown Veterans Affairs Medical Center, Northwestern University Feinberg School of Medicine, Department of Medicine, Chicago, IL, USA

K. Reed
Jesse Brown Veterans Affairs Medical Center, Women Veteran Health Center, Chicago, IL, USA

and contributes to the opioid crisis are discussed in the National Institute for Drug Abuse (NIDA) report [9]. This report shows that one in three Americans used prescription opioids in 2015. To address this growing opioid epidemic, President Obama signed into law the Comprehensive Addiction and Recovery Act (CARA) on July 22, 2016 [10].

One of the strategies proposed by CARA was expansion and delivery of complementary and integrative health (CIH) approaches to Veterans to maximize their access to nonpharmacological pain treatments [11]. In response to the CARA bill, the Veterans Health Administration's (VHA's) Integrative Health Clinical Coordinating Center was established, and the VHA Directive 1137 Provision of Complementary and Integrative Health was approved on May 19, 2017. It requires that each Veterans Affairs Medical Center (VAMC) offers evidence-based CIH interventions either on site or through community referrals. In 2018 the list of required CIH interventions includes acupuncture, massage therapy, yoga, tai chi, biofeedback, hypnosis, meditation, and guided imagery.

With the implementation of new CIH interventions, there is increased need to educate VHA and other providers on evidence-based indications, efficacy, expected therapeutic response, and safety. To address this growing need, this chapter will summarize evidence for CIH modalities that are used most commonly in pain management. A special emphasis is placed on CIH interventions that can be used by Veterans as active self-management and to foster patient engagement and self-efficacy. In conclusion, this chapter highlights fibromyalgia and migraines, two pain conditions that are particularly challenging to treat, to illustrate how providers can introduce CIH interventions in their clinical practice.

Evidence-Based CIH Interventions for Chronic Pain

Mindfulness Meditation and Mindfulness-Based Interventions

Mindfulness meditation is a regular practice that one uses to cultivate open, acceptant, nonjudgmental awareness of the present moment (i.e., mindfulness) by focusing her attention on her breathing. There are several types of mindfulness meditation that originated from different Buddhist monastic traditions (e.g., Zen, Vipassana, Shambhala meditations). To standardize care delivery, ancient Buddhist practices were adapted in the form of group-based meditation trainings.

These 6- to 8-week mindfulness-based interventions (MBIs) usually consist of weekly sessions with a certified instructor and daily practice of mindfulness or movement meditation at home. The goal is to develop a mindfulness practice and introduce a sustained health behavior change. Two MBIs that are used for pain most commonly are mindfulness-based stress reduction (MBSR) and the Mindfulness-Oriented Recovery Enhancement (MORE) program. These interventions are safe, and no serious adverse events were reported [12, 13].

Several recent systematic reviews suggest that MBSR effectively and durably reduces pain intensity, and associated depressive symptoms, while improving functional status and quality of life [12–14]. A recent systematic review of 37 randomized controlled trials (RCTs) ($n = 3536$) defines the quality of evidence as low, suggesting that larger studies with longer follow-up are needed [13]. However, the existing RCTs with longer follow-up show that when patients continued with regular meditation practice beyond an initial 8-week MBSR course, the therapeutic gain of feeling in control and accepting of pain, improved anxiety, depression, and quality of life maintained at 6-month follow-up [15].

MORE is different from MBSR in that it focuses on chronic opioid therapy for pain. When compared to a pain support group [16, 17], MORE participants reported significantly greater reductions in pain severity and improvement of functional status (e.g., general activity, walking ability, normal work) and psychological function (e.g., improvement in mood, relationships, sleep, and enjoyment of life). MORE group participants additionally demonstrated significantly less stress reactivity and desire for opioids and were significantly more likely to no longer meet the criteria for opioid use disorder immediately following treatment. Therapeutic gains in pain reduction and functional and psychological status were largely maintained at 3-month follow-up.

Mechanistic and neuroimaging findings are consistent with clinical research in providing evidence that MBIs are associated with reduction in chronic pain intensity and unpleasantness, decreased sensitivity to pain, and improved ability to observe and not react to pain. Meditators report better pain management compared to controls with reduction in pain intensity between 22% and 50%, decrease in pain unpleasantness by 57%, and decrease in anticipatory anxiety by 29% [18, 19]. MBIs also target neurocognitive mechanisms of addiction by reducing negative emotions and stress reactivity, promoting learning to uncouple drug-use triggers from conditioned responses to use, enhancing cognitive control over cravings, modulating impulse control, and increasing savoring to restore natural reward processing [20].

Finally, several systematic reviews suggest efficacy and safety of MBIs used adjunctively in the treatment of depression [21], smoking cessation [22], PTSD [23], substance use disorder [24], and sleep disturbance [25]. This wide-spectrum effectiveness of mindfulness meditation for several highly prevalent conditions in Veterans makes it an exceptionally versatile clinical tool. It's also one of the most effective self-management strategies in patients with chronic pain and mental health conditions because it is easy to learn, requires no equipment, can be done anywhere, is low to no cost, and requires minimal time investment (e.g., as little as 20 min a day).

Biofeedback for Chronic Pain

Biofeedback is a process in which electronic monitoring of involuntary bodily functions (e.g., muscle tension) is used to train patients to acquire voluntary control of these functions. A type of biofeedback that is most commonly used for pain is electromyography (EMG) biofeedback. EMG uses surface electrodes to detect change in skeletal muscle activity and provides feedback to a patient in the form of a visual or auditory signal. The patient is then trained to utilize this signal to facilitate relaxation of a spastic muscle. Usually, a course of biofeedback consists of 10 sessions, 45 min each. However, during this time, patients learn techniques that they can later use as self-care at home without the assistance of biofeedback technology.

In a 2017 meta-analysis ($N = 21$ RCTs, 1062 patients), Sielski et al. concluded that biofeedback sustainably decreases pain intensity, muscle tension, and coping. They reported no observed adverse events. Longer biofeedback courses were shown to be more effective for reducing disability and depressive symptoms [26]. The improvement was noted in the short and long term, with biofeedback used adjunctively to standard care or alone.

Several systematic reviews exist for specific pain conditions. The American College of Physicians Clinical Practice Guideline recommends biofeedback for chronic low back pain based on their systematic review [27, 28]. Another meta-analysis ($N = 53$ RCTs) found biofeedback effective for tension headaches, with stable therapeutic benefit for up to 15 months, and reduction of headache frequency, muscle tone, use of analgesic medication, and associated symptoms of anxiety and depression [29]. A meta-analysis of biofeedback for fibromyalgia ($N = 7$ RCTs, 321 patients) found significant reduction of pain, but only short-term studies were available [30].

Yoga

Yoga originated in ancient India. It combines three components: meditation (dhyana), breathing (pranayama), and transitioning through a sequence of physical postures (asanas). Yoga is commonly used therapeutically to help people manage stress, as well as symptoms of health conditions.

The 2017 clinical practice guideline developed by the American College of Physicians (ACP) makes a strong recommendation to offer nonpharmacologic approaches as a first-line treatment for chronic low back pain (cLBP) [27]. Yoga is included in the ACP's list of evidence-based interventions for cLBP. This recommendation is based on findings by three recent systematic reviews that demonstrate moderate strength of evidence that yoga is associated with greater effects on pain and function at 3 and 6 months compared to nonexercise controls (e.g., placebo, usual care, sham, wait list) [28, 31, 32]. There was no statistically significant difference between exercise versus yoga in function or pain.

According to several systematic reviews and meta-analyses, yoga was found to be beneficial for osteoarthritis [33, 34], neck pain [35], rheumatoid arthritis [33], kyphosis [33], and fibromyalgia [33], Furthermore, yoga was found to be beneficial in decreasing pain-related disability even when used short term [36] and improve fatigue, sleep, depression, and health-related quality of life (HRQL) [37]. Yoga's safety was found to be comparable to exercise, usual care, and physical therapy [38, 39]. Research also shows that among 52 different yoga styles, there was no advantage to a particular style when used for pain [40]. This finding is particularly useful in clinical practice, since it indicates that choice of yoga could be based on patient's preference and local availability.

Tai Chi

Tai chi is an ancient Chinese discipline of meditative movements. It was used as a form of martial art and a health practice. Tai chi practice consists of meditative focus on a sequence of slow, low-impact movements with the purpose of creating balance, integrating mind and body, and cultivating health. Because of its leisurely pace and low-impact on the joints, tai chi can be practiced by patients of all ages and levels of conditioning.

According to several recent systematic reviews and meta-analyses, moderate-quality evidence suggests that tai chi was more effective than usual care, wait list, or no treatment at reducing disability and pain related to osteoarthritis [41, 42], low back pain [28, 31, 41, 42], headache [41], and fibromyalgia [37]. One systematic review suggested that reduction of LBP may be nearly immediate but that valid duration of tai chi practice for osteoarthritis-related pain was about 5 weeks [42]. A systematic review of 153 trials shows that tai chi is unlikely to result in serious adverse events but may be associated with minor and self-limiting musculoskeletal aches and pains [43]. However, it also indicates that adverse events were not always monitored and reported in existing published trials and recommends more research in this area.

Acupuncture

Acupuncture takes its origin in traditional Chinese medicine (TCM) and has been in use for over 5000 years. It involves the insertion of very thin sterile needles at very precise strategically chosen points. These points may be located on the body and/or ear, hands, feet, or scalp. Some TCM-style acupuncture treatments may utilize additional techniques, such as electrical stimulation, application of infrared heat, manual therapy called tui na, moxibustion, cupping, or gua sha. Acupuncture is usually administered as a course of 6–12 treatment sessions that occur every 2–7 days.

Efficacy of acupuncture for chronic pain has been shown by Vickers et al. in their landmark 2012 and 2014 meta-analyses (29 RCTs, n = 17,992) [44, 45]. In addition to establishing acupuncture efficacy for several chronic pain conditions (e.g., LBP, neck and shoulder pain, knee osteoarthritis, and headaches) [44], they also demonstrated that, when used adjunctively to standard care, acupuncture results in 50% of pain reduction, while treatment as usual alone yields merely 30% pain reduction [45]. A more recent 2017 meta-analyses by MacPherson et al. confirmed earlier findings and additionally showed durability of this analgesic effect for up to 12 months, following a course of acupuncture treatment (e.g., 10–12 sessions) [46].

Several systematic reviews evaluated acupuncture for diverse types of headaches. A 2016 Cochrane systematic review investigated acupuncture for migraine prophylaxis (22 RCTs, n = 4485) [47]. It showed that acupuncture monotherapy is as effective as prophylactic meds at reducing migraine frequency. When used adjunctively, acupuncture was more effective than standard care alone. Another Cochrane systematic review (11 RCTs, n = 2349) suggests acupuncture efficacy for treating frequent episodic or chronic tension-type headaches and reducing their intensity, duration, and frequency [48]. Positive systematic reviews also exist for neurovascular headaches (16 RCTs, $n = 1535$) [49] and headaches of mixed etiology (31 RCTs, $n = 3916$) [50].

Trinh et al. concluded in their 2016 Cochrane systematic review (27 RCTs, $n = 10{,}098$) that moderate evidence suggests that acupuncture is more effective than sham, inactive treatments, or wait-list control at decreasing pain and disability for up to 13 weeks [51]. The types of neck pain evaluated are whiplash, myofascial neck pain, arthritis of cervical spine, neck pain with radiculopathy, and mechanical neck pain. A meta-analysis on low back pain (32 RCTs) shows that pain was effective at reducing pain and functional status [52]. When used adjunctively, it was more effective than standard care alone.

As monotherapy, acupuncture was only slightly statistically more effective than pharmacologic analgesics. Three systematic reviews and meta-analyses evaluated acupuncture for osteoarthritis of knee, hip, or both. Their consistent conclusions show that acupuncture was more effective than control (e.g., sham, wait-list, standard care) at improving short- and long-term physical function and pain relief [53–55].

According to multiple systematic reviews and prospective surveys, acupuncture is safe when performed by appropriately trained and licensed practitioners [56–61]. Infrequent minor side effects include itching at point of needle insertion and feeling relaxed, drowsy, or tired [62]. Serious complications such as infection or pneumothorax are rare and directly related to inadequate training [59, 60].

Massage Therapy

Massage therapy is manual manipulation of soft body tissues (i.e., muscle, connective tissue, tendons, and ligaments) to enhance a person's health and well-being. Such manual techniques may include applying fixed or movable pressure, holding, and/or causing passive movement of a joint or body part to achieve therapeutic outcomes such as muscle relaxation or increase in range of motion.

The 2017 systematic review by the American College of Physicians (13 TCTs, $n = 1596$) compared massage effectiveness with several noninvasive interventions (e.g., manipulation, exercise, physiotherapy, acupuncture, transcutaneous electrical nerve stimulation (TENS), etc.). It showed that massage had better effect on pain in 8 of 9 trials and short-term function in 4 of 5 trials [28]. These findings were echoed in the 2017 comparative effectiveness review conducted by the Agency of Healthcare Research and Quality (AHRQ) [31] and a 2015 systematic review by Bervoets et al. [63]. Although the AHRQ review concluded that evidence was generally better for acupuncture than massage, it clearly states that in head-to-head trials, no clear difference was found between the two.

Two recent systematic reviews evaluated massage for chronic low back pain (cLBP) (7 RCTs, $n = 1062$) [64, 65]. Both reviews suggest that massage compared to usual care resulted in modest improvement in function and decrease of cLBP at

Table 13.1 CIH Use for Specific Pain Conditions

Chronic Pain Condition	Effective CIH Approaches
Chronic pain syndrome	MBSR, biofeedback, acupuncture, massage
Chronic opioid therapy for pain	MORE
Chronic low back pain	MBSR, biofeedback, tai chi, yoga, massage
Osteoarthritis	MBSR, tai chi, yoga, massage
Fibromyalgia	Tai chi, yoga, qigong, acupuncture, guided imagery/hypnosis, EMG-biofeedback, balneotherapy
Tension-type headache	MBSR, biofeedback, tai chi, acupuncture
Migraine	MBSR, biofeedback, yoga, acupuncture, massage
Neurovascular and mixed etiology headaches	MBSR, acupuncture
Neck pain	MBSR, yoga, acupuncture, massage
Shoulder pain	MBSR, acupuncture, massage

10 weeks, but the benefit was not sustained at 52 weeks. Furlan et al. further reported that the effects of massage for cLBP improved when combined with exercise and education. Although most reviews report that massage benefits for pain are short-lived (up to 10 weeks), Furlan et al. suggest that beneficial effects of massage for cLBP may be up to 1 year if a full series of treatments is completed [64].

Summary

A selection of CIH approaches is available for any given pain condition. MBSR and acupuncture can be used almost universally, while other techniques have specific indications (see Table 13.1). We recommend emphasizing CIH interventions that can be used long term as self-management and giving priority to interventions consistent with patient preference. Since we focused this chapter on interventions that are required by the VHA Directive 1137, additional effective modalities, including some dietary supplements, may exist.

Clinical Case Scenarios

Fibromyalgia

Background
Fibromyalgia (FM) is a syndrome of widespread pain associated with sleep disturbance, fatigue, depression, headache, abdominal pain, and poor concentration [66, 67]. These symptoms lead to significant personal and socioeconomic cost, including limitations in work ability and high health-care utilization [68, 69]. The prevalence of FM among the general population in the United States is estimated to be between 1.1% and 6.4% [70]. FM is more common in both civilian and veteran women than men [71, 72].

The standard of care in the management of FM combines pharmacologic and nonpharmacologic therapy [73, 74]. Guideline-recommended nonpharmacologic therapies include education about the nature of the disorder, cognitive-behavioral therapy, aerobic exercise, and multicomponent therapy [74, 75]. However, the effect sizes of these pharmacologic and nonpharmacologic therapies on the outcomes of pain and quality of life in FM have been found to be moderate at best [76]. Therefore, clinical experts recommend an individualized approach based on disease severity, comorbidities, and patient preference [77].

CIH Evidence Synthesis and Clinical Guidelines

Complementary and integrative health (CIH) should be considered in the management of FM. Great interest exists in CIH therapies among patients with FM. It has been estimated that up to 91% of FM patients seek alternative therapies [78]. Several systematic reviews have attempted to consolidate the rapidly evolving evidence base for CIH therapies in FM, and comments on select CIH therapies have been incorporated into European League Against Rheumatism (EULAR) and Canadian, German, and Israeli treatment guidelines [73, 74, 79, 80].

Meditative movement therapies (MMT) include tai chi, yoga, and qigong. MMT have been found to improve both functional limitations and associated symptoms in FM and are recommended by multiple guidelines [73, 74]. In a systematic review of 7 RCTs ($N = 362$), MMT were found to provide short-term moderate improvements in health-related quality of life (HRQOL), sleep, and fatigue and a small improvement in depression. Although the subgroup analysis was underpowered, the benefit in these four symptom categories was maintained for a median of 4.5 months of follow-up following a yoga intervention, while tai chi only benefitted sleep at follow-up [37]. Qigong was found ineffective in subgroup analysis in this review [37].

A separate systematic review and meta-analysis of 4 homogenous RCTs ($N = 201$) of qigong in FM showed at least moderate benefit in pain, sleep, and physical and mental function after 6–8 weeks of practice, which lasted up to 4–6 months after the intervention period when practiced at least 5 h per week [81]. MMT offer several potential benefits to patients with FM, but the magnitude of benefit is likely mediated by the frequency of practice. MMT were found to have no serious adverse effects [37].

While EULAR guidelines do not currently recommend guided imagery or hypnosis (GI/H) due to flawed trials, a more recent systematic review of 7 RCTs ($N = 387$) found low-quality evidence that GI/H decreased pain by at least 50%, decreased psychological distress by a small amount, and improved sleep by a large amount in the short term [73, 82]. Hypnosis improved pain by at least 30% and improved sleep symptoms at 3-month follow-up as well [82]. The number needed to benefit from GI/H was 4 (95% CI 2–16) for pain relief of at least 30% and 6 (95% CI 3–50) for pain relief of at least 50% [82]. While additional research is necessary, the use of guided imagery is clinically appealing because it can be administered at home via the Internet, smartphone, and other audio applications.

Acupuncture has a well-established role in chronic pain management, as discussed above, but more sparse evidence in FM specifically. A Cochrane review of 9 trials ($N = 395$) found low-to-moderate quality evidence that acupuncture improves short-term pain and stiffness, but the effect was similar to that of sham acupuncture [83]. No serious adverse events were directly attributable to acupuncture in this review [83]. However, the scientific study of standardized acupuncture regimens has been problematic because acupuncture is traditionally a variable, personalized intervention.

A recent RCT ($N = 162$) evaluated acupuncture in a more naturalistic clinical setting [84]. In this study, women with FM were referred to TCM practitioners who applied customized acupuncture treatments in 20-min weekly sessions for 9 weeks based on the patient's TCM diagnosis. The control was the sham application of empty guide tubes without puncturing the skin. At 6-month follow-up, there was a small improvement in overall well-being, moderate improvement in pain, and moderate improvement in physical function [84]. Current EULAR and German guidelines recommend acupuncture for select patients with FM, although additional well-designed trials of acupuncture in its intended clinical context are warranted [73, 74].

Biofeedback may be effective in decreasing pain in FM, although the quality of evidence is limited. A meta-analysis of 7 RCTs ($N = 321$) found evidence for the reduction of pain in the short term, but included studies were of poor quality [30]. Also, in subgroup analysis, only EMG-biofeedback significantly reduced pain, whereas electroencephalographic biofeedback was ineffective.

Survey data indicate that water-based therapies are widely used among patients with FM [85]. A Cochrane review studied supervised group aquatic exercise and found low- to moderate-quality evidence of benefit in both pain and physical functioning [86]. The number needed to treat for aquatic exercise to affect clinically meaningful change in multidimensional functioning was 5 (95% CI 3–9) [86]. There was a suggestion that aquatic therapy was as effective and as well tolerated as land-based exercise, although the quality of evidence was low [86].

Balneotherapy or hydrotherapy refers to bathing in mineral or thermal water and has also been found to have moderate quality evidence of moderate to large benefit on pain and HRQOL in FM, but the effect size is uncertain due to methodological issues, including treatment heterogeneity and small sample sizes [87, 88]. Care should be taken when referring patients with frailty or certain medical comorbidities to exercise- or water-based therapies although hydrotherapy appears safe from limited data [87].

While higher-quality research regarding the role of CIH therapies in FM is needed, meditative movement therapies, guided imagery/hypnosis, acupuncture, supervised group aquatic exercise, and balneotherapy can improve key FM symptoms, including pain, sleep, HRQOL, and physical functioning. Eliciting the priorities and preferences of the patient can enhance engagement with recommended therapies and guide the choice among therapeutic alternatives.

Clinical Case

Mrs. EM is a 47-year-old female veteran. She has been diagnosed with fibromyalgia, post-traumatic stress disorder, and depression. She has undergone a cervical spinal laminectomy and fusion and has a chronic rotator cuff tear. She is on disability from her postmilitary career in law enforcement. She complains of pain in her neck, shoulders, hands, and feet, as well as headaches and abdominal upset. She finds that hot showers help her pain somewhat. She only leaves the house for medical appointments and has trouble with household tasks such as laundry and cooking due to pain and fatigue. She attends psychotherapy every 2 weeks. Medications include cyclobenzaprine and pregabalin. Duloxetine was previously stopped due to gastrointestinal upset. She is frustrated with her current functional status and inadequate sleep.

During a follow-up visit, it was discussed with Mrs. EM that no single intervention was likely to provide complete symptom relief, but a combination of therapies might alleviate them. Goals for improved function in daily life were set. Mrs. EM asked for reading material about fibromyalgia and was provided with a detailed printed handout. She also planned to continue psychotherapy as she had a strong therapeutic relationship with her therapist.

Because aerobic exercise is considered a component of standard therapy in FM, the addition of an exercise plan was prioritized. Since Mrs. EM had poorly tolerated land-based activity in the past and expressed interest in water-based therapy, she was referred to water aerobics through the VHA recreation therapy center.

In order to avoid overly taxing new physical demands and multiple appointments, MMT and acupuncture were not recommended at this visit. Also, GI was recommended because it could conveniently be practiced at home and would address the multiple symptom domains of pain, psychological symptoms, and sleep. It was explained that the benefit was more likely with regular practice and Mrs. EM was provided with a VHA website with a downloadable smartphone application. A follow-up appointment in 6 weeks was planned to assess initial responses to these interventions.

At 6-week follow-up, Mrs. EM had read the handout and felt reassured regarding the nature of the disease process. This helped motivate her to sign up for the water aerobics class and to download the guided imagery application. After another 6 weeks, she had attended a few water aerobics classes, which she enjoyed, and had tried guided imagery once or twice. She did not notice immediate changes in her sleep, energy, or pain. She was encouraged to continue participating in water aerobics as scheduled and to practice guided imagery daily. She was counseled regarding the incremental nature of the expected changes. Frequent follow-up was planned in order to enhance adherence with the treatment recommendations.

Migraine

Background

Migraine can present as an episodic or chronic headache disorder with or without aura and is typically characterized by severe unilateral, pulsating headache pain. Migraines can last 4–72 h. They worsen with activity and are often accompanied by photophobia, phonophobia, nausea, and/or vomiting [89].

Veterans with migraines are more likely to have a diagnosis of PTSD and combat-related injury [90]. Thus, Veterans are uniquely impacted by the complex relationship between physical and psychological trauma and headaches, including diagnosis of migraine. Migraine headache affects 12% of individuals in the general population in the United States (US) while disproportionately affecting women who experience migraines at about three times the rate of men [91].

Migraine headaches present an economic burden for sufferers and negatively impact functioning and quality of life. Conventional pharmacologic treatments of migraine have limitations, including side effects, lack of efficacy, and comorbidity [92]. For this reason, many patients with migraine seek out complementary and alternative therapies for migraine relief [93].

An integrative approach is important in improving self-efficacy and empowering patients in the self-management of migraines [92]. The current evidence and national guidelines support the use of CIH in the treatment of migraine. The development of an individualized treatment plan that incorporates CIH therapies can prevent migraine and improve quality of life for Veterans.

CIH Evidence Synthesis and Clinical Guidelines

The most frequently used CIH therapies by migraineurs include manipulative therapy, herbal supplementation, and mind-body therapy [93]. Additionally, most patients will not have improvement to headache measures unless lifestyle modifications are made, including sleep hygiene, stress management, regular aerobic exercise, and dietary modifications [94]. A synthesis of a literature review for the self-management and CIH therapies, including vitamins and supplements incorporating current clinical guidelines, will follow.

Koseoglu et al. suggested in their 2015 literature review that exercise is effective in migraine prophylaxis [95]. Although earlier RCTs focused on aerobic exercise, two recent RCTs suggest that high-intensity interval training (HIT) is also effective [96, 97]. After 12 weeks of training with twice a week exercise session, HIT was effective for migraine day reduction and improvement of cerebrovascular health compared to moderate continuous training [97].

Nutrition plays a role in managing migraines, but the role of specific dietary triggers is complex and clinical advice should be individualized. Patients should be encouraged to keep a detailed diet and headache diary over several months rather than be provided an extensive list of trigger foods to avoid, which can cause anxiety or limit healthy food options. Fasting or skipping meals has been reported as the most frequent food trigger [92].

There are no systematic reviews to provide definitive evidence for a specific diet that improves migraine symptoms; however, a 36-week randomized crossover trial divided 42 adults into 2 periods in which they received a placebo or were advised to follow a low-fat vegan diet [98]. Headache frequency declined in both periods, while the diet period had a greater decline in the worst headache pain in the last 2 weeks. While more research needs to be done on the optimal diet for migraineurs, in addition to considering a low-fat vegan diet, most patients can be recommended to follow a well-balanced diet incorporating whole foods and avoidance of fasting [98].

Sleep hygiene may decrease the frequency and duration of migraine attacks. While direct evidence in the adult population is lacking, a consistent sleep schedule of 7–8 h per night, and instructions on improving sleep hygiene, resulted in a decrease of migraine duration and frequency in a group of children and adolescents [99]. No effect on migraine severity was observed.

Stress management is important in reducing migraine symptoms, and MBSR, yoga, cognitive-behavioral therapy, and biofeedback can be considered. While more research is needed on MBSR and yoga, small trials show promising results with both as being equally or more beneficial than conventional treatments without the risk of side effects.

For example, 44 patients with chronic migraine and medication overuse withdrawal were randomized to a mindfulness-based approach or medication prophylaxis [100]. At 1-year follow-up, the mindfulness group had a similar reduction in headache frequency as the medication group. A small RCT of 19 patients with migraine were randomized to either 9 classes of MBSR of usual care [101]. MBSR had a beneficial effect on headache duration, disability, self-efficacy, and mindfulness compared to usual care, but the sample was too small to provide statistical significance. An RCT of 72 patients with migraine without aura were randomized to either yoga and meditation for 60 min 5 days weekly or self-care for 3 months [102]. The yoga group had significant reduction of frequency, severity of headache, and pain compared to self-care group. A 2006 meta-analysis of 55 studies (including RCTs) showed biofeedback, ranging from 3 to 24 sessions, was more effective than controls in improving frequency of headache and self-efficacy [103].

A 2015 systematic review of 10 studies using cognitive-behavioral therapy (CBT) for migraine and chronic headache may reduce physical symptoms of headache and migraine but show mixed support for use [104]. CBT was more effective than waiting list in reducing headache frequency and intensity. CBT plus relaxation was statistically more effective than the conventional prophylactic agent amitriptyline in reducing mean-level headache pain and increasing headache free days. However, there was no difference between CBT and biofeedback or self-managed CBT program at home.

CIH approaches such as massage, spinal and osteopathic manipulation, and acupuncture may also be considered in the integrative approach of the patient with migraine. A study of 47 patients randomized patients to either massage or control, without blinding [105]. The massage group received 45 min of massage for 6 of the 13 weeks and had significant improvements in migraine frequency.

A systematic review of 22 trials ($n = 4985$) showed acupuncture associated with a moderate reduction in migraine frequency when compared with no acupuncture [47]. One trial, included in this review, shows small but significant benefit after 12 months. Acupuncture was associated with headache reduction compared with sham acupuncture. Acupuncture also reduced migraine frequency significantly more than drug prophylaxis, but significance was not maintained at follow-up [47].

The 2012 American Academy of Neurology and American Headache Society (AAN/AHS) guidelines support the use of complementary treatments and certain nutritional supplements for headache prevention. The level of evidence in the AAN/

AHS guidelines will be provided for each supplement or vitamin discussed [106]. As with any daily prophylactic medication, supplements need to be used at the goal dose for 2–3 months before determining effectiveness [92]. Magnesium citrate 400–600 mg by mouth daily showed a 41.6% reduction in migraine attack frequency when compared with placebo [107]. Magnesium may be more effective for migraine with aura or menstrual migraine [92]. The AAN/AHS gave magnesium citrate an evidence grade level of B, which means that the therapy is probably effective and should be offered for migraine prevention.

Riboflavin or vitamin B2 400 mg by mouth daily decreased the number of migraines daily compared with placebo [108]. Another small RCT of 26 patients showed similar effects of riboflavin 400 mg once daily and metoprolol 200 mg once daily for migraine prophylaxis [109]. Riboflavin was also graded at level B evidence by AAN/AHS, and it should be offered in the prophylaxis of migraine. Coenzyme Q10 100 mg by mouth three times daily reduced migraine attacks compared to placebo in an RCT of 43 patients [110]. AAN/AHS graded coenzyme Q10 with evidence level C, meaning the therapy is possibly effective and should be considered for the prevention of migraine.

Feverfew (MIG-99 feverfew extract) 6.25 mg by mouth three times daily was graded at level B evidence by AAN/AHS in 2012. However, a more recent (2015) systematic review of 6 trials added some positive evidence to previously mixed and inconclusive results for the use of feverfew for migraine prevention. Feverfew was shown to significantly reduce the number of headache attacks per month when compared to placebo [111]. While more research is needed, there are already ample data and evidence-based guidelines to recommend the multiple modalities of established and safe CAM therapies for migraine prevention.

Clinical Case

Ms. LP is a 54-year-old noncombat veteran with a diagnosis of hypertension, asthma, sleep apnea, obesity, and migraine. She has had episodic migraines since her twenties, which have increased in the last few months to three to four times weekly. She is missing a few days of work per month. Her neurology work-up is insignificant, including brain imaging, and she uses her equipment for sleep apnea nightly. However, her job is relatively new, and she has only been sleeping 4–5 h per night due to stress. She has used a combination of butalbital, acetaminophen, and caffeine with some headache relief and takes metoprolol for hypertension, which has the adjunct benefit of being a conventional prophylaxis agent for migraine. Additionally, she has tried magnesium oxide 420 mg once daily for the last few months without much change to her migraine pattern.

During her next follow-up visit, Ms. LP was recommended to discontinue a combination of butalbital, acetaminophen, and caffeine as a rescue agent due to concerns for rebound headaches and dependency [112]. Instead, she was offered mindfulness meditation classes available at the VA. She was encouraged to keep a detailed headache diary, including information on sleep, diet, triggers, and specifics about the headache (e.g., length, severity). She was recommended to maintain a regular sleep pattern, which may improve her headaches. A trial of riboflavin

400 mg by mouth daily was offered. At her 3-month follow-up, she reports that after discontinuation of a rescue agent and addition of riboflavin, her headaches are greatly improved, occurring once per month or less.

Conclusion

Evidence-based CIH interventions offer a cost-effective nonpharmacologic approach to pain management. Because of the VHA Directive 1137, CIH interventions will become more and more accessible at every VA medical center either on-site or through community referrals. It is important for primary care and mental health providers to be aware of the safety and efficacy of these offerings. We recommend to always start with active self-management interventions and add other modalities (e.g., acupuncture, massage) later to achieve adequate pain control.

References

1. Toblin R, Quartana P, Riviere L, Walper K, Hoge C. Chronic pain and opioid use in US soldiers after combat deployment. JAMA Intern Med. 2014;174(8):1400–1.
2. Gironda R, Clark M, Massengale J, Walker R. Pain among veterans of Operations Enduring Freedom and Iraqi Freedom. Pain Med. 2006;7(4):339–43.
3. Bosco MA, Gallinati JL, Clark ME. Conceptualizing and treating comorbid chronic pain and PTSD. Pain Res Treat. 2013;2013:174728.
4. Gureje O, Von Korff M, Simon G, Gater R. Persistent pain and well-being: a World Health Organization study in primary care. JAMA. 1998;280(2):147–51.
5. Bosco M, Murphy J, Peters W, Clark M. Post-deployment multi-symptom disorder rehabilitation: an integrated approach to rehabilitation. Work. 2015;50(1):143–8.
6. Von Korff M, Dworkin S, Le Resche L, Kruger A. An epidemiologic comparison of pain complaints. Pain. 1988;32(2):173–83.
7. Gerrits M, van Oppen P, Leone S, van Marwijk H, van der Horst H, Penninx B. Pain, not chronic disease, is associated with the recurrence of depressive and anxiety disorders. BMC Psychiatry. 2014;14(187):1–9.
8. Davis M, Lin L, Liu H, Sites B. Prescription opioid use among adults with mental health disorders in the United States. J Am Board Fam Med. 2017;30(4):407–14.
9. Han B, Compton W, Blanco C, Crane E, Lee J, Jones C. Prescription opioid use, misuse, and use disorders in U.S. Adults: 2015 National Survey on Drug Use and Health. Ann Intern Med. 2017;167:293–301.
10. The Comprehensive Addiction and Recovery Act of 2016 [Internet]. 2016 [cited February 27, 2018]. Available from: https://www.congress.gov/114/plaws/publ198/PLAW-114publ198.pdf.
11. Veterans Health Administration. VHA Directive 1137, Provision of Complementary and Integrative Health (CIH) [Internet]. 2017 [cited February 27, 2018]. Available from: https://www.va.gov/VHAPUbLICAtIons/ViewPublication.asp?pub_ID=5401.
12. Anheyer D, Haller H, Barth J, Lauche R, Dobos G, Cramer H. Mindfulness-based stress reduction for treating low back pain: a systematic review and meta-analysis. Ann Intern Med. 2017;166(11):799–807.
13. Hilton L, Hempel S, Ewing B, Apaydin E, Xenakis L, Newberry S, et al. Mindfulness meditation for chronic pain: systematic review and meta-analysis. Ann Behav Med. 2017;51(2):199–213.

14. Chiesa A, Serretti A. Mindfulness-based interventions for chronic pain: a systematic review of the evidence. J Altern Complement Med. 2011;17(1):83–93.
15. la Cour P, Petersen M. Effects of mindfulness meditation on chronic pain: a randomized controlled trial. Pain Med. 2015;16(4):641–52.
16. Garland E, Thomas E, Howard M. Mindfulness-oriented recovery enhancement ameliorates the impact of pain on self-reported psychological and physical function among opioid-using chronic pain patients. J Pain Symptom Manag. 2014;48(6):1091–9.
17. Garland E. Disrupting the downward spiral of chronic pain and opioid addiction with mindfulness-oriented recovery enhancement: a review of clinical outcomes and neurocognitive targets. J Pain Palliat Care Pharmacother. 2014;28(2):122–9.
18. Gard T, Hölzel BK, Sack AT, Hempel H, Lazar SW, Vaitl D, et al. Pain attenuation through mindfulness is associated with decreased cognitive control and increased sensory processing in the brain. Cereb Cortex. 2011;22(11):2692–702.
19. Zeidan F, Grant J, Brown C, McHaffie J, Coghill R. Mindfulness meditation-related pain relief: evidence for unique brain mechanisms in the regulation of pain. Neurosci Lett. 2012;520(2):165–73.
20. Garland E, Froeliger B, Howard M. Mindfulness training targets neurocognitive mechanisms of addiction at the attention-appraisal-emotion interface. Front Psych. 2014;4:173.
21. Sorbero M, Ahluwalia C, Reynolds K, Lovejoy S, Farris C, Sloan J, et al. Meditation for depression: a systematic review of mindfulness-based cognitive therapy for major depressive disorder. Santa Monica: RAND Corporation; 2015.
22. de Souza I, de Barros V, Gomide H, Miranda T, Menezes V, Kozasa E, et al. Mindfulness-based interventions for the treatment of smoking: a systematic literature review. J Altern Complement Med. 2015;21(3):129–40.
23. Polusny M, Erbes C, Thuras P, Moran A, Lamberty G, Collins R, et al. Mindfulness-based stress reduction for posttraumatic stress disorder among veterans: a randomized clinical trial. JAMA. 2015;314(5):456–65.
24. Grant S, Hempel S, Cplaiaco B, Motala A, Shanman R, Booth M, et al. Mindfulness-based relapse prevention for substance use disorders: a systematic review [Internet]. 2015 Available from: http://www.rand.org/pubs/research_reports/RR1031.html.
25. Winbush N, Gross C, Kreitzer M. The effects of mindfulness-based stress reduction on sleep disturbance: a systematic review. Explore (NY). 2007;3(6):585–91.
26. Sielski R, Rief W, Glombiewski J. Efficacy of biofeedback in chronic back pain: a meta-analysis. Int J Behav Med. 2017;24(1):25–41.
27. Qaseem A, Wilt T, McLean R, Forciea M. Noninvasive treatments for acute, subacute, and chronic low back pain: a clinical practice guideline from the American College of Physicians. Ann Intern Med. 2017;166(7):514–30.
28. Chou R, Deyo R, Friedly J, et al. Nonpharmacological therapies for low back pain: a systematic review for an American College of Physicians clinical practice guideline. Ann Intern Med. 2017;166:493–505.
29. Nestoriuc Y, Rief W, Martin A. Meta-analysis of biofeedback for tension-type headache: efficacy, specificity, and treatment moderators. J Consult Clin Psychol. 2008;76(3):379–96.
30. Glombiewski J, Bernardy K, Häuser W. Efficacy of EMG- and EEG-Biofeedback in Fibromyalgia Syndrome: a meta-analysis and a systematic review of randomized controlled trials. Evid Based Complement Alternat Med. 2013;2013:962741.
31. Chou R, Deyo R, Friedly J, Skelly A, Hashimoto R, Weimer M, et al. Prepared by the Pacific Northwest Evidence-based Practice Center under Contract No. 290-2012-00014-I. AHRQ Publication No. 16-EHC004-EF., editor. Noninvasive Treatments for Low Back Pain. Comparative Effectiveness Review No. 169. Agency for Healthcare Research and Quality: Rockville; 2016.
32. Wieland L, Skoetz N, Pilkington K, Vempati R, D'Adamo C, Berman B. Yoga treatment for chronic non-specific low back pain. Cochrane Database Syst Rev. 2017;1:10.

33. Ward L, Stebbings S, Cherkin D, Baxter G. Yoga for functional ability, pain and psychosocial outcomes in musculoskeletal conditions: a systematic review and meta-analysis. Musculoskeletal Care. 2013;11(4):203–17.
34. Kan L, Zhang J, Yang Y, Wang P. The effects of yoga on pain, mobility, and quality of life in patients with knee osteoarthritis: a systematic review. Evid Based Complement Alternat Med. 2016;2016:6016532.
35. Kim S. Effects of yoga on chronic neck pain: a systematic review of randomized controlled trials. J Phys Ther Sci. 2016;28(7):2171–4.
36. Büssing A, Ostermann T, Lüdtke R, Michalsen A. Effects of yoga interventions on pain and pain-associated disability: a meta-analysis. J Pain. 2012;13(1):1–9.
37. Langhorst J, Klose P, Dobos G, Bernardy K, Häuser W. Efficacy and safety of meditative movement therapies in fibromyalgia syndrome: a systematic review and meta-analysis of randomized controlled trials. Rheumatol Int. 2013;33(1):193–207.
38. Saper R, Lemaster C, Delitto A, Sherman K, Herman P, Sadikova E, et al. Yoga, physical therapy, or education for chronic low back pain: a randomized noninferiority trial. Ann Intern Med. 2017;167(2):85–94.
39. Cramer H, Ward L, Saper R, Fishbein D, Dobos G, Lauche R. The safety of yoga: a systematic review and meta-analysis of randomized controlled trials. Am J Epidemiology. 2015;182(4):281–93.
40. Cramer H, Lauche R, Langhorst J, Dobos G. Is one yoga style better than another? A systematic review of associations of yoga style and conclusions in randomized yoga trials. Complement Ther Med. 2016;25:178–87.
41. Hall A, Copsey B, Richmond H, Thompson J, Ferreira M, Latimer J, et al. Effectiveness of tai chi for chronic musculoskeletal pain conditions: updated systematic review and meta-analysis. Phys Ther. 2017;97(2):227–38.
42. Kong L, Lauche R, Klose P, Bu J, Yang X, Guo C, et al. Tai chi for chronic pain conditions: a systematic review and meta-analysis of randomized controlled trials. Sci Rep. 2016;6:25325.
43. Wayne P, Berkowitz D, Litrownik D, Buring J, Yeh G. What do we really know about the safety of tai chi: a systematic review of adverse event reports in randomized trials. Arch Phys Med Relabel. 2014;95(12):2470–83.
44. Vickers A, Cronin A, Maschino A, Lewith G, MacPherson H, Foster N, et al. Acupuncture for chronic pain: individual patient data meta-analysis. Arch Intern Med. 2012;172(19):1444–53.
45. Vickers A, Linde K. Acupuncture for chronic pain. JAMA. 2014;311(9):955–6.
46. MacPherson H, Vertosick E, Foster N, Lewith G, Linde K, Sherman K, et al. The persistence of the effects of acupuncture after a course of treatment: a meta-analysis of patients with chronic pain. Pain. 2017;158(5):784–93.
47. Linde K, Allais G, Brinkhaus B, Fei Y, Mehring M, Vertosick E, et al. Acupuncture for the prevention of episodic migraine. Cochrane Database Syst Rev. 2016;10.
48. Linde K, Allais G, Brinkhaus B, Fei Y, Mehring M, Shin B, et al. Acupuncture for the prevention of tension-type headache. Cochrane Database Syst Rev. 2016;4:CD007587.
49. Zhao L, Guo Y, Wang W, Yan LJ. Systematic review on randomized controlled clinical trials of acupuncture therapy for neurovascular headache. Chin J Integr Med. 2011;17(8):580–6.
50. Sun Y, Gan T. Acupuncture for the management of chronic headache: a systematic review. Anesth Analg. 2008;107(6):2038–47.
51. Trinh K, Graham N, Irnich D, Cameron I, Forget M. Acupuncture for neck disorders. Cochrane Database Syst Rev. 2016 4;(5):CD004870.
52. Lam M, Galvin R, Curry P. Effectiveness of acupuncture for nonspecific chronic low back pain: a systematic review and meta-analysis. Spine (Phila Pa 1976). 1976;38(24):2124–38.
53. Cao L, Zhang X, Gao Y, Jiang Y. Needle acupuncture for osteoarthritis of the knee. A systematic review and updated meta-analysis. Saudi Med J. 2012;33(5):526–32.
54. Lin X, Huang K, Zhu G, Huang Z, Qin A, Fan S. The effects of acupuncture on chronic knee pain due to osteoarthritis: a meta-analysis. J Bone Joint Surg Am. 2016;98(18):1578–85.
55. Manheimer E, Cheng K, Linde K, Lao L, Yoo J, Wieland S, et al. Acupuncture for peripheral joint osteoarthritis. Cochrane Database Syst Rev. 2010 20;(1):CD001977.

56. MacPherson H, Thomas K, Walters S, Fitter M. A prospective survey of adverse events and treatment reactions following 34,000 consultations with professional acupuncturists. Acupunct Med. 2001;19(2):93–102.
57. Bergqvist D. Vascular injuries caused by acupuncture. A systematic review. Int Angiol. 2013;32(1):1–8.
58. Ernst E, White A. Prospective studies of the safety of acupuncture: a systematic review. Am J Med. 2001;110(6):481–5.
59. Yamashita H, Tsukayama H, White A, Tanno Y, Sugishita C, Ernst E. Systematic review of adverse events following acupuncture: the Japanese literature. Complement Ther Med. 2001;9(2):98–104.
60. White A. A cumulative review of the range and incidence of significant adverse events associated with acupuncture. Acupunct Med. 2004;22(3):122–33.
61. Yamashita H, Tsukayama H. Safety of acupuncture practice in Japan: patient reactions, therapist negligence and error reduction strategies. Evid Based Complement Alternat Med. 2008;5(4):391–8.
62. MacPherson H, Thomas K. Short term reactions to acupuncture--a cross-sectional survey of patient reports. Acupunct Med. 2005;23(3):112–20.
63. Bervoets D, Luijsterburg P, Alessie J, Buijs M, Verhagen A. Massage therapy has short-term benefits for people with common musculoskeletal disorders compared to no treatment: a systematic review. J Physiother. 2015;61(3):106–16.
64. Furlan A, Giraldo M, Baskwill A, Irvin E, Imamura M. Massage for low-back pain. Cochrane Database Syst Rev. 2015 1;(9):CD001929.
65. Nahin R, Boineau R, Khalsa P, Stussman B, Weber W. Evidence-based evaluation of complementary health approaches for pain management in the United States. Mayo Clin Proc. 2016;91(9):1292–306.
66. Clauw D. Fibromyalgia: a clinical review. JAMA. 2014;311(15):1547–55.
67. Wolfe F, Clauw D, Fitzcharles M, Goldenberg D, Katz R, Mease P, et al. The American College of Rheumatology preliminary diagnostic criteria for fibromyalgia and measurement of symptom severity. Arthritis Care Res (Hoboken). 2010;62(5):600–10.
68. Berger A, Sadosky A, Dukes E, Edelsberg J, Zlateva G, Oster G. Patterns of healthcare utilization and cost in patients with newly diagnosed fibromyalgia. Am J Manag Care. 2010;16(5 Suppl):S126–37.
69. Palstam A, Mannerkorpi K. Work ability in fibromyalgia: an update in the 21st Century. Curr Rheumatol Rev. 2017;13(3):180–7.
70. Vincent A, Lahr B, Wolfe F, Clauw D, Whipple M, Oh T, et al. Prevalence of fibromyalgia: a population-based study in Olmsted County, Minnesota, utilizing the Rochester Epidemiology Project. Arthritis Care Res (Hoboken). 2013;65(5):786–92.
71. Marques A, Santo A, Berssaneti A, Matsutani L, Yuan S. Prevalence of fibromyalgia: literature review update. Rev Bras Reumatol Engl Ed. 2017;57(4):356–63.
72. Higgins D, Fenton B, Driscoll M, Heapy A, Kerns R, Bair M, et al. Gender differences in demographic and clinical correlates among veterans with musculoskeletal disorders. Womens Health Issues. 2017;27(4):463–70.
73. Macfarlane G, Kronisch C, Dean L, Atzeni F, Häuser W, Flu E, et al. EULAR revised recommendations for the management of fibromyalgia. Ann Rheum Dis. 2017;76(2):318–28.
74. Ablin J, Fitzcharles M, Buskila D, Shir Y, Sommer C, Häuser W. Treatment of fibromyalgia syndrome: recommendations of recent evidence-based interdisciplinary guidelines with special emphasis on complementary and alternative therapies. Evid Based Complement Alternat Med. 2013;2013:485272.
75. Häuser W, Ablin J, Perrot S, Fitzcharles M. Management of fibromyalgia: practical guides from recent evidence-based guidelines. Pol Arch Intern Med. 2017;127(1):47–56.
76. Nüesch E, Häuser W, Bernardy K, Barth J, Jüni P. Comparative efficacy of pharmacological and non-pharmacological interventions in fibromyalgia syndrome: network meta-analysis. Ann Rheum Dis. 2013;72(6):955–62.

77. Häuser W, Perrot S, Clauw D, Fitzcharles M. Unravelling fibromyalgia-steps toward individualized management. J Pain. 2018;19(2):125–34.
78. Pioro-Boisset M, Esdaile J, Fitzcharles M. Alternative medicine use in fibromyalgia syndrome. Arthritis Care Res. 1996;9(1):13–7.
79. Lauche R, Cramer H, Häuser W, Dobos G, Langhorst J. A systematic overview of reviews for complementary and alternative therapies in the treatment of the fibromyalgia syndrome. Evid Based Complement Alternat Med. 2015;2015:610615.
80. Perry R, Leach V, Davies P, Penfold C, Ness A, Churchill R. An overview of systematic reviews of complementary and alternative therapies for fibromyalgia using both AMSTAR and ROBIS as quality assessment tools. Syst Rev. 2017;6(1):97.
81. Sawynok J, Lynch ME. Qigong and fibromyalgia circa 2017. Medicines (Basel). 2017;4(2):E37
82. Zech N, Hansen E, Bernardy K, Häuser W. Efficacy, acceptability and safety of guided imagery/hypnosis in fibromyalgia - A systematic review and meta-analysis of randomized controlled trials. Eur J Pain. 2017;21(2):217–27.
83. Deare J, Zheng Z, Xue C, et al. Acupuncture for treating fibromyalgia. Cochrane Database of Syst Rev. 2013;(5):CD007070.
84. Vas J, Santos-Rey K, Navarro-Pablo R, Modesto M, Aguilar I, Campos M, et al. Acupuncture for fibromyalgia in primary care: a randomised controlled trial. Acupunct Med. 2016;34(4):257–66.
85. Bennett R, Jones J, Turk D, Russell I, Matallana L. An internet survey of 2,596 people with fibromyalgia. BMC Musculoskelet Disord. 2007;8:27.
86. Bidonde J, Busch A, Webber S, et al. Aquatic exercise training for fibromyalgia. Cochrane Database Syst Rev. 2014;(10):CD011336.
87. Langhorst J, Musial F, Klose P, Häuser W. Efficacy of hydrotherapy in fibromyalgia syndrome--a meta-analysis of randomized controlled clinical trials. Rheumatology (Oxford). 2009;48(9):1155–9.
88. Naumann J, Sadaghiani C. Therapeutic benefit of balneotherapy and hydrotherapy in the management of fibromyalgia syndrome: a qualitative systematic review and meta-analysis of randomized controlled trials. Arthritis Res Ther. 2014;16(4):R141.
89. Headache C. The International Classification of Headache Disorders, 3rd edition (beta version). Cephalalgia. 2013;33(9):629–808.
90. Afari N, Harder L, Madra N, Heppner P, Moeller-Bertram T, King C, et al. PTSD, combat injury, and headache in Veterans Returning from Iraq/Afghanistan. Headache. 2009;49(9):1267–76.
91. Living with Migraine | American Migraine Foundation [Internet]. 2018 [cited 3/11/2018]. Available from: https://americanmigrainefoundation.org/living-with-migraines/.
92. Wells R, Baute V, Wahbeh H. Complementary and integrative medicine for neurologic conditions. Med Clin North Am. 2017;101(5):881–93.
93. Zhang Y, Dennis J, Leach M, Bishop F, Cramer H, Chung V, et al. Complementary and alternative medicine use among US adults with headache or migraine: results from the 2012 National Health Interview Survey. Headache. 2017;57(8):1228–42.
94. Sun-Edelstein C, Mauskop A. Foods and supplements in the management of migraine headaches. Clin J Pain. 2009;25(5):446–52.
95. Koseoglu E, Yetkin M, Ugur F, Bilgen M. The role of exercise in migraine treatment. J Sports Med Phys Fitness. 2015;55(9):1029–36.
96. Hanssen H, Minghetti A, Magon S, Rossmeissl A, Papadopoulou A, Klenk C, et al. Superior effects of high-intensity interval training vs. moderate continuous training on arterial stiffness in episodic migraine: a randomized controlled trial. Front Physiol. 2017;8:1086.
97. Hanssen H, Minghetti A, Magon S, Rossmeissl A, Rasenack M, Papadopoulou A, et al. Effects of different endurance exercise modalities on migraine days and cerebrovascular health in episodic migraineurs: a randomized controlled trial. Scand J Med Sci Sports. 2018;28(3):1103–12.
98. Bunner A, Agarwal U, Gonzales J, Valente F, Barnard N. Nutrition intervention for migraine: a randomized crossover trial. J Headache Pain. 2014;15:69.

99. Bruni O, Galli F, Guidetti V. Sleep hygiene and migraine in children and adolescents. Cephalalgia. 1999;25:57–9.
100. Grazzi L, Sansone E, Raggi A, D'Amico D, De G, Leonardi M, et al. Mindfulness and pharmacological prophylaxis after withdrawal from medication overuse in patients with Chronic Migraine: an effectiveness trial with a one-year follow-up. J Headache Pain. 2017;18(1):15.
101. Wells R, Burch R, Paulsen R, Wayne P, Houle T, Loder E. Meditation for migraines: a pilot randomized controlled trial. Headache. 2014;54(9):1484–95.
102. John P, Sharma N, Sharma C, Kankane A. Effectiveness of yoga therapy in the treatment of migraine without aura: a randomized controlled trial. Headache. 2007;47(5):654–61.
103. Nestoriuc Y, Martin A. Efficacy of biofeedback for migraine: a meta-analysis. Pain. 2007;128(1–2):111–27.
104. Harris P, Loveman E, Clegg A, Easton S, Berry N. Systematic review of cognitive behavioural therapy for the management of headaches and migraines in adults. Br J Pain. 2015;9(4):213–24.
105. Lawler S, Cameron L. A randomized, controlled trial of massage therapy as a treatment for migraine. Ann Behav Med. 2006;32(1):50–9.
106. Holland S, Silberstein S, Freitag F, Dodick D, Argoff C, Ashman E. Evidence-based guideline update: NSAIDs and other complementary treatments for episodic migraine prevention in adults: report of the Quality Standards Subcommittee of the American Academy of Neurology and the American Headache Society. Neurology. 2012;78(17):1346–53.
107. Peikert A, Wilimzig C, Köhne-Volland R. Prophylaxis of migraine with oral magnesium: results from a prospective, multi-center, placebo-controlled and double-blind randomized study. Cephalalgia. 1996;16(4):257–63.
108. Schoenen J, Jacquy J, Lenaerts M. Effectiveness of high-dose riboflavin in migraine prophylaxis. A randomized controlled trial. Neurology. 1998;50(2):466–70.
109. Sándor P, Afra J, Ambrosini A, Schoenen J. Prophylactic treatment of migraine with beta-blockers and riboflavin: differential effects on the intensity dependence of auditory evoked cortical potentials. Headache. 2000;40(1):30–5.
110. Sándor P, Di C, Coppola G, Saenger U, Fumal A, Magis D, et al. Efficacy of coenzyme Q10 in migraine prophylaxis: a randomized controlled trial. Neurology. 2005;64(4):713–5.
111. Wider B, Pittler M, Ernst E. Feverfew for preventing migraine. Cochrane Database Syst Rev. 2015;4:CD002286.
112. Feeney R. Medication overuse headache due to Butalbital, Acetaminophen, and Caffeine Tablets. J Pain Palliat Care Pharmacother. 2016;30(2):148–9.

Traumatic Brain Injury

14

Blessen C. Eapen and Bruno Subbarao

Overview of TBI in the Military/Veterans

Traumatic brain injuries (TBIs) within the military are considered one of the "signature injuries" of the recent US military conflicts in the Middle East including Operation Enduring Freedom/Operation Iraqi Freedom and Operation New Dawn (OEF/OIF/OND) [1]. Given the advancements in protective armor and battlefield medicine, many service members are surviving their injuries when compared to previous combat operations. These war heroes may return stateside with polytraumatic injuries. Polytrauma is defined by the Department of Veterans Affairs (VA) as TBI plus "two or more injuries, one of which may be life threatening, sustained in the same incident that affect multiple body parts or organ systems and result in physical, cognitive, psychological, or psychosocial impairments and functional disabilities [2]." TBI can co-occur in this unique population along with pain, amputations, spinal cord injury, burns, visual disturbances, and other psychological conditions such as anxiety, depression, and posttraumatic stress disorder (PTSD), thus making this complex polymorbid population a challenge to treat.

B. C. Eapen (✉)
Chief, Physical Medicine and Rehabilitation, VA Greater Los Angeles Health Care System, Associate Professor, David Geffen School of Medicine
at UCLA, Los Angeles, CA, USA
e-mail: blessen.eapen2@va.gov

B. Subbarao
Medical Director, Polytrauma/Transition and Care Management Programs, Phoenix Veterans Healthcare System, Physical Medicine and Rehabilitation, Phoenix, AZ, USA

© Springer Nature Switzerland AG 2019
E. C. Ritchie, M. D. Llorente (eds.), *Veteran Psychiatry in the US*,
https://doi.org/10.1007/978-3-030-05384-0_14

Definition of TBI

The Veterans Affairs/Department of Defense (VA/DoD) defines TBI as a "traumatically induced structural injury and/or physiological disruption of brain function as a result of an external force and is indicated by new onset or worsening of at least one of the following clinical signs immediately following event: any period of loss of or decreased level of consciousness; any loss of memory for events immediately before or after the injury; any alteration in mental state at the time of the injury (confusion, disorientation, slowed thinking, etc.); neurological deficits (weakness, loss of balance, change in vision, praxis, paresis/plegia, sensory loss, aphasia, etc.) that may or may not be transient; [an] intracranial lesion [3] Table 14.1."

It is important to note that while external forces include any object striking the head or vice versa, it also encompasses penetrating injury, blast forces, and acceleration/deceleration movement without direct external trauma. Furthermore, the event itself without manifestation of altered consciousness, altered mentation, memory loss, or the aforementioned clinical signs does not constitute a TBI [3].

There are significant challenges associated with diagnosing TBI retrospectively, as often is the case when service members return from deployment and screen positive as a veteran. The diagnosis is usually based solely on the veterans' recollection of events, sometimes occurring many years ago. Highlighting these difficulties is one 2012 study that demonstrated that service members who reported loss of consciousness with their mild TBI were significantly less likely to have abnormal neuroimaging than those who suffered a mild TBI and did not report loss of consciousness [4].

Another concern in correctly establishing a diagnosis is the difficulty in teasing out whether alteration of consciousness occurred as a result of the physical or psychological trauma. Furthermore, the high prevalence of PTSD in the military population, as well as the overlapping nature of symptomatology with TBI, also hinders the ability to establish a firm diagnosis.

Table 14.1 TBI severity grading

	Mild	Moderate	Severe
Loss of consciousness	0–30 min	30 min–24 h	>24 h
Alteration of consciousness	Up to 24 h	>24 h	>24 h
Posttraumatic amnesia	0–1 day	1–7 days	>1 week
Structural imaging	Normal	Normal or abnormal	Normal or abnormal

Adapted from the VA/DoD Clinical Practice Guidelines 2016

Epidemiology with Causes of TBI Including Blast Wave Physics

The Defense and Veterans Brain Injury Center (DVBIC) reports that since the year 2000, there have been 379,519 service members worldwide who have received a first-time diagnosis of traumatic brain injury, 82.3% of which were graded as mild (Fig. 14.1).

Explosions during OEF/OIF were responsible for 78% of the injuries suffered, accenting the importance of research into blast wave physics and the brain [5]. Blast waves are a unique phenomenon that can lead to brain injury through four distinct mechanisms. The primary mechanism is through direct effect of the blast wave itself on the vasculature and soft tissue components of the brain. The secondary aspect involves the debris that is launched through the air as a result of the blast and includes rocks, shrapnel, or any other projectile that may result in blunt or penetrating injury. The tertiary mechanism involves the force of the blast throwing the entire individual against a blunt object, the ground, or a wall, for example. Lastly, the quaternary effect of a blast relates to the inhalation injuries, burns, and/or potential toxic exposures that compound the traumatic nature of this event [6].

The primary mechanism of injury through blast wave exposure deserves special mention as debate exists as to the underlying physics of the event. Two leading hypotheses are as follows: (1) the blast wave itself is transmitted through intracranial structures resulting in direct deformation closely resembling acceleration-deceleration-type injurious motion [7]. (2) The blast wave impacts the torso, pressurizing the underlying vasculature and large cavities resulting in oscillations of the fluid within. These oscillations carry with them the kinetic energy of the blast wave to the intracranial structures, thus culminating in injury and initiation of the inflammatory cascade [8].

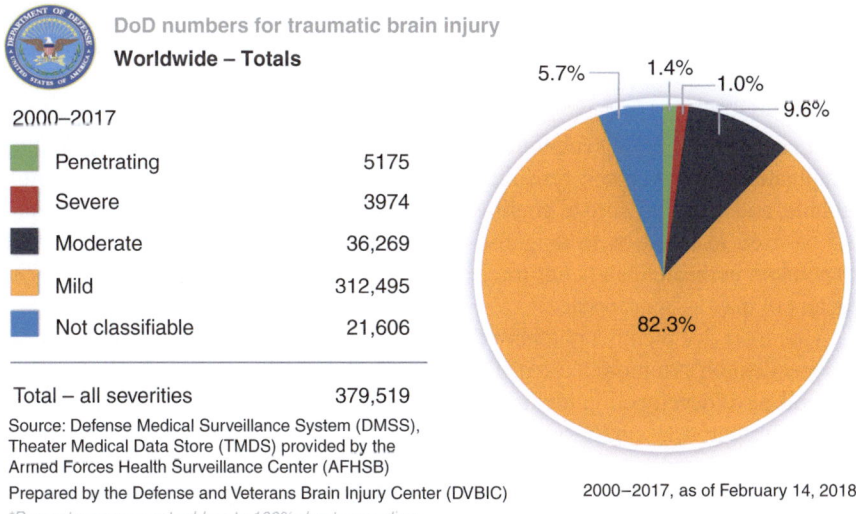

Fig. 14.1 Total number of Department of Defense traumatic brain injuries reported by the Defense and Veterans Brain Injury Centers (DVBIC). (Reprinted with permission from public domain: http://dvbic.dcoe.mil/)

The mechanisms for injury in blunt head trauma are more straightforward. Acceleration-deceleration motion within the skull affects the brain itself as its motion within the skull is independent from the more rigid structures. Beyond the direct distortion of the brain through translational forces, this motion can cause a coup-contrecoup injury, in which the brain impacts one side of the skull and bounces backward, impacting the opposite side as well. Ultimately, contusions and swelling may result at polar ends of the brain [9]. A second mechanism is that of rotational acceleration. Rotational acceleration can cause damage secondary to the shearing forces on tissues of different densities within the brain. These shearing forces cause what is known as diffuse axonal injury (DAI), or, in other words, widespread injury to the white matter tracts, and are hypothesized as the cause of persistent deficits in mild TBI [10, 11].

Initial In-Theater Evaluation and Management of Mild TBI

As mentioned previously, objective identification of mild traumatic brain injuries is difficult, as symptoms may resolve quickly, there may be entangling of psychological trauma, and there is yet to be a worldwide standard for diagnosis. Within the VA/DoD system, diagnosis is made by identifying loss of consciousness, alterations of consciousness, or posttraumatic amnesia due to disruption of brain function secondary to external forces.

To further aid in diagnosis, some federal agencies have opted to mandate predeployment testing utilizing the Automated Neuropsychological Assessment Metric (ANAM). The ANAM is a battery of neurocognitive tests that help establish a baseline predeployment and can identify decline in the postdeployment setting [12].

Once in theater, a screening for potential concussion after an inciting event is through the use of the Military Acute Concussion Evaluation (MACE). The MACE test is a measure developed by the Defense and Veterans Brain Injury Center (DVBIC) in 2006. The MACE is designed to help obtain a detailed history of the event and identify acute symptomatology through history and brief neurocognitive examinations. Independent research has shown that the MACE exam is a useful, reliable, and valid measure of cognitive dysfunction after mild TBI, although it cannot be used in isolation to diagnose concussion [13]. Through this method, first responders in theater can better triage those with suspected brain injuries to higher centers of care as appropriate.

After a service member obtains a diagnosis of concussion, their recovery process is dependent on symptom burden. The DVBIC and the Office of the Army Surgeon General have developed guidelines for return to activity in the military setting. A step-wise approach, similar to that seen in return-to-play guidelines in the sports world, is advocated.

Service members are progressed through six different stages of activity, the first of which is a 24-h mandatory rest period. Additional time for recovery may be warranted but is determined through clinical examination and symptomatology. Of note, if this is a service member's first concussion, and symptoms resolve within 24 h, exertional testing may be trialed without having to undergo the six steps for full return to activity. Individuals could conceivably return to activity afterward if they successfully remain asymptomatic.

A second concussion obtained within a year of the first automatically mandates a rest period of 1 week after resolution of symptoms. A third concussion within 1 year necessitates a full neurological examination, including neuroimaging, a functional assessment, and neuropsychological testing.

Progression within the return-to-activity guidelines involves daily subjective scoring through the Neurobehavioral Symptom Inventory (NSI), which helps elicit severity of physical and cognitive symptom burden perceived after TBI, and Borg's Rate of Perceived Exertion (RPE), which quantifies the self-assessed perception of physical exertion exhibited by the service member. For objective measures, theoretical maximum heart rate (TMHR), calculated using 220 minus years of age, and blood pressure are tracked. A score of 2 or higher on the NSI for any symptom, resting heart rate of greater than 100, and resting blood pressure of greater than 140/90 mm Hg will warrant another 24 h at the service member's current stage [14]. Even with these activity guidelines, many service members return stateside with lingering effects of their TBI and other comorbid conditions.

Polytrauma System of Care

Assessment of all severities of brain injury is accomplished through the VA Polytrauma System of Care which is a tiered comprehensive network of rehabilitation care comprised of the Polytrauma Rehabilitation Centers (PRCs), Polytrauma Network Sites (PNSs), Polytrauma Support Clinic Teams (PSCTs), and Polytrauma Point of Contacts (PPOCs). There are five PRCs nationwide: San Antonio, Tampa, Palo Alto, Minneapolis, and Richmond [15]. The PRCs are regional hubs for clinical care, education, and research.

Colocated at each PRC are residential brain injury programs, robust outpatient programs, VA Amputee System of Care, VA Spinal Cord Injury Centers, and Assistive Technology Centers of Excellence. Each PRC is staffed with a full interdisciplinary team trained to handle these complex conditions, as well as a wide array of consultative services. Several of the inpatient beds are also dedicated for emerging consciousness programs, which are specifically designed to help service members with disorders of consciousness [16]. In addition, all of the PRCs are accredited by the Commission on Accreditation of Rehabilitation Facilities (CARF).

The Polytrauma Transitional Rehabilitation Programs are located at each of the PRCs and are designed as a residential rehabilitation program to monitor and optimize the ability of service members to live independently and successfully reintegrate into the community [17]. Residents typically continue physical, cognitive, and behavioral therapies in a subacute setting under 24-h supervision by licensed practical nurses. Other aspects of the program involve focus on living skills, home maintenance, shopping, food preparation, return to drive, money management, community social skills, and vocational training among other aspects of independent living [15].

PNS's are postacute outpatient sites containing both Commission on Accreditation of Rehabilitation Facilities (CARF) accredited inpatient facilities and outpatient facilities for medically stabilized service members. They are 23 PNSs sites which assist in coordinating care across all of the Veterans Integrated Service Networks (VISNs), which consist of regional PSCTs and PPOCs. PNSs can additionally help as a first-line triage facility for service members with polytrauma to determine the need for referral into a PRC or PTRP [18].

PSCTs continue the interdisciplinary approach to management but through outpatient facilities that help manage and monitor veterans with any long-term, chronic needs. Referrals stem from PNSs and PRCs as veterans continue to functionally improve. These centers can also refer back if they identify any new or worsening conditions that may be related to polytrauma or TBI.

Finally, PPOCs typically consist of social workers or case managers knowledgeable about the Polytrauma System of Care. Their roles are to assist with the monitoring of long-term needs in this patient population and to refer to higher levels of care when necessary. Direct treatment at PPOCs is generally limited in scope [19–21] (Fig. 14.2).

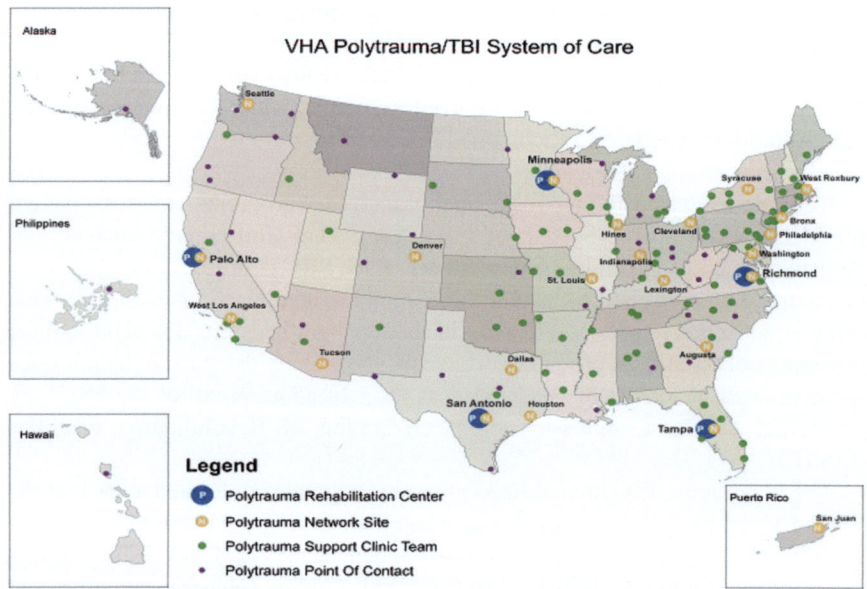

Fig. 14.2 Polytrauma System of Care locations. (Reprinted with permission from public domain: www.polytrauma.va.gov)

Assessment of TBI in the VA

In 2007, the VA has implemented a TBI screening measures for all veterans returning from the conflicts in Iraq and Afghanistan to identify and treat those with possible TBI, which may have gone unreported and untreated [22]. The initial screening consists of four questions assessing any exposure to an inciting event that could cause a TBI and the resultant symptoms that the veteran experienced and continues to experience [23] Table 14.2.

A positive screen results in the veteran undergoing a comprehensive VHA TBI evaluation (CTBIE) which includes full history and physical examination and history of TBI events with persistent sequelae, administration of the Neurobehavioral Symptom Inventory (NSI), and providing a diagnosis and treatment plan which is typically through the interdisciplinary polytrauma rehabilitation teams [24]. Since April 2007, over 1.1 million OEF/OIF/OND Veterans have been screened for possible mild traumatic brain injury (mTBI) with over 154,000 completed CTBIEs.

Table 14.2 VA/DoD TBI clinical reminder

Traumatic brain injury screening
The patient reports service in Operation Iraqi Freedom, Operation Enduring Freedom, Operation New Dawn, Operation Inherent Resolve or Operation Freedom's Sentinel.
Section 1: The veteran experienced the following events during OIF/OEF deployment:
Blast or explosion – IED (improvised explosive device), RPG (rocket-propelled grenade), land mine, grenade, etc.
Vehicular accident/crash (any vehicle, including aircraft)
Fragment wound or bullet wound above the shoulders
Fall
Section 2: The veteran had the following symptoms immediately afterwards:
Losing consciousness/"knocked out"
Being dazed, confused or "seeing stars"
Not remembering the event
Concussion
Head injury
Section 3: The veteran states the following problems began or got worse afterward:
Memory problems or lapses
Balance problems or dizziness
Sensitivity to bright light
Irritability
Headaches
Sleep problems
Section 4: The veteran relates he/she is currently having or has had the following symptoms within the past week:
Memory problems or lapses
Balance problems or dizziness
Sensitivity to bright light
Irritability
Headaches
Sleep problems

Table 14.3 Common symptoms of postconcussive syndrome

Potential symptomatology in postconcussive syndrome		
Physical	Cognitive	Behavioral
Headache	Impaired memory	Sleep disturbances
Sensory deficits	Attention/concentration deficits	Irritability and anger
Visual disturbances	Difficulty with executive functions	Anxiety
Nausea/vomiting	Impaired processing speeds	Depression
Balance problems	Impaired communication	Isolation
Phono/photophobia		
Tinnitus		

Postconcussive Symptoms

Postconcussive syndrome is an umbrella term used to describe any number of nonspecific symptoms occurring at a nonspecific time after a TBI and persisting beyond a nonspecific time frame for recovery [25]. Of note, the 5th international conference on concussion in sport held in Berlin recently proffered that normal recovery be defined as greater than 10–14 days in adults and greater than 4 weeks in children [26]. Regardless of timing, symptoms to be aware of include physical ailments such as headaches, sensory deficits, and balance problems; cognitive issues such as difficulty with attention and concentration, memory problems, and executive dysfunction; and emotional/behavioral difficulties such as sleep disturbances, depression, and anxiety.

Risk factors for persistent postconcussive syndrome include lower education, lower rank, female sex, secondary gain, and psychiatric comorbidities [27]. The single most effective strategy for treatment after mild traumatic brain injury has been found to be early education about concussion, potential symptoms and their management, and the natural expected course of recovery [28] Table 14.3.

Evaluation and Management of Common Symptoms After TBI

Posttraumatic Headache

With one of the highest incidences of any postconcussive symptom, and as the most common secondary headache disorder, posttraumatic headaches (PTH) should be screened for appropriately [29]. The International Classification of Headache Disorders version 3 criteria label PTH as a "headache attributed to trauma or injury to the head and/or neck." Although they admit the time frame is arbitrary, requirements for diagnosis remain a headache that develops within 1 week of the concussion, arousal from coma, or attainment of the ability to sense or report pain. PTH is termed "persistent PTH" when headaches continue for greater than 3 months [30]. In some individuals, PTH can continue for years, leading to a decrease in the quality of life and potential loss of work [31]. Risk factors for prolonged PTH include female gender, multiple TBIs, and premorbid migraine history [32].

There are no clinical characteristics that distinguish PTH from a primary headache, such as migraines. Treatment, therefore, follows the same principles as for the primary headache phenotype it most closely resembles in that individual. Some of the frequently encountered primary headache types are migraines, which present as unilateral and throbbing in nature, often time accompanied by an aura; cervicogenic headache, which stems from the cervical spine and is associated with neck pain and limited range of motion; tension-type headache, which is associated with stress and presents in a band-like fashion, described as tightness; and neuralgic headache, which occurs with irritation of the occipital nerves, producing pain distributed along the path of the nerves, and can often be reproduced through palpation [33].

Identifying triggers, optimizing sleep, limiting caffeine and alcohol intake, and reducing stress are all personal measures that a service member can focus on to help reduce the frequency of PTH [34, 35]. Consideration of ice, heat, physical therapy, acupuncture, and cognitive behavioral therapy is appropriate to lessen dependence on pharmaceuticals [36]. If headaches are unresponsive to environmental and behavioral modifications, the next consideration will be between medications and procedural interventions, depending on the headache type and frequency.

If medications are warranted, a decision between abortive and prophylactic treatment must be made. Prophylactic medications include beta-blockers, antidepressants, and antiepileptics and are used to reduce headache frequency to less than 10 per month [37]. Abortive therapies are used for breakthrough headache relief and include acetaminophen, nonsteroidal anti-inflammatory drugs, and triptans. A selection of a few common choices is listed in the table below.

Sleep Disturbances

Sleep disturbances are also highly prevalent after TBI and can disrupt or prolong natural recovery if not effectively addressed. Inadequate sleep quality has been implicated as an independent risk factor for persistent neurobehavioral conditions [38]. One study of veterans who had committed suicide highlighted that those with sleep disturbances were quicker to commit suicide than those veterans without sleep complaints, estimating a 57% loss of survival time [39].

Insomnia is one of the most common sleep disturbances encountered and has been reported to occur in 30–60% of individuals after a concussion [40]. It has been found to be associated with decreased quality of life, fatigue, pain, suicidal ideation, PTSD, and depression [41–43]. Other sleep disturbances encountered after TBI include hypersomnia, obstructive sleep apnea, periodic limb movement, and narcolepsy [44].

Ideally, this condition will respond to behavioral interventions, such that pharmacological treatments may not be needed. This entails that the provider obtains a good history that includes pre- and postinjury sleep habits, caffeine use, alcohol use, nicotine use, diet, exercise habits, current medications, comorbid conditions, mood, TV and cellphone habits, history of nightmares, and any other potential contributors to poor sleep in general.

The American College of Physicians (ACP) now recommend cognitive behavioral therapy for insomnia (CBT-I) as the first-line treatment [45]. In fact, a recent randomized controlled trial of 151 active duty army members found CBT-I to be effective in not only treating insomnia but also improving mental health, curbing caffeine and nicotine use, and reducing daytime fatigue [46]. Pharmaceutical options for when CBT-I is not available include melatonin and melatonin-receptor agonists, z-drugs (sedative/hypnotics), and medications within the antidepressant family.

Cognitive Dysfunction

Cognitive impairments can be seen in the immediate aftermath of concussion and may affect any cognitive domain, including processing speeds, attention, memory, and executive function [47]. Executive function is a term that describes the combined behavioral and cognitive functions, controlled through the prefrontal cortex, that is needed to accomplish higher order tasks by way of planning, adequate judgment, memory retrieval, and motivation [48]. When executive function is impaired, individuals are more likely to have disorganized memory encoding, such that they will conflate or misremember events [49, 50].

Generally, most individuals with cognitive complaints will report resolution within a 6-month period, although about 15% will describe persistent difficulties [51, 52]. In fact, this was further confirmed in one study comparing 902 service member's ANAM scores pre- and postdeployment for those reporting TBI vs no TBI. Seventy percent of those who suffered a TBI did not show a deviation from their predeployment baseline, and only those with active symptomatology and TBI were shown to be at highest risk for cognitive dysfunction [53].

Management should include a comprehensive history to assess other causes of cognitive clouding including alcohol and/or drug use, sleep disorders, mental health conditions, and medication side effects. After those conditions are addressed, referral for neuropsychological testing will assist in identifying the cognitive domains affected in service members with persistent impairments, thus helping guide efforts in cognitive rehabilitation.

Although research is divided at present in regard to the efficacy of cognitive rehabilitation, several small studies successfully demonstrated improvements in attention, processing speeds, memory, and executive dysfunction [48, 54–56]. Thus, it may be a worthwhile effort, as current pharmaceutical options carry with them a host of side effects. Methylphenidate, for instance, has been studied in the moderate to severe TBI population and has shown benefits in improving processing speed but has a side effect profile that includes emotional lability, aggression, headaches, insomnia, psychosis, arrhythmias, and a high potential for abuse and dependence [57–59].

Dizziness/Vestibular

Balance is achieved through coordination of the vestibular, visual, and proprioceptive systems chiefly through the brainstem. The vestibular system is composed of the semicircular canals, which recognize angular acceleration, and otolithic organs, which recognize linear acceleration [60]. Insult to these systems, by way of blunt or blast trauma to the head, can result in vertigo, dizziness, and/or postural instability and cause prolonged issues if more systems are involved, as is the case in polytrauma patients [61].

Initial assessment should involve a detailed history, to include onset, frequency, duration, characterization, worsening and alleviating factors, and associations to be able to target better appropriate treatments. The differential should initially remain broad and include orthostasis, vertigo, ataxia, benign paroxysmal positional vertigo (BPPV), Meniere's disease, and other causes of impaired balance. Additionally, a thorough review of medications is warranted as dizziness as a side effect is quite common with many drugs [35].

Management and treatment differ among the etiologies of dizziness. For example, a diagnosis of BPPV can be treated by repositioning maneuvers; a diagnosis of orthostasis with hydration, medication review, and salt tablets; or a diagnosis of peripheral or central vertigo with physical therapy and consideration of short-term vestibular suppressant medications [62]. Of special mention is vestibular physical therapy, which has shown efficacy in the treatment of unilateral peripheral vertigo and chronic Meniere's disease and significant symptom reduction in central vertigo [61].

Depression

There is an increased risk of suicide in military members that have suffered multiple TBIs, with one study reporting a three- to fourfold increase in risk as compared to the normal population [63, 64]. Screening for depression is essential as prevalence after TBI is high, estimated at about 30% [65]. In addition, emotional distress may lead to a heavier symptom burden in postconcussive syndrome if not effectively treated [19758488]. However, screening should occur at variable times even though prevalence is highest in the first year post-TBI, as lifetime risk is increased in general after TBI, and some studies demonstrate development of depressive symptoms in the second year and beyond [66].

Risk factors for depression after TBI have been postulated to include premorbid history of alcohol or substance abuse, premorbid depression, location of brain injury, and older age, but there is an overall lack of consistent data in this population [67–70]. Assessment of these depressive disorders under the *Diagnostic and Statistical Manual of Mental Disorders*, 5th Edition, may most appropriately be within the criteria for mood disorders due to another medical condition [American Psychiatric Association. (2013). *Diagnostic and statistical manual of mental disorders* (5th ed.)]. Utilization of psychiatric scales including the Beck Depression Inventory, Hamilton Depression Scale, and the Neurobehavioral Functioning Inventory Depression Scale has been found as valid and reliable options for assessment [66].

Nonpharmaceutical options such as psychotherapy and psychoeducation are preferred treatment methods in this population in order to avoid side effects carried by medications that may interfere with cognition or recovery. Unfortunately, a 2015 systematic review of cognitive and behavioral rehabilitation interventions only found limited support for these methods, but more research is certainly warranted and underway [48]. If treatment with medications is necessary, selective serotonin reuptake inhibitors (SSRIs) have been considered first-line treatment secondary to their generally favorable side effect profile [71]. However, many pharmaceutical options exist, and careful selection should be made to optimize benefits and limit side effects.

Posttraumatic Stress Disorder and TBI

Concurrent posttraumatic stress disorder (PTSD) with mild TBI is to be expected considering the context of military injuries [72]. Prevalence of PTSD among military service members and veterans with TBI spans anywhere from 12% to 89% [73]. Symptom burden is more severe in individuals with coexisting mild TBI and PTSD than those with PTSD alone, and unfortunately, there is significant overlap in experienced symptoms with both diagnoses, making it challenging to determine a best pathway for treatment [74]. Shared symptoms include depression, anxiety, sleep disturbances, emotional lability, and cognitive dysfunction [75].

Management for those suffering with PTSD and TBI is difficult, as research in this specialized population is limited and some treatments may be of benefit to one pathological entity while simultaneously a detriment to the other. For example, the use of benzodiazepines may help in the treatment of PTSD, but is relatively contraindicated in TBI, as studies have shown that benzodiazepines may hinder neuroplasticity [76]. Similarly, prescribing neurostimulants to help cognitive functioning in TBI patients may worsen anxiety and insomnia in PTSD.

Current strategies include the use of evidence-based psychotherapies to help not only treat PTSD but also to potentially disentangle which symptoms can be attributed to either diagnosis. Cognitive processing therapy and prolonged exposure therapy have shown promise in decreasing symptom burden in individuals with TBI and PTSD [77, 78]. The VA/DoD Clinical Practice Guidelines for PTSDs state if pharmaceutical management is needed, first-line medications for the treatment of PTSD include sertraline, paroxetine, fluoxetine, and venlafaxine, but close monitoring and judicious use are essential.

Lastly, and potentially most ideal, comprehensive treatment with an interdisciplinary team may help tackle the complexities of such patients, as was shown in a 2014 study of twenty-four veterans with PTSD and TBI. After an 8-week intervention, researchers found a reduction of overall symptom burden and improvements in quality of life and occupational performance [79].

Neurodegeneration/CTE in Veterans

Chronic traumatic encephalopathy (CTE) is an insidious, progressive neurodegenerative process that is hypothesized to occur secondary to sustaining repetitive traumatic brain injuries, as no evidence to date exists that a single TBI can lead to this diagnosis [80]. CTE is only diagnosed posthumously through autopsy [81]. At autopsy, neuropathologists observe a characteristic distribution of hyperphosphorylated tau protein distinct from other neurodegenerative processes, with a propensity to accumulate in the depths of the cerebral sulci in an irregular pattern [82, 83]. Of note, CTE has been described in individuals without history of concussion. Therefore, CTE is deemed a product of repetitive head injuries and subconcussive blows, but not necessarily concussions [84].

Clinical presentation is similar to that of persistent postconcussion syndrome and can include nonspecific symptoms from a vast array of domains. Behavioral symptoms like explosivity, impulsivity, and paranoia, cognitive symptoms like memory loss and impaired attention, and physical symptoms like headaches and dysarthria have all been described in this setting [85].

Most studies to date are in large part focused on sports athletes. However, in a 2012 study by Goldstein et al., a postmortem comparison of the neuropathology of four military veterans with a history of blast exposure and/or blunt concussion and four sports athletes with a history of blunt concussion was made and found to be remarkably similar. CTE-linked tau neuropathology was indistinguishable among the brains and deposited in the characteristic distribution pattern as would be expected with development of CTE. This study was indeed intriguing, although limited by the small sample size, inherent selection bias, inability to account for confounding factors, and difficulty establishing causality through postmortem analysis [86].

Although research is blossoming quickly to better understand this unique disease entity, at present there lacks large, longitudinal prospective studies to guide prevention, education, and management strategies, especially in the military population. Additionally, as diagnosis is only made at autopsy, controversy still exists as to how to identify this process in the living. As we await further research, a holistic approach and symptom-focused treatment remain the mainstay of management.

Pharmacology in Mild TBI

If physical therapies, psychotherapies, environmental and behavioral modifications, and education are insufficient in controlling persistent symptoms following mild TBI, pharmaceuticals may be indicated to provide relief. As previously alluded to in the antecedent sections, pharmacotherapy in the TBI population necessitates careful consideration as to not hinder recovery or cause additional complications secondary to side effects. In fact, many medications carry with them a side effect profile that resembles the symptoms experienced after a TBI. Thus, a medication review is warranted first and foremost, and optimization is advised prior to enlisting any new drug.

It is important to remember that, as with all medications, the approach should be to start low and go slow. Educate the patient as to the medication, the intended use, and potential side effects they may experience so they can alert their providers if issues arise. Be wary of polypharmacy, especially in a population with a multitude of symptomatology, and attempt to define an appropriate but finite length of time for the medication. Finally, in the TBI population, try to avoid or use extreme caution with any medication that may lower the seizure threshold [35] Table 14.4.

Table 14.4 Selection of common pharmaceutical options in the treatment of postconcussive syndrome

Medication	Classification	Dosage	Side effects	Notes
Headaches (abortive medications)				
Naproxen	Nonsteroidal anti-inflammatory drug	Initial: 750 mg PO as needed; max dose: 1250 mg/day	Abdominal pain, constipation, dizziness, headache, nausea, GI bleed, cardiovascular risk	
Acetaminophen	Analgesic	Initial: 325–650 mg PO as needed q4hours; max dose: 3250 mg/day	Dizziness, disorientation, rash, Stevens-Johnson syndrome, agranulocytosis	
Sumatriptan	Serotonin 5-HT-receptor agonist	Initial: 25 mg PO as needed; max dose: 200 mg/day	Paresthesias, dizziness, warm/hot sensation, chest pressure, diaphoresis	
Headaches (prophylactic medications)				
Amitriptyline	Tricyclic antidepressant	Initial: 10–25 mg PO daily	Headache, sedation, constipation, confusion	Anticholinergic effects, may worsen cognition
Topiramate	Antiepileptic	Titrate over 4 weeks to a dose of 50 mg PO BID	Decrease in serum bicarbonate, dizziness, fatigue, nausea, nervousness	
Propranolol	Beta-blocker	Initial: 80 mg/day PO	Bradycardia, hypotension, depression, fatigue, insomnia, nausea	Also effective in treating aggression and agitation
Depression				
Sertraline	SSRI	Initial: 50 mg PO daily	Decreased sex drive, diarrhea, nausea	SSRIs are generally considered first-line treatment
Amitriptyline	Tricyclic antidepressant	Initial: 25–50 mg PO daily	Headache, sedation, constipation, confusion	Anticholinergic effects, may worsen cognition
Venlafaxine	SNRI	Initial: 75 mg PO daily	Insomnia, hypertension, contraindicated in narrow-angle glaucoma	

Bupropion	Aminoketone	Initial: (immediate-release) 100 mg PO q12h	Headache, dry mouth, nausea, insomnia, agitation, dizziness	Lowers seizure threshold
Insomnia				
Melatonin	Pineal hormone	Initial: 5 mg PO 3–4 h before sleep	Daytime fatigue, dizziness, drowsiness, headache, irritability	Found to improve daytime alertness
Trazodone	Antidepressant	Initial: 50 mg/PO qDay	Blurred vision, dizziness, dry mouth, headache, nausea, constipation, QT prolongation	Concern for QT prolongation exists, but in general, medication is well tolerated
Zolpidem	Sedative/hypnotic	Initial: (immediate-release) 5 mg PO qHS	Should be avoided for long-term use in TBI. Dizziness, headache, hallucinations, memory disorder, visual disturbances	May impair cognitive recovery with long-term use
Cognitive impairments				
Methylphenidate	Stimulant	Initial: (immediate-release) 20 mg/day PO divided q12h, 30 min before meals	Headache, seizures, arrhythmia, psychosis, angina, tachycardia, agitation	Found to improve cognitive complaints and posttraumatic stress symptoms in a study of patients with PTSD, TBI, or both
Donepezil	Acetylcholinesterase inhibitor	Initial: 5 mg PO qHS	Nausea, diarrhea, insomnia, headache, hallucinations, confusion	Studies are only in moderate to severe TBI patients but demonstrate improvement in short-term memory
Amphetamine/dextroamphetamine	Stimulant	Initial: 5 mg PO qDay	Anorexia, headache, insomnia, anxiety, tachycardia, nausea, emotional lability, dizziness	Risk for substance abuse

Adapted from Bhatnagar et al. [37]

Conclusion

Mild traumatic brain injuries continue to be a highly prevalent and hotly researched topic, but much work still needs to be done to adequately assess and manage the service members afflicted. Education remains the most important and effective treatment, especially in the early stages of injury. Reassurance and support are enough for most as symptoms are expected to resolve in a short time. However, for those suffering with persistent postconcussive syndrome, a holistic approach and symptomatic treatment, first with nonpharmaceuticals, are ideal. A judicious and finite use of medications may be warranted for the few who require them.

References

1. Snell FI, Halter MJ. A signature wound of war: mild traumatic brain injury. J Psychosoc Nurs Ment Health Serv. 2010;48(2):22–8. https://doi.org/10.3928/02793695-20100107-01.
2. VHA Handbook 1172.01, Polytrauma System of Care - ViewPublication.asp. http://www.va.gov/vhapublications/ViewPublication.asp?pub_ID=2875. Accessed 2 April 2013.
3. Management of Concussion/mTBI Working Group. VA/DoD clinical practice guideline for management of concussion/mild traumatic brain injury. J Rehabil Res Dev. 2009;46(6):CP1–68.
4. Xydakis MS, Ling GSF, Mulligan LP, Olsen CH, Dorlac WC. Epidemiologic aspects of traumatic brain injury in acute combat casualties at a major military medical center: a cohort study. Ann Neurol. 2012;72(5):673–81. https://doi.org/10.1002/ana.23757.
5. Owens BD, Kragh JF, Wenke JC, Macaitis J, Wade CE, Holcomb JB. Combat wounds in operation Iraqi Freedom and operation Enduring Freedom. J Trauma. 2008;64(2):295–9. https://doi.org/10.1097/TA.0b013e318163b875.
6. Chandra N, Sundaramurthy A. Acute pathophysiology of blast injury—from biomechanics to experiments and computations: implications on head and polytrauma. In: Kobeissy FH, editor. Brain neurotrauma: molecular, neuropsychological, and rehabilitation aspects. Frontiers in Neuroengineering. Boca Raton: CRC Press/Taylor & Francis; 2015. http://www.ncbi.nlm.nih.gov/books/NBK299229/. Accessed 3 May 2018.
7. Magnuson J, Leonessa F, Ling GSF. Neuropathology of explosive blast traumatic brain injury. Curr Neurol Neurosci Rep. 2012;12(5):570–9. https://doi.org/10.1007/s11910-012-0303-6.
8. Cernak I, Noble-Haeusslein LJ. Traumatic brain injury: an overview of pathobiology with emphasis on military populations. J Cereb Blood Flow Metab. 2010;30(2):255–66. https://doi.org/10.1038/jcbfm.2009.203.
9. King AI. Fundamentals of impact biomechanics: part I--biomechanics of the head, neck, and thorax. Annu Rev Biomed Eng. 2000;2:55–81. https://doi.org/10.1146/annurev.bioeng.2.1.55.
10. Young L, Rule GT, Bocchieri RT, Walilko TJ, Burns JM, Ling G. When physics meets biology: low and high-velocity penetration, blunt impact, and blast injuries to the brain. Front Neurol. 2015;6:89. https://doi.org/10.3389/fneur.2015.00089.
11. Browne KD, Chen X-H, Meaney DF, Smith DH. Mild traumatic brain injury and diffuse axonal injury in swine. J Neurotrauma. 2011;28(9):1747–55. https://doi.org/10.1089/neu.2011.1913.
12. PubMed entry. http://www.ncbi.nlm.nih.gov/pubmed/22360064. Accessed 3 May 2018.
13. McCrea M, Guskiewicz K, Doncevic S, Helmick K, Kennedy J, Boyd C, Asmussen S, Ahn KW, Wang Y, Hoelzle J, Jaffee M. Day of injury cognitive performance on the military acute concussion evaluation (MACE) by U.S. military service members in OEF/OIF. Mil Med. 2014;179(9):990–7. https://doi.org/10.7205/MILMED-D-13-00349.
14. McCulloch KL, Goldman S, Lowe L, Radomski MV, Reynolds J, Shapiro R, West TA. Development of clinical recommendations for progressive return to activity after military

mild traumatic brain injury: guidance for rehabilitation providers. J Head Trauma Rehabil. 2015;30(1):56–67. https://doi.org/10.1097/HTR.0000000000000104.
15. Eapen BC, Jaramillo CA, Tapia RN, Johnson EJ, Cifu DX. Rehabilitation care of combat related TBI: veterans health administration polytrauma system of care. Curr Phys Med Rehabil Rep. 2013;1:151. https://doi.org/10.1007/s40141-013-0023-0.
16. Eapen BC. Emerging consciousness program. In: Kreutzer J, DeLuca J, Caplan B, editors. Encyclopedia of clinical neuropsychology. Cham: Springer International Publishing; 2017. p. 1–2. https://doi.org/10.1007/978-3-319-56782-2_9222-1.
17. Duchnick JJ, Ropacki S, Yutsis M, Petska K, Pawlowski C. Polytrauma transitional rehabilitation programs: comprehensive rehabilitation for community integration after brain injury. Psychol Serv. 2015;12(3):313–21. https://doi.org/10.1037/ser0000034.
18. Sigford BJ. "To care for him who shall have borne the battle and for his widow and his orphan" (Abraham Lincoln): the Department of Veterans Affairs polytrauma system of care. Arch Phys Med Rehabil. 2008;89(1):160–2. https://doi.org/10.1016/j.apmr.2007.09.015.
19. Evans CT, St Andre JR, Pape TL-B, Steiner ML, Stroupe KT, Hogan TP, Weaver FM, Smith BM. An evaluation of the veterans affairs traumatic brain injury screening process among operation enduring freedom and/or operation Iraqi freedom veterans. PM R. 2013;5(3):210–20.; quiz 220. https://doi.org/10.1016/j.pmrj.2012.12.004.
20. Mernoff ST, Correia S. Military blast injury in Iraq and Afghanistan: the veterans health administration's polytrauma system of care. Med Health R I. 2010;93(1):16–18, 21.
21. Belanger HG, Uomoto JM, Vanderploeg RD. The veterans health administration's (VHA's) polytrauma system of care for mild traumatic brain injury: costs, benefits, and controversies. J Head Trauma Rehabil. 2009;24(1):4–13. https://doi.org/10.1097/HTR.0b013e3181957032.
22. Vanderploeg RD, Groer S, Belanger HG. Initial developmental process of a VA semistructured clinical interview for TBI identification. J Rehabil Res Dev. 2012;49(4):545–56.
23. Belanger HG, Vanderploeg RD, Soble JR, Richardson M, Groer S. Validity of the veterans health administration's traumatic brain injury screen. Arch Phys Med Rehabil. 2012;93(7):1234–9. https://doi.org/10.1016/j.apmr.2012.03.003.
24. Belanger HG, Powell-Cope G, Spehar AM, McCranie M, Klanchar SA, Yoash-Gantz R, Kosasih JB, Scholten J. The veterans health administration's traumatic brain injury clinical reminder screen and evaluation: practice patterns. J Rehabil Res Dev. 2016;53(6):767–80. https://doi.org/10.1682/JRRD.2015.09.0187.
25. Leddy JJ, Baker JG, Willer B. Active rehabilitation of concussion and post-concussion syndrome. Phys Med Rehabil Clin N Am. 2016;27(2):437–54. https://doi.org/10.1016/j.pmr.2015.12.003.
26. McCrory P, Meeuwisse W, Dvořák J, Aubry M, Bailes J, Broglio S, Cantu RC, Cassidy D, Echemendia RJ, Castellani RJ, Davis GA, Ellenbogen R, Emery C, Engebretsen L, Feddermann-Demont N, Giza CC, Guskiewicz KM, Herring S, Iverson GL, Johnston KM, Kissick J, Kutcher J, Leddy JJ, Maddocks D, Makdissi M, Manley GT, McCrea M, Meehan WP, Nagahiro S, Patricios J, Putukian M, Schneider KJ, Sills A, Tator CH, Turner M, Vos PE. Consensus statement on concussion in sport-the 5th international conference on concussion in sport held in Berlin, October 2016. Br J Sports Med. 2017;51(11):838–47. https://doi.org/10.1136/bjsports-2017-097699.
27. Lange RT, Brickell TA, Kennedy JE, Bailie JM, Sills C, Asmussen S, Amador R, Dilay A, Ivins B, French LM. Factors influencing postconcussion and posttraumatic stress symptom reporting following military-related concurrent polytrauma and traumatic brain injury. Arch Clin Neuropsychol. 2014;29(4):329–47. https://doi.org/10.1093/arclin/acu013.
28. Ponsford J, Willmott C, Rothwell A, Cameron P, Kelly A-M, Nelms R, Curran C. Impact of early intervention on outcome following mild head injury in adults. J Neurol Neurosurg Psychiatry. 2002;73(3):330–2.
29. D'Onofrio F, Russo A, Conte F, Casucci G, Tessitore A, Tedeschi G. Post-traumatic headaches: an epidemiological overview. Neurol Sci. 2014;35(Suppl 1):203–6. https://doi.org/10.1007/s10072-014-1771-z.

30. Headache Classification Committee of the International Headache Society (IHS). The international classification of headache disorders, 3rd edition (beta version). Cephalalgia. 2013;33(9):629–808. https://doi.org/10.1177/0333102413485658.
31. Lucas S. Posttraumatic headache: clinical characterization and management. Curr Pain Headache Rep. 2015;19(10):48. https://doi.org/10.1007/s11916-015-0520-1.
32. Couch JR, Lipton RB, Stewart WF, Scher AI. Head or neck injury increases the risk of chronic daily headache: a population-based study. Neurology. 2007;69(11):1169–77. https://doi.org/10.1212/01.wnl.0000276985.07981.0a.
33. Brown AW, Watanabe TK, Hoffman JM, Bell KR, Lucas S, Dikmen S. Headache after traumatic brain injury: a national survey of clinical practices and treatment approaches. PM R. 2015;7(1):3–8. https://doi.org/10.1016/j.pmrj.2014.06.016.
34. Obermann M, Naegel S, Bosche B, Holle D. An update on the management of post-traumatic headache. Ther Adv Neurol Disord. 2015;8(6):311–5. https://doi.org/10.1177/1756285615605699.
35. Tapia RN, Eapen BC. Rehabilitation of persistent symptoms after concussion. Phys Med Rehabil Clin N Am. 2017;28(2):287–99. https://doi.org/10.1016/j.pmr.2016.12.006.
36. Puledda F, Shields K. Non-pharmacological approaches for migraine. Neurother J Am Soc Exp Neurother. 2018;15:336. https://doi.org/10.1007/s13311-018-0623-6.
37. Bhatnagar S, Iaccarino MA, Zafonte R. Pharmacotherapy in rehabilitation of post-acute traumatic brain injury. Brain Res. 2016;1640(Pt A):164–79. https://doi.org/10.1016/j.brainres.2016.01.021.
38. Sullivan KA, Berndt SL, Edmed SL, Smith SS, Allan AC. Poor sleep predicts subacute postconcussion symptoms following mild traumatic brain injury. Appl Neuropsychol Adult. 2016;23(6):426–35. https://doi.org/10.1080/23279095.2016.1172229.
39. Pigeon WR, Britton PC, Ilgen MA, Chapman B, Conner KR. Sleep disturbance preceding suicide among veterans. Am J Public Health. 2012;102(Suppl 1):S93–7. https://doi.org/10.2105/AJPH.2011.300470.
40. Ouellet M-C, Beaulieu-Bonneau S, Morin CM. Sleep-wake disturbances after traumatic brain injury. Lancet Neurol. 2015;14(7):746–57. https://doi.org/10.1016/S1474-4422(15)00068-X.
41. Swinkels CM, Ulmer CS, Beckham JC, Buse N, Calhoun PS. The association of sleep duration, mental health, and health risk behaviors among U.S. Afghanistan/Iraq era veterans. Sleep. 2013;36(7):1019–25. https://doi.org/10.5665/sleep.2800.
42. Lang KP, Veazey-Morris K, Andrasik F. Exploring the role of insomnia in the relation between PTSD and pain in veterans with polytrauma injuries. J Head Trauma Rehabil. 2014;29(1):44–53. https://doi.org/10.1097/HTR.0b013e31829c85d0.
43. Ribeiro JD, Pease JL, Gutierrez PM, Silva C, Bernert RA, Rudd MD, Joiner TE. Sleep problems outperform depression and hopelessness as cross-sectional and longitudinal predictors of suicidal ideation and behavior in young adults in the military. J Affect Disord. 2012;136(3):743–50. https://doi.org/10.1016/j.jad.2011.09.049.
44. Mathias JL, Alvaro PK. Prevalence of sleep disturbances, disorders, and problems following traumatic brain injury: a meta-analysis. Sleep Med. 2012;13(7):898–905. https://doi.org/10.1016/j.sleep.2012.04.006.
45. Koffel E, Bramoweth AD, Ulmer CS. Increasing access to and utilization of cognitive behavioral therapy for insomnia (CBT-I): a narrative review. J Gen Intern Med. 2018;33:955. https://doi.org/10.1007/s11606-018-4390-1.
46. Taylor DJ, Peterson AL, Pruiksma KE, Hale WJ, Young-McCaughan S, Wilkerson A, Nicholson K, Litz BT, Dondanville KA, Roache JD, Borah EV, Brundige A, Mintz J, STRONG STAR Consortium. Impact of cognitive behavioral therapy for insomnia disorder on sleep and comorbid symptoms in military personnel: a randomized clinical trial. Sleep. 2018;41 https://doi.org/10.1093/sleep/zsy069.
47. Soble JR, Cooper DB, Lu LH, Eapen BC, Kennedy JE. Symptom reporting and management of chronic post-concussive symptoms in military service members and veterans. Curr Phys Med Rehabil Rep. 2018;6:62. https://doi.org/10.1007/s40141-018-0173-1.
48. Cooper DB, Bunner AE, Kennedy JE, Balldin V, Tate DF, Eapen BC, Jaramillo CA. Treatment of persistent post-concussive symptoms after mild traumatic brain injury: a systematic

review of cognitive rehabilitation and behavioral health interventions in military service members and veterans. Brain Imaging Behav. 2015;9(3):403–20. https://doi.org/10.1007/s11682-015-9440-2.
49. Rabinowitz AR, Levin HS. Cognitive sequelae of traumatic brain injury. Psychiatr Clin North Am. 2014;37(1):1–11. https://doi.org/10.1016/j.psc.2013.11.004.
50. Dikmen SS, Corrigan JD, Levin HS, Machamer J, Stiers W, Weisskopf MG. Cognitive outcome following traumatic brain injury. J Head Trauma Rehabil. 2009;24(6):430–8. https://doi.org/10.1097/HTR.0b013e3181c133e9.
51. Elder GA. Update on TBI and cognitive impairment in military veterans. Curr Neurol Neurosci Rep. 2015;15(10):68. https://doi.org/10.1007/s11910-015-0591-8.
52. Bigler ED, Farrer TJ, Pertab JL, James K, Petrie JA, Hedges DW. Reaffirmed limitations of meta-analytic methods in the study of mild traumatic brain injury: a response to Rohling et al. Clin Neuropsychol. 2013;27(2):176–214. https://doi.org/10.1080/13854046.2012.693950.
53. Roebuck-Spencer TM, Vincent AS, Twillie DA, Logan BW, Lopez M, Friedl KE, Grate SJ, Schlegel RE, Gilliland K. Cognitive change associated with self-reported mild traumatic brain injury sustained during the OEF/OIF conflicts. Clin Neuropsychol. 2012;26(3):473–89. https://doi.org/10.1080/13854046.2011.650214.
54. Tiersky LA, Anselmi V, Johnston MV, Kurtyka J, Roosen E, Schwartz T, Deluca J. A trial of neuropsychologic rehabilitation in mild-spectrum traumatic brain injury. Arch Phys Med Rehabil. 2005;86(8):1565–74. https://doi.org/10.1016/j.apmr.2005.03.013.
55. Niemeier JP, Kreutzer JS, Marwitz JH, Gary KW, Ketchum JM. Efficacy of a brief acute neurobehavioural intervention following traumatic brain injury: a preliminary investigation. Brain Inj. 2011;25(7–8):680–90. https://doi.org/10.3109/02699052.2011.573520.
56. Cantor J, Ashman T, Dams-O'Connor K, Dijkers MP, Gordon W, Spielman L, Tsaousides T, Allen H, Nguyen M, Oswald J. Evaluation of the short-term executive plus intervention for executive dysfunction after traumatic brain injury: a randomized controlled trial with minimization. Arch Phys Med Rehabil. 2014;95(1):1–9.e3. https://doi.org/10.1016/j.apmr.2013.08.005.
57. Whyte J, Hart T, Vaccaro M, Grieb-Neff P, Risser A, Polansky M, Coslett HB. Effects of methylphenidate on attention deficits after traumatic brain injury: a multidimensional, randomized, controlled trial. Am J Phys Med Rehabil. 2004;83(6):401–20.
58. Willmott C, Ponsford J. Efficacy of methylphenidate in the rehabilitation of attention following traumatic brain injury: a randomised, crossover, double blind, placebo controlled inpatient trial. J Neurol Neurosurg Psychiatry. 2009;80(5):552–7. https://doi.org/10.1136/jnnp.2008.159632.
59. Sivan M, Neumann V, Kent R, Stroud A, Bhakta BB. Pharmacotherapy for treatment of attention deficits after non-progressive acquired brain injury. A systematic review. Clin Rehabil. 2010;24(2):110–21. https://doi.org/10.1177/0269215509343234.
60. Khan S, Chang R. Anatomy of the vestibular system: a review. NeuroRehabilitation. 2013;32(3):437–43. https://doi.org/10.3233/NRE-130866.
61. Chandrasekhar SS. The assessment of balance and dizziness in the TBI patient. NeuroRehabilitation. 2013;32(3):445–54. https://doi.org/10.3233/NRE-130867.
62. Bronstein AM, Lempert T. Management of the patient with chronic dizziness. Restor Neurol Neurosci. 2010;28(1):83–90. https://doi.org/10.3233/RNN-2010-0530.
63. Bryan CJ, Clemans TA. Repetitive traumatic brain injury, psychological symptoms, and suicide risk in a clinical sample of deployed military personnel. JAMA Psychiat. 2013;70(7):686–91. https://doi.org/10.1001/jamapsychiatry.2013.1093.
64. Gordon WA, Zafonte R, Cicerone K, Cantor J, Brown M, Lombard L, Goldsmith R, Chandna T. Traumatic brain injury rehabilitation: state of the science. Am J Phys Med Rehabil. 2006;85(4):343–82. https://doi.org/10.1097/01.phm.0000202106.01654.61.
65. John M. Eisenberg center for clinical decisions and communications science. Depression following a traumatic brain injury. In: Comparative Effectiveness Review Summary Guides for Policymakers. AHRQ Comparative Effectiveness Reviews. Rockville: Agency for Healthcare Research and Quality (US); 2011. http://www.ncbi.nlm.nih.gov/books/NBK379843/. Accessed 14 May 2018.

66. Jorge RE, Arciniegas DB. Mood disorders after TBI. Psychiatr Clin North Am. 2014;37(1):13–29. https://doi.org/10.1016/j.psc.2013.11.005.
67. Osborn AJ, Mathias JL, Fairweather-Schmidt AK. Depression following adult, non-penetrating traumatic brain injury: a meta-analysis examining methodological variables and sample characteristics. Neurosci Biobehav Rev. 2014;47:1. https://doi.org/10.1016/j.neubiorev.2014.07.007.
68. Bombardier CH, Fann JR, Temkin NR, Esselman PC, Barber J, Dikmen SS. Rates of major depressive disorder and clinical outcomes following traumatic brain injury. JAMA J Am Med Assoc. 2010;303(19):1938–45. https://doi.org/10.1001/jama.2010.599.
69. Fann JR, Jones AL, Dikmen SS, Temkin NR, Esselman PC, Bombardier CH. Depression treatment preferences after traumatic brain injury. J Head Trauma Rehabil. 2009;24(4):272–8. https://doi.org/10.1097/HTR.0b013e3181a66342.
70. Albrecht JS, Kiptanui Z, Tsang Y, Khokhar B, Liu X, Simoni-Wastila L, Zuckerman IH. Depression among older adults after traumatic brain injury: a national analysis. Am J Geriatr Psychiatry. 2015;23(6):607–14. https://doi.org/10.1016/j.jagp.2014.07.006.
71. Silver JM, McAllister TW, Arciniegas DB. Depression and cognitive complaints following mild traumatic brain injury. Am J Psychiatry. 2009;166(6):653–61. https://doi.org/10.1176/appi.ajp.2009.08111676.
72. Koren D, Norman D, Cohen A, Berman J, Klein EM. Increased PTSD risk with combat-related injury: a matched comparison study of injured and uninjured soldiers experiencing the same combat events. Am J Psychiatry. 2005;162(2):276–82. https://doi.org/10.1176/appi.ajp.162.2.276.
73. Bahraini NH, Breshears RE, Hernández TD, Schneider AL, Forster JE, Brenner LA. Traumatic brain injury and posttraumatic stress disorder. Psychiatr Clin North Am. 2014;37(1):55–75. https://doi.org/10.1016/j.psc.2013.11.002.
74. Brenner LA, Ivins BJ, Schwab K, Warden D, Nelson LA, Jaffee M, Terrio H. Traumatic brain injury, posttraumatic stress disorder, and postconcussive symptom reporting among troops returning from Iraq. J Head Trauma Rehabil. 2010;25(5):307–12. https://doi.org/10.1097/HTR.0b013e3181cada03.
75. Chen Y, Huang W, Constantini S. Concepts and strategies for clinical management of blast-induced traumatic brain injury and posttraumatic stress disorder. J Neuropsychiatry Clin Neurosci. 2013;25(2):103–10. https://doi.org/10.1176/appi.neuropsych.12030058.
76. Larson EB, Zollman FS. The effect of sleep medications on cognitive recovery from traumatic brain injury. J Head Trauma Rehabil. 2010;25(1):61–7. https://doi.org/10.1097/HTR.0b013e3181c1d1e1.
77. Chard KM, Schumm JA, McIlvain SM, Bailey GW, Parkinson RB. Exploring the efficacy of a residential treatment program incorporating cognitive processing therapy-cognitive for veterans with PTSD and traumatic brain injury. J Trauma Stress. 2011;24(3):347–51. https://doi.org/10.1002/jts.20644.
78. Wolf GK, Strom TQ, Kehle SM, Eftekhari A. A preliminary examination of prolonged exposure therapy with Iraq and Afghanistan veterans with a diagnosis of posttraumatic stress disorder and mild to moderate traumatic brain injury. J Head Trauma Rehabil. 2012;27(1):26–32. https://doi.org/10.1097/HTR.0b013e31823cd01f.
79. Speicher SM, Walter KH, Chard KM. Interdisciplinary residential treatment of posttraumatic stress disorder and traumatic brain injury: effects on symptom severity and occupational performance and satisfaction. Am J Occup Ther. 2014;68(4):412–21. https://doi.org/10.5014/ajot.2014.011304.
80. Montenigro PH, Corp DT, Stein TD, Cantu RC, Stern RA. Chronic traumatic encephalopathy: historical origins and current perspective. Annu Rev Clin Psychol. 2015;11:309–30. https://doi.org/10.1146/annurev-clinpsy-032814-112814.
81. Stein TD, Alvarez VE, McKee AC. Chronic traumatic encephalopathy: a spectrum of neuropathological changes following repetitive brain trauma in athletes and military personnel. Alzheimers Res Ther. 2014;6(1):4. https://doi.org/10.1186/alzrt234.
82. McKee AC, Alosco ML, Huber BR. Repetitive head impacts and chronic traumatic encephalopathy. Neurosurg Clin N Am. 2016;27(4):529–35. https://doi.org/10.1016/j.nec.2016.05.009.

83. Cifu DX, Carne W, Eapen BC. Chronic Traumatic Encephalopathy (CTE): overview, background, timeline and history of CTE. April 2016. http://emedicine.medscape.com/article/2500042-overview. Accessed 19 April 2016.
84. McKee AC, Stein TD, Nowinski CJ, Stern RA, Daneshvar DH, Alvarez VE, Lee H-S, Hall G, Wojtowicz SM, Baugh CM, Riley DO, Kubilus CA, Cormier KA, Jacobs MA, Martin BR, Abraham CR, Ikezu T, Reichard RR, Wolozin BL, Budson AE, Goldstein LE, Kowall NW, Cantu RC. The spectrum of disease in chronic traumatic encephalopathy. Brain. 2013;136(1):43–64. https://doi.org/10.1093/brain/aws307.
85. Stern RA, Daneshvar DH, Baugh CM, Seichepine DR, Montenigro PH, Riley DO, Fritts NG, Stamm JM, Robbins CA, McHale L, Simkin I, Stein TD, Alvarez VE, Goldstein LE, Budson AE, Kowall NW, Nowinski CJ, Cantu RC, McKee AC. Clinical presentation of chronic traumatic encephalopathy. Neurology. 2013;81(13):1122–9. https://doi.org/10.1212/WNL.0b013e3182a55f7f.
86. Goldstein LE, Fisher AM, Tagge CA, Zhang X-L, Velisek L, Sullivan JA, Upreti C, Kracht JM, Ericsson M, Wojnarowicz MW, Goletiani CJ, Maglakelidze GM, Casey N, Moncaster JA, Minaeva O, Moir RD, Nowinski CJ, Stern RA, Cantu RC, Geiling J, Blusztajn JK, Wolozin BL, Ikezu T, Stein TD, Budson AE, Kowall NW, Chargin D, Sharon A, Saman S, Hall GF, Moss WC, Cleveland RO, Tanzi RE, Stanton PK, McKee AC. Chronic traumatic encephalopathy in blast-exposed military veterans and a blast neurotrauma mouse model. Sci Transl Med. 2012;4(134):134ra60. https://doi.org/10.1126/scitranslmed.3003716.

Homeless Veterans and Mental Health

15

Kaitlin Slaven and Maria D. Llorente

Background and Historical Perspective

Homelessness among military veterans has been reported as far back as the Revolutionary War [1]. Following the Civil War, Congress established the National Home for Disabled Volunteer Soldiers. By 1900, more than 100,000 Union soldiers had received care in federal institutions as they struggled to reintegrate into civilian life.

Similar to homeless veterans today, residents of these institutions were often single, widowed or divorced, lacked family support and had some type of disability. Many of these facilities evolved into Veterans Affairs (VA) residential treatment centers [2].

Within the past decade, there has been a concerted and collaborative effort to address veteran homelessness.

A surge in the US homeless population that occurred in the 1970s led to an increased academic study of this social phenomenon. This surge was primarily caused by deinstitutionalization of the state mental hospital system, the demolition of single-occupancy residences (primarily low-income housing options for single men), and social changes in family makeup and structure. Understanding and addressing the risk factors that lead to homelessness can have a significant impact on prevention and reduction of homelessness.

K. Slaven (✉)
George Washington University, Department of Psychiatry, Washington, DC, USA
e-mail: kaitlinbudnik@gwu.edu

M. D. Llorente
Georgetown University School of Medicine, Washington DC VA Medical Center, Department of Psychiatry, Washington, DC, USA

Demographics of the Homeless Veteran Population

Homeless veterans are predominantly single men residing in urban centers. More than half have either a mental or physical disability [3]. While Blacks represent 11% of the veteran population, they account for 39% of homeless veterans. Most homeless men served during the Vietnam era, although did not necessarily serve in combat.

Veterans are at increased risk, compared to the civilian population, for homelessness [4]. Risk factors include lower socioeconomic status and having a psychiatric disorder and/or substance use disorder.

As a result of military occupational exposures, veterans are also at higher risk of exposure to traumatic brain injuries and post-traumatic stress disorder (PTSD). The prevalence of homelessness has also been found to be extremely high among veterans with an opioid use disorder.

The experience of military sexual trauma is an additional risk factor for homelessness. Veterans may experience unique risk factors, including difficulty adapting to civilian life, which often lacks the social support and structure of the military.

Risk factors for chronic versus first-time homelessness may vary. Those who are chronically or repeatedly homeless have more traditional risk factors, including substance abuse and mental illness, specifically bipolar disorder. First-time homelessness, in contrast, is associated with high housing costs, recent incarceration, self-reported diagnosis of mental illness other than bipolar disorder (TBI or psychotic disorders), and medical issues. Treatment interventions therefore may need to vary between chronic and more acute homeless individuals.

Demographics are shifting as more women enter the military [2]. Since 2005, the VA has seen a 154% increase in the number of women veterans accessing VHA mental health services. In fiscal year (FY) 2015, 182,107 women veterans received VA mental health care [5]. Female veterans are 4 times more likely to be homeless than their male counterparts [6].

Mental Illness in Homeless Veterans

Mental illness is highly prevalent among homeless veterans. Approximately 50% of homeless veterans have a serious mental illness, including mood and psychotic disorders, such as bipolar disorder, major depressive disorder, and schizophrenia. However, PTSD is the most common mental health diagnosis [7, 8]. Often, PTSD is comorbid with other psychiatric disorders [9], and among US military personnel and combat veterans who have been deployed in Afghanistan and Iraq, PTSD co-occurs with mild traumatic brain injury (TBI) in 48% of cases [10].

Research thus far is inconclusive as to whether PTSD is a risk factor for homelessness. Most homeless veterans served during peacetime eras and were thus not exposed to combat [11]. Combat exposure, at least among Vietnam veterans, was not found to be a risk factor for homelessness. This could potentially be because these veterans were able to access VA compensation, pensions, and health benefits

[12]. Factors outside of military experience may modify risk for PTSD, including previous life experiences and genetics. Studies have demonstrated that paternal history of PTSD may be a risk factor for PTSD among veterans [13].

Among homeless mentally ill veterans in one study by Mares and Rosenheck (2004), two thirds believed that their homelessness had nothing to do with their military service. Of those who felt that being homeless did have to do with their military experience, 75% believed that this was related to substance abuse issues that started in the military. Those who believed that being in the military increased their risk of homelessness were almost twice as likely to have endured childhood problems, such as abuse or tumultuous family relationships [14].

Of grave concern is the high suicide rate among veterans. In 2014, the rate of suicide among all veterans was 35.6 per 100,000, which is 22% higher than the general population [6]. Veterans experiencing housing instability have been found to be at greater risk for mental distress and suicidal ideation compared with veterans who have stable housing [15]. One study by Schinka and Schinka et al. (2012) found that 12% of older homeless veterans in a housing program [16] reported suicidal ideation. Depression and violent behavior have been found to be the strongest predictors of suicidal behavior among homeless veterans [17].

Both homelessness and severe mental illness are associated with early mortality [18]. Homeless individuals are at greater risk of mortality, as they are often exposed to the elements, are more likely to abuse substances, are more likely to have untreated medical problems, and are at greater risk of exposure to violence. Those at greatest risk of death are generally older and have been homeless for shorter periods of time [19]. Regardless of psychiatric diagnosis, homeless veterans die at younger ages than non-homeless veterans [18].

Homeless female veterans are more likely to have serious mental illness than their male counterparts, particularly schizophrenia, other psychotic spectrum illnesses, or mood disorders [20]. Women are less likely than men to abuse alcohol/drugs or to be dual diagnosed with substance abuse and mental illness. Female veterans may be more susceptible to secondary traumatization, which occurs when an individual hears about a firsthand account of a trauma experience and then subsequently develops PTSD symptoms themselves [21].

Mental Health Treatment Challenges in Homeless Veterans

While there are many challenges to appropriate treatment of mentally ill veterans, one of the most difficult is the management of co-occurring substance use. Individuals may use substances to self-medicate or as a coping strategy. Substance use in homeless veterans decreases opportunities for obtaining housing or employment. Use also increases levels of interpersonal conflict, increases risk for HIV infection and other serious health problems, and increases exposure to criminal behavior [21–25], all of which may directly impact homelessness.

Similarly, negative beliefs about mental health care and perceptions of decreased support are associated with increased stigma. Service members who report stigma associated with psychiatric disorders are more likely to report embarrassment, being perceived as weak, not knowing where to get help, and having difficulties scheduling a mental health appointment [26].

Substance use disorders and psychosis among homeless veterans can limit follow-up care in the ambulatory setting, thus leading to more frequent emergency room visits and inpatient admissions. Access to consistent care is thus difficult with homeless populations. Often homeless individuals have difficulty attending medical appointments due to barriers such as access to reminders, reliable transportation, and cost. Because of this lack of regular health care, homeless veterans are more likely to use emergency services than their nonveteran counterparts and less likely to use outpatient resources [27].

The addition of integrated primary care services into homeless programs is a potential model to offer one-stop services for homeless veterans. Homeless mentally ill peers may offer a unique support. Those who have peer support are more likely to follow up with appointments and have better overall outcomes [28].

Medication adherence among homeless veterans is a major challenge. One study by Hermes and Rosenheck (2016) found that homeless veterans were 16.2% less likely to fill psychotropic prescriptions than their matched counterparts. Those in residential programs were more likely to fill their prescriptions, suggesting that these settings, which provide stability and structured routines, could improve outcomes [29]. Additional identified barriers to receiving mental health and primary care services include not knowing where to go for services (32.4% of homeless veterans), not being able to afford services, too much confusion, hassles, long wait times, and having been denied services previously [30].

This highlights the importance of enhancing and facilitating access to affordable and comprehensive services that offer housing, substance use disorder and mental health treatment, and primary care services. For those veterans who reside in rural areas, the use of telemental health services is expanding. The VA has made telemental health one of their initiatives to address gaps in care with the establishment of 10 telemental health hubs across the VA system [6].

Addressing relationships is another strategy to address homelessness. The majority of homeless veterans are single, either never married or divorced. The lack of social supports may be a factor that interferes with access to care. Families may not know how to address psychiatric conditions. Increasingly, services are including services to family members of veterans, such as support groups or crisis lines, to minimize burnout and keep families involved in the lives of veterans. Keeping families engaged with veterans improves outcomes.

Another contributory factor for both psychiatric and substance abuse disorders, as well as homelessness among veterans, is recent incarceration [12, 25]. Many incarcerated veterans will ultimately reenter the community. The Department of Veterans Affairs has established the Health Care for Re-Entry Veterans (HCRV) to promote success and prevent homelessness among veterans returning home after incarceration. HCRV services include outreach, health-care assessments during the 6 months just prior to release, and referrals to medical, mental health, employment, and other social services.

Additional problems for which veterans seek services include application for VA benefits, housing, and family issues. Addressing these issues prevents recidivism and is more cost effective than the financial burden of chronic homelessness. Veterans who received medical-legal partnership services showed significantly better outcomes in both mental health and housing [30].

Similarly, the Veterans Justice Outreach Program was established by the VA to prevent the unnecessary criminalization of mental illness and extended incarceration. This program ensures that eligible, justice-involved veterans receive access to indicated VA services. The program staff provide outreach, assessment, and case management for justice-involved veterans, working with local courts, jails, public defenders, and judges.

A new challenge is the increasing number of women veterans returning from Iraq and Afghanistan (Operation Iraqi Freedom and Operation Enduring Freedom – OEF/OIF) [33]. The USA has never had to deal with the large number of returning female troops, who performed varied assignments beyond nursing. Women veterans are at three to four times increased risk compared to their civilian counterparts for homelessness [31]. Because previous generations of veterans were predominantly men, services for women have had to be developed quickly. In particular, services for military sexual trauma are highly needed. Among female veterans experiencing homelessness, treatment related to military sexual trauma was three times higher than among non-homeless veteran females. Approximately 29% of non-OEF/OIF homeless female veterans and 34% of OEF/OIF homeless female veterans received treatment related to MST from the VA health system [32].

If providers do not know how to screen for or manage the treatment of military sexual trauma (MST), women veterans may feel marginalized. To address this issue, VA has mandated MST training for all providers and has hired primary care providers who have specialty training in women's health concerns through the Designated Women's Health program. These providers exist at all VA Medical Centers and 90% of community-based outpatient clinics [6].

If these women do not seek care within the VA, however, community providers need to be sensitive to the possibility that they may have experienced MST and should obtain specialty training to inquire about MST and offer appropriate services. Residential care options are important for women veterans. Homeless female veterans who entered a 30-day residential treatment program had better outcomes in terms of community functioning, psychiatric symptoms, and drug and alcohol abstinence. They also did better in terms of employment, social support, and housing status [31].

Veteran Administration Initiatives to End Veteran Homelessness

In 2009, the VA established a national priority to end veteran homelessness. Services expanded over time to include residential programs and transitional housing and Compensated Work Therapy. Opening Doors, the nation's first federal strategy to address this important issue, outlined strategies that included partnerships among federal, state, and local agencies to prevent veteran homelessness and to stably house those who are homeless as urgently as possible [34]. The VA adopted the Housing First model, in which veterans are assisted in obtaining stable housing first, and other problems, such as abstinence from substances of abuse or engagement in mental health services are addressed later.

The VA, together with the Department of Housing and Urban Development (HUD), developed a joint supportive housing program [5]. HUD provides Section Housing Choice vouchers for eligible veterans, and the VA provides case management and supportive housing services. More than 85,000 vouchers have been awarded since 2008. A national call center was also developed to provide 24/7 assistance for homeless veterans. In fiscal year 2016, the center received more than 128,000 calls. In 2012, the VA established the Supportive Services for Veteran Families (SSVF) program which provides time-limited services and financial assistance. The program has served more than 150,000 individuals, including 34,000 children. Only 15% of those who were rehoused returned to homelessness after 2 years.

As a result of these initiatives, homelessness among veterans has been reduced by nearly 50% since 2010. The average length of stay in temporary VA housing has been reduced to 179 days, the lowest length of stay since 2009. Almost a half million veterans and their families have been assisted in obtaining or maintaining stable housing.

Conclusions

There are many challenges for homeless veterans. Some of the most significant barriers to care within this population include comorbid substance abuse, shifting demographics (including more homeless female veterans than ever before) with unique needs, challenges in access to care, limited social supports, and justice involvement. The Housing First model is working to address housing problems. During the past decade, a concerted effort between the Departments of Housing and Urban Development and Veterans Affairs, in collaboration with US Interagency Council on Homelessness and state and local agencies, has significantly reduced homelessness among veterans. While these efforts continue, they can serve as a model to address the problem of chronic homelessness. It is imperative that the elimination of homelessness among veterans remain a societal priority.

References

1. Llorente MD, Morton K, Boughton S, Crawford PA. A real welcome home: permanent housing for homeless veterans. Fed Pract. 2016;33(5):26–31.
2. Estrine S. Service delivery for vulnerable populations: new directions in behavioral health [e-book]. New York: Springer Publishing Company; 2011.
3. National Alliance to End Homelessness. Veteran homelessness. 2015. Available at: https://endhomelessness.org/resource/veteran-homelessness/. Accessed 7 April 2018.

4. US Department of Housing and Urban Development and the US Department of Veterans' Affairs. Veteran homelessness: a supplemental report to the annual homeless assessment report to Congress. 2009. Available at: https://www.va.gov/homeless/docs/2010aharveteransreport.pdf. Accessed 7 April 2018.
5. U.S. Department of Veterans Affairs. Office of Mental Health and Suicide Prevention (OMHSP). Facts About Veteran Suicide: August 2017. https://www.mentalhealth.va.gov/docs/VA-Suicide-Prevention-Fact-Sheet.pdf. Revised August 2017. Accessed 23 Feb 2018.
6. Gamache G, Rosenheck R, Tessler R. Overrepresentation of women veterans among homeless women. Am J Public Health. 2003;93(7):1132–6.
7. 100,000 Homes Campaign. National Survey of Homeless Veterans in 100,000 Homes Campaign Communities. November 2011. Available at: https://www.va.gov/homeless/docs/nationalsurveyofhomelessveterans_final.pdf. Accessed 7 April 2018.
8. Kasprow WJ, Cuerdon T, DiLella D, et al. Health care for homeless veterans programs: twenty-third annual report. West Haven: Department of Veterans Affairs; 2010.
9. American Psychiatric Association. Diagnostic and statistical manual of mental disorders (5th ed.). Washington DC: American Psychiatric Association.; 2013.
10. Schell TL, Marshall GN. Survey of individuals previously deployed for OEF/OIF. In: Tanielian T, Jaycox LH, editors. Invisible wounds of war: psychological and cognitive injuries, their consequences, and services to assist recovery. Santa Monica: RAND Corporation; 2008. p. 87–115.
11. Rosenheck R, Frisman L, Chung AM. The proportion of veterans among homeless men. Am J Public Health. 1994;84(3):466–9.
12. Tsai J, Rosenheck RA. Risk factors for homelessness among US veterans. Epidemiol Rev. 2015;37(1):177–95.
13. Shepherd-Banigan M, Goldstein K, Fecteau T, et al. Paternal history of mental illness associated with posttraumatic stress disorder among veterans. Psychiatry Res. 2017;256:461–8.
14. Mares A, Rosenheck R. Perceived relationship between military service and homelessness among homeless veterans with mental illness. J Nerv Ment Dis. 2004;192(10):715–9.
15. Bossarte RM, Blosnich JR, Piegari RI, et al. Housing instability and mental distress among US veterans. Am J Public Health. 2013;103:S213–6.
16. Schinka JA, Schinka KC, Casey RJ, et al. Suicidal behavior in a national sample of older homeless veterans. Am J Public Health. 2012;102:S147–53.
17. Goldstein G, Luther J, Haas G. Medical, psychiatric and demographic factors associated with suicidal behavior in homeless veterans. Psychiatry Res. 2012;199:37–43.
18. Birgenheir D, Zongshan L, Kilbourne A. Trends in mortality among homeless VA patients with severe mental illness. Psychiatr Serv. 2013;64(7):608.
19. Kasprow W, Rosenheck R. Mortality among homeless and nonhomeless mentally ill veterans. J Nerv Ment Dis. 2000;188(3):141–7.
20. Leda C, Rosenheck R, Gallup P. Mental illness among homeless female veterans. Hosp Community Psychiatry. 1992;43(10):1026–8.
21. Baum N, Rahav G, Sharon M. Heightened susceptibility to secondary traumatization: a meta-analysis of gender differences. Am J Orthopsychiatry. 2014;84:111–22.
22. Coumans M, Spreen M. Drug use and the role of homelessness in the process of marginalization. Subst Use Misuse. 2003;38:311–38.
23. Devine JA, Wright JD. Losing the housing game: the leveling effects of substance abuse. Am J Orthopsychiatry. 1997;67:618–31.
24. Zlotnick C, Tam T, Robertson MJ. Disaffiliation, substance use, and exiting homelessness. Subst Use Misuse. 2003;38:577–99.
25. Tsai J, Rosenheck RA. Risk factors for ED use among homeless veterans. Am J Emerg Med. 2013;31:855–8.
26. Hoge CW, Castro CA, Messer SC, et al. Combat duty in Iraq and Afghanistan, mental health problems, and barriers to care. N Engl J Med. 2004;351:13–22.
27. Desai M, Rosenheck R, Kasprow W. Determinants of receipt of ambulatory medical care in a national sample of mentally ill homeless veterans. Med Care. 2003;41(2):275–87.

28. Weissman E, Covell N, Kushner M, Irwin J, Essock S. Implementing peer-assisted case management to help homeless veterans with mental illness transition to independent housing. Community Ment Health J. 2005;41(3):267–76.
29. Hermes E, Rosenheck R. Psychopharmacologic services for homeless veterans: comparing psychotropic prescription fills among homeless and non-homeless veterans with serious mental illness. Community Ment Health J. 2016;52(2):142–7.
30. Rosenheck R, Lam JA. Client and site characteristics as barriers to service use by homeless persons with serious mental illness. Psychiatr Serv. 1997;48(3):387–90.
31. Tsai J, Middleton M, Rosenheck R, et al. Medical-legal partnerships at veterans affairs medical centers improved housing and psychosocial outcomes for vets. Health Aff. 2017;36(12):2195–203.
32. Harpaz-Rotem I, Rosenheck R, Desai R. Residential treatment for homeless female veterans with psychiatric and substance use disorders: effect on 1-year clinical outcomes. J Rehabil Res Dev. 2011;48(8):891–9.
33. Department of Veterans Affairs Office of Inspector General. Homeless incidence and risk factors for becoming homeless in veterans. Report No. 11–03428-173. May 2012. https://www.va.gov/oig/pubs/VAOIG-11-03428-173.pdf.
34. USICH. Opening Doors. 2015. Available at: https://www.usich.gov/opening-doors Accessed 7 April 2018.

Contextual Frameworks for Addressing Risk and Fostering Resilience Among Sexual and Gender Minority Veterans

16

Rebecca Gitlin and Michael R. Kauth

Sexual and gender minority (SGM) veterans are no longer a hidden population. Healthcare providers can expect to see SGM veterans in their practice, whether as solo practitioners or within specialty care programs or integrated care teams in the VHA or civilian healthcare systems. In particular, mental health professionals play a crucial role in addressing risk and resilience factors of SGM veterans. In this chapter, we employ a minority stress lens as a framework for identifying and addressing contributors to distress and resilience in SGM veterans. We will provide an overview of SGM veteran health disparities and outline strategies for promoting a welcoming clinical environment for SGM veterans. We will describe how to provide patient-centered, culturally informed, and affirming mental healthcare, including treatment considerations for transgender veterans seeking transition-related care. For a thorough review of comprehensive transgender care for mental health professionals, see Adult Transgender Care: An Interdisciplinary Approach for Training Mental Health Professionals (2018) by Kauth and Shipherd [2].

Sexual and gender minorities have become increasingly visible and socially accepted in broader society in recent years. Population-based surveys [3] estimate that over eight million (3.5%) adults in the United States (US) identify as a sexual minority. The actual number varies by whether one counts identity, behavior,

---

R. Gitlin (✉)
Los Angeles County Department of Mental Health, Los Angeles, CA, USA
e-mail: rgitlin@dmh.lacounty.gov

M. R. Kauth
VHA LGBT Health Program, Washington, DC, USA

VA South Central Mental Illness Research, Education, and Clinical Center, Houston, TX, USA

Department of Psychiatry, Baylor College of Medicine, Michael E. DeBakey Veterans Affairs Medical Center, Houston, TX, USA

attraction, or relationships. Some population-based surveys indicate that twice as many people report same-sex sexual behavior than self-identify as a sexual minority [3]. Similarly, estimates of gender minorities vary by self-identity, gender expression, and clinical versus community sample. Almost 700,000 American adults identify as transgender, making up 0.6% of the adult population.

Among the 23 million US veterans, it is estimated that there are over one million sexual and gender minority (SGM) veterans; the exact number, however, is unknown [3, 4]. Neither the Department of Defense nor VHA routinely collect data on sexual orientation identity or gender identity, although the VHA has implemented the first phase of a self-identified gender identity field. Like their heterosexual and cisgender counterparts, most SGM veterans seek care outside the VHA. However, if SGM veterans came to the VHA at the same rate as other veterans, we could expect several hundred thousand SGM veterans receiving healthcare in VHA.

Many community providers also fail to routinely assess sexual orientation identity, gender identity, and veteran status, increasing the difficulty of accurately capturing the number of SGM veterans. It is also worth noting that not assessing for veteran status also ignores potential risks for health conditions associated with service in the military.

Among the more than one million SGM veterans, around 71,000 sexual minority individuals are currently serving in the military, representing about 2.2% of current service members [5]. Sexual minority women are overrepresented in the military. Approximately 6.2% of women serving in the military self-identify as sexual minorities compared with 5.2% of sexual minority women in the general population. Although women make up only 14% of active duty military personnel, sexual minority women represent more than 43% of sexual minorities currently on active duty [5].

However, sexual minority men are underrepresented among current military personnel. Approximately 1.5% of men serving in the military self-identify as sexual minorities compared with 3.3% of men in the general population. That is, self-identified gay men are significantly less prevalent in the military personnel than in the general population. Of note, when sexual identity and behavior are assessed together among men, civilian and military personnel self-report identifying as gay, bisexual, or other MSM at similar rates [6]. In other words, although sexual minority identity may be less common among men in military samples when compared with civilian samples, rates of same-sex sexual behavior are comparable between the two groups.

Transgender individuals are overrepresented in the military. Gates and Herman [4] calculated that 21.4% of transgender people have served in the military versus 10.4% of the general population. While transgender individuals may join the service for many of the same reasons as others, some may seek to suppress their gender dysphoria within an ultra-masculine environment, referred to as a "flight into hypermasculinity" [7].

> **Box 16.1 Did You Know?**
> The exact number of sexual and gender minority veterans is unknown. If sexual and gender minority veterans get care within the VHA at rates comparable to other veterans, that would make the VHA the largest provider of SGM healthcare in the world [8].

Because VHA medical records do not include self-identified gender, identifying transgender individuals within the VHA is only possible by using alternative methods. These include International Classification of Diseases (ICD) diagnostic codes (e.g., gender identity disorder) or codes related to transgender care services (e.g., hormone therapy). Using this method, more than 9,000 unique transgender veterans could be identified through VHA records. Recently, an electronic self-identified gender identity field was implemented within the Master Veteran Index. This data will be invaluable in determining the numbers of transgender veterans accessing some VA benefits; however, only the first phase implementation of the gender identity field has been completed, and it will take several years to populate this field for the millions of veterans who receive VHA services.

Before going further, we need to distinguish identity labels from behavior and define several important terms used throughout this chapter.

Identity labels and categories are ever-evolving in response to social environments, increased visibility, and cultural and political change. As our vocabulary expands, so does our understanding of the diversity and complexity within sexual and gender minority communities. For sexual and gender minorities, using the label or pronoun that an individual identifies with communicates respect and affirmation. This is critical for establishing rapport. Hence, we begin with a brief overview of language and common terms. While this discussion is by no means exhaustive, it provides a foundation for understanding specific identities within the sexual and gender minority communities.

Sexual orientation identity or just *sexual identity* refers to a person's identification of their sexual or romantic orientation or attractions. *Lesbian*, *gay*, and *bisexual* are among the most common sexual identities. However, mental health professionals may also hear people identify as queer, ambisexual, pansexual, omnisexual, asexual, and others, which may require some definition from the individual. See Table 16.1 for more examples.

Gender identity refers to how a person identifies their internal sense of masculinity (or being a man or male) or femininity (or being a woman or female). A person's gender identity may also incorporate both masculinity and femininity (e.g., androgynous), neither masculinity nor femininity (e.g., agender), or another experience of gender entirely (e.g., genderqueer).

When referring to SGM communities, the acronym *LGBT* (lesbian, gay, bisexual, transgender) or *LGBTQ* (lesbian, gay, bisexual, transgender, queer or questioning) is often used. However, because the number and diversity of sexual and gender identity categories are constantly expanding, variations on these acronyms or alternative terms are common. For example, the phrase *sexual and gender minorities* (SGM) refers to those whose sexual identities are nonheterosexual and individuals whose gender identity does not correspond with their sex assigned at birth. In this chapter, we use SGM both as a noun to refer to individuals whose identities lie outside heterosexual and cisgender societal norms or expectations and as an adjective as in SGM veterans.

It is important to remember that sexual identity, sexual attractions, and sexual behavior may not be congruent [10, 11]. This may be due to avoidance of discrimination, internalized stigma toward one's sexual behaviors or attractions, personal

Table 16.1 Helpful terms for provider-patient interactions

Common Terms (and Some to Avoid) [9]
Sexual (Orientation) Identities
Gay *(adjective)* – a person who is attracted to people of their own gender; most commonly used in reference to men
Lesbian *(adjective/noun)* – a woman who is attracted to other women
Bisexual *(adjective)* – a person who is attracted to same-gender and other-gender individuals
Queer *(adjective)* – often used as a more inclusive or umbrella term, rather than having a sexual identity inherently defined by/within a gender binary. Once a derogatory slur, this term has been reclaimed and used by many (though not all) individuals and communities
Questioning *(adjective)* – a person who is currently exploring their identity
Gender Identities
Transgender *(adjective)* – umbrella term for a person whose current gender identity is not congruent with their sex assigned at birth
Transgender man/transman *(noun)* – a person assigned female at birth who now identifies as a man
Transgender woman/transwoman *(noun)* – a person assigned male at birth who now identifies as a woman
Cisgender *(adjective)* – a person whose current gender identity corresponds with their sex assigned at birth
Intersex *(adjective, noun)* – a category of conditions where sex-related anatomical or chromosomal development occurs differently from what is expected. Some intersex conditions may not be evident at birth
Genderqueer/nonbinary/gender variant *(adjective)* – a person whose gender identity does not align with the gender binary (man/masculine and woman/feminine)
Two-spirit *(adjective)* – a gender identity that integrates masculine and feminine energies, most commonly used in Native American communities
Medical/Public Health Terminology
Sex assigned at birth *(noun)* – the sex categorization (male or female) assigned to a person at the time of birth. This designation is most commonly made by the appearance of the infant's genitals. Abbreviations include *AMAB (assigned male at birth)* and *AFAB (assigned female at birth)*
Men who have sex with men (MSM) or women who have sex with women (WSW) *(noun)* – refers to sexual behavior, which may or may not correspond with a person's sexual identity
Gender confirmation surgery/gender affirmation surgery *(noun)* – surgical procedures conducted to modify a person's body to increase congruence with their gender identity, formerly sex reassignment surgery
Terms to Avoid as Outdated and/or Offensive
Transgendered/tranny or using "Transgender" as a noun – see above
Hermaphrodite – "intersex" is the appropriate term
Sexual preference – "sexual identity" is the appropriate term
Sex change – "gender confirmation surgery" or "gender affirmation surgery" are appropriate terms

decisions against disclosing sexual identity or behavior to a provider, or other factors.

Professional health organizations have long encouraged patients to disclose their sexual identity. However, recently, the VHA (*Directive 1340* [12]) directed providers to ask veterans about their sexual identity in order to determine potential health risks associated with sexual minority status and conduct a history of sexual health to assess sexual risk. These developments are not unique to the VHA; in late 2017, Britain's National Health Service recommended healthcare providers ask patients about sexual identity [13]. The VHA has also directed providers to ask veterans about their self-identified gender identity in order to respectfully address the individual and assess potential health risks associated with gender minority status.

Case Example
Felicity is a 24-year-old biracial (White and Black) Air Force veteran who is seeking treatment for panic attacks, which occur once or twice per month with unidentified triggers. She identifies as a lesbian and came out at the age of 17. Felicity has been with her girlfriend for 3 years. While discussing medication options, Felicity asks whether there might be any interactions between the suggested psychotropic medications and oral contraceptives. Upon further inquiry, Felicity reveals that she has been taking oral contraceptives since adolescence. She further reports that it is important for her to stay on her oral contraceptives since she and her girlfriend are occasionally sexually intimate with a close male friend of her girlfriend's. Even though Felicity wants to use condoms during these encounters, both her girlfriend and their male friend dismiss her concerns because Felicity is on oral contraceptives, "so there's nothing to worry about."

From this initial interaction, several key points emerge:

- Felicity identifies as a lesbian and has been in a relationship for several years. A provider may incorrectly assume that she is in a monogamous partnership and/or only sexually engages with other women. This scenario underscores the importance of inquiring about behavior as well as identity. In addition, a brief assessment of sexual health risk behaviors is also warranted.
- Engaging patients in discussions about sexual behavior can reveal information that is clinically relevant for further inquiry as well as subsequent treatment. Especially within the context of case conceptualization and treatment planning, Felicity's story presents an opportunity to:
  - Explore possible relationships between her sexual encounters and panic attacks.
  - Discuss strategies for self-advocacy.
  - Further probe for dynamics around consent.
  - Assess for emotional or physical abuse occurring within her sexual or romantic relationships.

Health Disparities and Social Determinants of Health

Marked systemic and health disparities experienced by SGM individuals are well documented. Compared with their heterosexual counterparts, sexual minority women and men tend to have higher rates of depression, anxiety, and problematic alcohol and drug use [10, 11, 14] as well as a greater prevalence of childhood and adult victimization [15]. Bisexual individuals show particularly elevated rates of most psychiatric symptoms, problematic substance use, and lifetime victimization.

Health disparities experienced by SGM individuals are often framed through the lens of *minority stress* [1]. Minority stress theory posits that daily stresses associated with stigma, discrimination, and navigating hostile social contexts contribute to elevated rates of distress, anxiety, depression, and maladaptive ways of coping such as smoking, binge drinking, drug use, not exercising, and not seeking healthcare when needed. The end result is chronic health conditions and poor mental health outcomes.

Distal and *proximal* stressors work together within the minority stress model to produce SGM health disparities. Distal stressors refer to institutional or societal dynamics that perpetuate stigma against SGM communities, including customs, belief systems, legislation, media representation, and invisibility (i.e., lack of training for providers about SGM healthcare). Prejudice, rejection (e.g., refusal to treat), and violence are further manifestations of distal stress. Proximal stressors include interpersonal experiences, such as demeaning looks, name-calling or jokes, or expressed prejudice (e.g., "I don't know why gay people feel they deserve special programs. They already got gay marriage, right?"). Cumulative distal and proximal stressors lead to internalized stigma, shame, and expectations of discrimination or rejection.

Identity-related factors (e.g., prominence of minority identity) as well as social and coping resources can have additional effects on the relationship between minority stressors and mental health outcomes. Testa and colleagues [16] adapted Meyer's work in a conceptualization of *gender minority stress* to explain the systemic health disparities faced by gender minorities.

The disparities faced by SGM communities may be exacerbated by veteran-specific risk factors. This includes medical and psychiatric risk factors (e.g., traumatic brain injury, posttraumatic stress) as well as sociocultural stressors (e.g., stigmatization of veteran identity). Intersectionality theory [17] provides a framework for understanding how holding multiple identities associated with marginalized groups may affect overall risk. Identifying oneself as a member of multiple vulnerable communities (e.g., woman, bisexual, transgender, ethnic minority) does not necessarily result in additive risks and disparities. An individual's risk and resilience factors are influenced by the unique intersections of their multiple identities. Holding both veteran and SGM identities may exacerbate risks for some and promote resilience for others.

Compared with a control (presumed heterosexual) group of veterans seeking care within VHA, sexual minority veterans report higher rates of depression, PTSD, and alcohol use [18]. Depressive and PTSD symptoms were partially predicted by concealment of lesbian, gay, or bisexual identity during military service. Further, nearly 15% of sexual minority veterans had made a serious suicide attempt.

Compared to (presumed heterosexual) women veterans, sexual minority women report higher rates of childhood and adult sexual abuse, current problematic substance use including smoking, and lifetime diagnoses of mood disorders, anxiety disorders, and PTSD [19–22]. Blosnich and colleagues [19] found that sexual minority women veterans reported significantly higher levels of distress, lower life satisfaction, and poorer physical health than women veterans generally.

Though the literature on gender minority veterans is small, notable physical and mental health disparities experienced by gender minority veterans have been found relative to cisgender veterans and gender minority civilians. In a comprehensive case-controlled study examining VHA patients with and without charted transgender-related ICD diagnostic codes (e.g., gender identity disorder, transsexualism), Brown and Jones [23] reported that transgender veterans had significantly higher rates of all psychiatric disorders and most medical disorders examined, including depression, severe mental illness, PTSD, alcohol use disorder, tobacco use disorder, obesity, and HIV.

Transgender veterans were also more likely to report a history of military sexual trauma, homelessness, and incarceration. Blosnich et al. [24] found that transgender veterans in VHA (identified by diagnostic codes) reported suicidal or self-harm events at a rate more than 20 times that of the general VHA patient population. However, increased rates of suicidality among transgender veterans was comparable to rates among transgender individuals without military service [25].

Impact of Policy and Legislation on SGM Veteran Health

Anti-SGM policy and legislation as well as the absence of nondiscrimination policies can be viewed as distal minority stressors. Examples include the absence of federal policies that protect SGM individuals from job or housing discrimination and state laws prohibiting same gender marriage prior to the 2015 US Supreme Court decision declaring those laws unconstitutional and legalizing same-gender marriage. For SGM veterans, the Department of Defense policy "Don't Ask, Don't Tell" (DADT), earlier bans on gay and lesbian service members, and the ban on transgender service members represent distal minority stressors and ultimately serve as barriers to healthcare for SGM veterans.

Supporting Meyer's framework [1] of how distal minority stressors impact health outcomes, Hatzenbuehler and colleagues, using national probability samples, found that sexual minority men and women living in states with nondiscrimination policies reported better health outcomes than sexual minorities living in states without civil rights protections [26, 27]. Further, Blosnich and colleagues [28], using VHA data, found that transgender veterans (identified by diagnostic codes) living in states with employment nondiscrimination protections for gender identity had lower rates of mood disorders and self-harm behaviors. Interestingly, positive health outcomes were not found for transgender veterans who lived in states with hate crime protection laws.

Most major healthcare organizations have nondiscrimination patient policies that include sexual orientation and gender identity and expression, although frontline clinical practices may not always be responsive to SGM patients. The VHA also has nondiscrimination patient policies inclusive of sexual orientation and gender identity and expression. In addition, the VHA has two healthcare policies that directly address the needs of SGM veterans.

Since 2011, the VHA has had a national policy establishing healthcare services for transgender veterans (originally, VHA *Directive 2011-024*: Provision of Health Care for Transgender and Intersex Veterans; later *Directive 2013-003*; now *Directive 1341*) [29]. This *Directive* specifies that gender minority veterans are able to access gender counseling and hormone therapy for gender transitioning and should be addressed by their self-identified gender identity. Gender minority veterans may also receive mental health/readiness assessments in preparation for hormone therapy or gender-confirming surgeries performed outside of the VHA. At present, the VHA cannot conduct or pay for gender-confirming surgical procedures. VHA mental health professionals conducting these assessments may write letters of support on behalf of veterans who are eligible for and ready to receive gender-confirming services. In addition, the VHA will provide medically necessary postoperative care for complications (e.g., infection, pain, loss of function) following gender confirmation surgeries but not cosmetic procedures.

The second VHA health policy, released in 2017, established care guidelines for sexual minority veterans (*VHA Directive 1340: Provision of Health Care for Veterans Who Identify as Lesbian, Gay, or Bisexual*) [12]. This *Directive* mandates that providers ask patients about their sexual identity, update this information at least annually, and conduct a brief sexual health history and update at least annually. This information allows providers to then follow up on potential health risks based on health disparity data and respond to sexual health risk. In addition, this *Directive* prohibits VHA staff from attempts to change the sexual orientation of veterans (i.e., so-called reparative or conversion therapy).

Barriers to Healthcare Among SGM Veterans

SGM experience a number of barriers to accessing healthcare within VHA as well as in community settings. These include difficulty acquiring health insurance, cost, few culturally competent providers in SGM health, and providers who refuse to treat SGM [30–33]. In a large national survey, nearly 1 in 5 transgender respondents reported being refused care by a healthcare provider.

Identity-related stigma also negatively impacts SGM veteran healthcare utilization. Stigma associated with one's SGM identity or veteran status may affect identity disclosure within a healthcare setting, which may prevent an SGM veteran from obtaining culturally informed care. As noted above, SGM veterans may not be identified as veterans within community health settings (either due to lack of provider inquiry or patient disclosure).

As noted earlier, there is no reliable data about the proportion of SGM veterans who receive healthcare at the VHA. Some SGM veterans may avoid seeking care at VHA facilities due to a perception that prohibitory military policies like DADT or the ban on transgender service members apply to veterans as well as active duty personnel.

While veterans with a dishonorable discharge are denied VA healthcare benefits [31, 34], the VHA has never restricted access to healthcare for SGM veterans due to disclosed identity or behavior. One study of SGM veterans at two VHA facilities reported that the top-ranked potential barrier for SGM veterans seeking care at the VHA was "hurtful, rejecting experiences in the military" [32].

An online survey of SGM veterans found that one-third of sexual minority veterans [35] and one-quarter of gender minority veterans [27] had not disclosed their identities to their VHA providers. It is worth noting, however, that the majority of SGM veterans surveyed did feel safe enough to disclose their identities to their providers.

A separate recent national survey of SGM veterans reported that a larger proportion of SGM veterans had disclosed their identities to their VHA provider than in past surveys, and many respondents viewed the current VHA environment as welcoming [36]. This provides suggestive evidence that VHA efforts to raise awareness about SGM veteran health and train providers to deliver respectful, culturally competent care may be working. Yet, transgender men were least likely among SGM veterans to report feeling comfortable disclosing their gender identity or feeling welcome at the facility.

Considerations for Diverse Populations Among SGM Veterans

This section focuses on the unique health needs of specific populations of SGM veterans.

Aging SGM veterans As with heterosexual and cisgender people, the number of aging SGM individuals in the US is growing at a rapid rate [37]. However, considerations for the unique needs of aging SGM communities have been largely absent in the healthcare programs addressing older adults. Few programs for aging SGM communities exist. Although there is little research on aging SGM veterans, Monin and colleagues [38] found that older sexual minority veterans had significantly smaller social networks than younger sexual minority veterans, potentially putting them at risk of social isolation and depression. However, older sexual minority veterans also showed more resilience to psychiatric symptoms, suggested by lower rates of depression and PTSD compared with younger sexual minority veterans.

Another study found that older transgender adults who served in the military reported fewer depressive symptoms than older transgender adults without military service [39]. While older SGM veterans may have several health risk factors, these veterans may also have developed adaptive coping strategies in response to minority stress.

Homeless SGM veterans SGM veterans in particular have high rates of homelessness. Housing instability is compounded by high rates of substance dependence and psychiatric symptoms among SGM veterans, as well as the lack of employment and housing nondiscrimination protections [14]. In addition, SGM individuals often have weaker ties to natal families who can provide some support compared with heterosexual and cisgender people. In discussing potential referrals and resources with homeless SGM veterans, safety and discrimination protections at the referral sites are critical.

SGM veterans of color For SGM veterans of color, racial and ethnic disparities may affect access to and engagement in treatment. Within veteran and civilian samples, SGM people of color report high levels of lifetime victimization and many psychiatric symptoms of distress [40, 41]. Yet, Black and Latinx veterans are less likely to receive individual psychotherapy compared with White veterans [42], and Latinx veterans are less likely to receive psychotherapy within mental health settings (as opposed to primary care clinics or other settings). Indeed, SGM veterans of color may experience clinician bias in diagnosis and treatment offerings [40, 43]. For example, Black transgender veterans have a higher prevalence of severe mental illness diagnoses but a lower prevalence of depressive disorders in comparison to White transgender veterans [40].

Given the historic barriers faced by those with marginalized identities, it is vital that mental health professionals take an affirmative and multicultural approach when working with SGM veterans of color [44]. Mental health professionals are encouraged to remember that different identities may have various levels of prominence or importance to a particular patient, leading to unique strengths and integration of communities that are difficult to predict. For example, some SGM veterans of color may be less involved with SGM communities [45], which may reflect the importance of their ethnic or racial community relative to the broader SGM community.

SGM veterans in rural areas SGM veterans who live in rural or small communities may be in environments that are less affirming or accepting of SGM individuals and may have more difficulty accessing healthcare [46]. For gay male veterans, living in a rural or small community is associated with greater depressive and anxiety symptoms and lower levels of community-related identification compared to living in urban settings. However, for lesbian or transgender veterans, community size is unrelated to depression or anxiety [46, 47]. Living in rural or small communities is also associated with higher levels of tobacco use among gay male and transgender veterans compared to urban settings [46, 47].

For SGM veterans with PTSD, rural or small town environments may serve as a protective factor against certain triggers [47], although the downside may be less social connectedness to SGM communities [46]. Specifically, gay male veterans living in urban areas report significantly higher levels of LGBT community-related identity relative to gay male veterans in rural areas. For lesbian and transgender veterans, LGBT community identity is unrelated to community size.

Resilience Factors Among SGM Veterans

While it is important to identify and address health risks, assessment of resilience factors and well-being is also important. Adaptive coping strategies, for example, significantly contribute to the successful navigation of distressing situations, relationships, and societal level stigma. The process of coming out to oneself or to another person – that is, accepting and disclosing one's SGM identity – can increase self-esteem and decrease distress in the face of institutional discrimination [48]. However, decisions to not come out or remain closeted may be adaptive within hostile, anti-SGM environments, such as the military during DADT or previous bans on gay/lesbian and transgender service members [18, 48].

Acceptance and pride in one's SGM identity is a critical resiliency factor, and it is the most cited identity-associated strength in one sample of transgender veterans [49]. Greater self-acceptance and positive self-esteem contribute to adaptive coping strategies such as values-driven living, emotional regulation skills, harm reduction, engagement in affirming activities, and stress management for SGM veterans.

Additional contributors to adaptability and resilience include positive relationships with friends and intimate partners, which can function as a buffer against stress and health risk factors [45, 49–51]. Integrating into SGM communities, with its sense of chosen family and safety, can be especially helpful to mitigate distress associated with rejection by family or peer groups after coming out. Building upon community connectedness, SGM advocacy and activism [49, 50] can serve to demonstrate pride in oneself and create a sense of personal meaning by helping others. Advocacy may take the form of overt political activism or one-on-one education with peers and family in response to microaggressions [48, 49].

Case Example
Rae is a 29-year-old White lesbian-identified Air Force veteran who was seen for a mental health intake. She received an honorable discharge 2 years ago. Six months later, she sustained a spinal fracture in an accident and is now using a wheelchair. Rae reported being in a committed monogamous romantic relationship, but she is otherwise socially isolated. She described symptoms consistent with mild depression, including anhedonia, low self-esteem, and low motivation. Rae expressed some reticence in taking psychotropic medication to address her symptoms. She ultimately agreed to make some behavioral and lifestyle changes and scheduled a follow-up appointment in 3 months.

At follow-up, Rae acknowledged reluctantly joining a co-ed wheelchair basketball team at her girlfriend's encouragement. From her first practice session, she began to form connections with women teammates, some of whom were also sexual minorities. Rae eventually noticed a marked improvement in her mood, energy, and motivation. She recognized that part of her improvement was related to integrating into a community of other young, active individuals who used wheelchairs. Inspired by the meaningfulness of this community involvement, Rae has begun looking into opportunities to volunteer with a local LGBTQ organization. She ultimately wants to work with this agency to improve its services for LGBTQ-identifying veterans.

What can be gleaned from this vignette about the role of resilience for Rae?

- Rae's demonstrated resilience appears to be tied to community connectedness, perhaps in addition to more straightforward behavioral activation.
- Rae's community involvement does not explicitly center on her lesbian identity; rather, she has integrated into a community defined by another aspect of difference.
- Rae's future goals involve promoting resilience and inclusiveness for others who share her intersecting sexual minority and veteran identities.

Assessment and Treatment with SGM Veterans: Cultivating Affirming and Culturally Competent Care

Assessment of Identity, Pronouns, and Sexual Risk

Earlier we recommended that providers assess SGM identity in addition to sexual health and behavior. Everyone has a sexual and gender identity, and SGM identity is linked to population-based health disparities. As we reviewed in the previous section, many of these disparities are likely driven by minority stress. Routinely asking all patients about sexual and gender identity in the context of a healthcare assessment reinforces the relationship of identity to health and can facilitate disclosure [52].

Although providers may be uncomfortable asking about sexual and gender identity, and even sexual behavior, it gets easier with practice. Routinely asking all patients about sexual and gender identity also conveys to patients that you are open to discussing any concerns related to sexuality or gender and will likely affirm one's having an SGM identity.

Effective approaches to assessing sexual and gender identity include taking an open, affirmative, and direct stance. Most often these questions can be integrated with other questions about identities and behavior. Providers might first ask about a patient's sex assigned at birth and then ask about gender identity, not assuming the answer to these questions in advance. Asking separately about sex assigned at birth and current gender identity communicates an awareness of their differences.

Example: "I'm going to ask several questions to better understand you who as person. I don't want to make any assumptions. What sex was listed on your original birth certificate – male or female? How do you identify your gender – man, woman, transgender man, transgender woman, or do you use another term? … How do you identify your race or ethnicity? …."

In the context of asking about gender identity, it is important to ask which pronouns the patient uses. While many patients use masculine (he/him/his) or feminine (she/her/hers) pronouns, others may use gender-neutral pronouns. Gender-neutral pronouns include the singular they/them (e.g., My patient reported that they are feeling depressed). Other gender-neutral pronouns have been created within SGM communities to convey a nonbinary approach to language, such as ze/hir (e.g., My patient reported that ze is feeling depressed, which has impacted hir life tremendously). Asking about preferred gender pronouns conveys that one's gender expression is a preference rather than a core aspect of identity; hence, we discourage the use of the word "prefer" in these inquiries.

Example: "OK. You identify your gender as a transgender woman. Which gender pronoun(s) do you use?"

While sexual identity may be viewed as a demographic characteristic, providers may find it convenient to incorporate assessment of sexual identity with routine questions about sexual partners and sexual behaviors.

Example: "Do you have sex with men, women, or both? How would you describe your sexual identity – gay, lesbian (if the patient identifies as a woman), bisexual, straight or heterosexual, or do you use another term? ...."

Example: "Are you currently involved in any significant romantic or sexual relationships? How long have you been together? Are your sexual relationships with men, women, or both? How would you describe your sexual identity – gay, lesbian (if the patient identifies as a woman), bisexual, straight or heterosexual, or do you use another term? ...."

Based on the patient's response, a mental health professional will want to assess for population-based health disparities and sexual health risks. There is not sufficient space here to do justice to a sexual health risk assessment. However, a useful, brief model for sexual health assessment is the Five P's recommended by the Centers for Disease Control and Prevention [53]. The Five P's are *Partners, sexual Practices, Protection from sexually transmitted infections (STI), Past history of STI, and Pregnancy prevention/planning.* While asking about sexual behavior can be uncomfortable, like asking about sexual and gender identity, it gets easier with practice.

Culturally Responsive Assessment and Treatment

Cultivating an affirming, responsive treatment environment for SGM veterans includes recognizing the complex interplay between multiple identities. For example, a 23-year-old Latino gay man who served in the Army and was stationed in Germany from 2013 to 2016 likely had a very different experience navigating his identities than a 93-year-old White Jewish gay man who served in the Army in western Europe during World War II. That these two men, even with shared commonalities, will present with distinct culturally relevant histories, risks, and strengths may seem obvious but should not be underestimated. Thoughtful consideration of each veteran's many identities serves to communicate affirmation, empathy, and a keen awareness of a patient's unique experience.

One helpful framework to identify and examine multiple cultural influences in a patient's lived experience is Pamela Hays' *ADDRESSING model* [54] (see Table 16.2). In addition to identifying dominant and nondominant social identities, the ADDRESSING framework is most effective when further probing or reflection is needed. Using the two Army veterans mentioned previously as an example, a provider might consider (a) significant events (e.g., wars, cultural phenomena) experienced by different generations, (b) policy and legislation (within and outside of the military) aimed toward the disclosure of an SGM identity, and (c) language and its meaning (e.g., the use of the word "queer" may have very different meanings for these two individuals).

Providers can use the ADDRESSING model as a cultural self-assessment tool to become more aware of their own cultural identities.

Healthcare has been moving toward a holistic, patient-centered model of care. Rather than simply identifying and treating specific symptoms, providers are encouraged to help patients achieve maximum functioning and optimal overall well-being. Through this lens, patients are viewed as more than their symptoms; they are understood as whole, complex individuals whose needs extend beyond the immediate reason for their medical visit. Establishing a comprehensive treatment plan includes engaging patients in a discussion about their overall health and wellness goals. This patient-centered concept is especially relevant for SGM veterans because it serves as a counterpoint to the historic trend of pathologizing SGM. Legitimizing SGM veterans' perspectives in defining their own health goals is central to a welcoming, affirming clinical environment.

Table 16.2 Hays' ADDRESSING Framework [54]

Cultural influences	Dominant group	Nondominant/minority group
Age & generational influences	Young/middle aged adults	Children & older adults
Disabilities (Developmental & Acquired)	People without disabilities	People with disabilities (cognitive, sensory, physical, and/or psychiatric)
Religion & spirituality	Christian & secular people	Muslim, Jewish, Hindu, Buddhist & other people of minority religious faith
Ethnic & racial identity	European Americans & White people	Asian, South Asian, Latino, Pacific Islander, African, Arab, Middle Eastern, & people of color
Socioeconomic status	Upper & middle class	People of lower socioeconomic status by occupation, education, income, or habitat (rural/inner city)
Sexual orientation/identity	Heterosexual people	Sexual minorities (people who identify as lesbian, gay, bisexual, queer, or related identities)
Indigenous heritage	European Americans	Native & indigenous people
National origin	USA-born Americans	Immigrants, refugees, & international students
Gender	Men & cisgender people	Women & transgender people

From Hays [54]. Reprinted with permission

Affirming Clinical Practice with SGM Veterans

What makes a clinical environment affirming for SGM veterans? Many SGM individuals find that healthcare environments treat them as invisible at best, or they are dismissive. Other SGM individuals, unfortunately, experience healthcare environments as rejecting and hostile. Consequently, SGM individuals may come to healthcare environments expecting providers to be uninformed, disrespectful, and prejudiced [32]. SGM veterans may be particularly sensitive to perceived stigma and disrespect.

Affirming mental healthcare not only accepts that SGM veterans exist and seek care in all healthcare systems; it prioritizes SGM patients' feelings of safety and validates their experiences and preferences. SGM patients recognize signs in the environment that signal SGM individuals are expected and welcome.

Inherent to affirming healthcare for SGM veterans are mental health professionals who explicitly convey positive views of SGM identities and relationships, including veteran status. Affirming mental health professionals recognize and openly address the effect of social and institutional discrimination affecting SGM veteran patients, such as homophobia, transphobia, and heterosexism. Indeed, affirming mental health treatment with SGM veterans may focus in part on thoughtfully and empathically exploring the intersection of multiple identities as well as the effect of chronic social stigma and prejudice.

Case Example
Shirley is a 48-year-old transgender woman. She presents for a mental health intake after being referred by her primary care provider. Shirley describes moderate-to-severe depressive symptoms, attributed to multiple life stressors that have emerged since leaving her marriage and coming out as transgender (e.g., employment, housing, and financial insecurity). She reports being diagnosed with gender identity disorder (DSM-IV-TR) by a community provider 8 years ago in order to begin hormone therapy. She is happy with the physical changes that resulted from hormone therapy. Shirley has since transferred her transition-related care to VHA and has a current diagnosis of gender dysphoria (DSM-5). In addition to depressive symptoms, she reports severe social anxiety that results in avoiding activities that are necessary for navigating daily tasks such as riding the public bus.

In treatment with Shirley, an affirming mental health professional will:

- Explore Shirley's anticipated responses from others while riding public transit.
- Acknowledge common, ingrained societal and interpersonal transphobia that make even routine activities difficult.
- Prioritize affirming Shirley's identity and maintaining safety over altering cognitive distortions or examining evidence for/against Shirley's anxious cognitions.
- Help Shirley cultivate adaptive coping skills to manage her anxiety and depressive symptoms in order to live a life that is congruent with her goals and values.

Integrated Psychosocial Assessments

Given identified health disparities faced by SGM veterans, mental health professionals should assess for mood and anxiety symptoms, suicidality, problem drinking, problematic substance use, trauma and abuse, experiences of discrimination, and poor health behaviors (e.g., overeating, not exercising) as well as SGM identity development, outness, social support, intimate relationships, and coping skills.

As noted earlier, chronic minority stress can contribute to internalized homophobia or transphobia, low self-esteem, concealment, isolation, and maladaptive patterns of coping. Depending on depth of rapport and the mental health professional's personal style, these experiences may be directly assessed (e.g., "Have you ever experienced discrimination, harassment, or abuse that you believe was in response to your identifying as _____?") or elicited by open-ended inquiry (e.g., "Were you out during your time in the military? What was that like for you?" or "Tell me about your coming out experience").

It is important to know that SGM identity development and the coming out process are not linear processes but certainly multidimensional. SGM veterans may be out to some but not all people in their lives or out in some but not all situations. Some SGM veterans may choose to conceal their SGM identity in situations where they do not feel safe.

Minority stress and its contribution to low self-esteem and shame also help to explain the higher rates of intimate partner violence among SGM communities, especially for bisexual and transgender men and women [55]. Veterans also have higher rates of intimate partner violence than civilians [56], with SGM veterans showing particularly elevated rates in some samples [57]. Unfortunately, low self-esteem and shame also result in SGM patients not voluntarily disclosing violence or abuse in an intimate relationship, even if asked about past trauma experiences.

Specific inquiries targeting dynamics within an intimate relationship may be more effective in revealing this information (e.g., "Do you feel safe in your current relationship?" while specifying that "safety" refers to physical, emotional, and financial security). Another way of asking is, "What happens when you and your partner fight?" or "Has your partner ever pushed, slapped, punched, or hit you?"

Assessment of intimate partner relationships also entails evaluation of the value and meaningfulness of the relationship and other sexual partners. Marriage or commitment to a relationship should not be taken to mean monogamy. Some SGM people in committed relationships have other sexual partners, either alone or together by agreement.

Discussion about sexual partners is a good time to talk about sexual risk behaviors. Some sexually transmitted infections are more prevalent among veterans and SGM individuals than among civilians and cisgender and heterosexual people. In one sample of VHA users [23], transgender veterans were five times more likely to have HIV than cisgender veterans. As noted previously, the Five P's [53] are a useful model for assessing sexual health and risk.

Transgender Care and Resources

Within VHA, *Directive 1341* [29] outlines the transition-related services for transgender veterans. These services are provided in VHA facilities or, if unavailable on-site, outsourced to the community and covered by VHA. Mental health professionals play an integral role in transgender veterans' healthcare in VHA.

Within and outside VHA, mental health professionals can conduct readiness assessments for transgender veterans seeking transition-related services (e.g., hormone therapy, surgeries). These readiness assessments include a clinical interview of the patient's psychosocial and clinical background, a history of gender dysphoria, information about a patient's identity development and coming out process, and expectations or treatment goals [58]. Table 16.3 outlines the main areas of evaluation covered during a readiness assessment for hormone treatment or surgical procedures.

Table 16.3 Assessment of Readiness for Gender Confirmation Treatment

History and development of gender dysphoria
Process in deciding to pursue gender confirmation treatment
Gender identity development
Background/psychosocial information
Living situation
Employment/school environment
Social environment
General social support system(s)
Significant relationships (friends, family, romantic/intimate partners)
Goals for hormone treatment
Steps already taken toward masculinization/feminization
Changes in appearance, voice, and/or mannerisms
Support seeking or community involvement
Patient's knowledge of process/procedures involved in treatment
Understanding risks and benefits
Realistic expectations for outcome
Cognitive ability to make informed decision
Psychosocial implications of engaging in gender confirmation treatment
Preparation for managing psychosocial domains
Living situation
Employment/school environment
Social environment and specific relationships
History of adherence to medical care treatment
Mental status
Psychiatric history
Assessment and diagnosis of gender dysphoria
Recommendations to enhance readiness for successful gender confirmation treatment

Historically, mental health professionals have been regarded as "gatekeepers" by transgender individuals seeking transition-related care [58]. That is, mental health professionals have frequently played the role of deciding whether and when a transgender patient merited access to hormones or surgery. More recently, mental health professionals have shifted to an "informed consent model," whereby readiness assessments serve to explore patients' goals and expectations, understanding of treatment risks and benefits, and plan for managing the social effects of transitioning and refer to resources for support.

After completing a readiness assessment, the mental health professional may write a letter of support for the patient's physician facilitating the particular gender confirmation treatment (e.g., a primary care provider, an endocrinologist, or a surgeon) [34, 58]. Readiness assessments and a letter of support are usually required by physicians who follow the World Professional Association for Transgender Health's (WPATH's) Standards of Care [59] and/or the clinical practice guidelines published by the US Endocrine Society [60]. Table 16.4 briefly summarizes the WPATH's Standards of Care, 7th edition (www.wpath.org), that are relevant for mental health professionals.

Table 16.4 WPATH Standards of Care: Criteria for Transition-Related Services [59]

WPATH Standards of Care: Criteria for Gender Affirmation Procedures
For adult patients seeking hormone therapy or chest reconstructive surgery:
One assessment or referral is required by a mental health professional, in which the below is described:
Diagnosed and documented gender dysphoria
Capacity to consent to treatment and make informed healthcare-related decisions
Age of majority in country where services are provided
Any significant medical or mental health issues are reasonably addressed or monitored
For mastectomy in AFAB patients:
Hormone therapy not required before undergoing surgery
For breast augmentation in AMAB patients:
At least 1 year of feminizing hormone therapy is recommended before undergoing surgery (not required)
For adult patients seeking genital reconstructive surgery:
Two assessments or referrals are required by separate mental health professionals (a current treatment provider and an objective evaluator), in which the below is described:
Diagnosed and documented gender dysphoria
Capacity to consent to treatment and make informed healthcare-related decisions
Age of majority in country where services are provided
Any significant medical or mental health issues are reasonably addressed or monitored
For hysterectomy, ovariectomy, or orchiectomy:
At least 1 year of hormone therapy in accordance with patient's goals for gender affirmation (unless the patient is unable or unwilling to do so)
For metoidioplasty, phalloplasty, or vaginoplasty:
At least 1 year of hormone therapy in accordance with patient's goals for gender affirmation (unless the patient is unable or unwilling to do so)
At least 1 year of living in a gender role that is congruent with patient's gender identity

The WPATH Standards of Care are intended as minimum guidelines for medical and mental health professionals; individual clinics or providers may adapt them in response to a patient's individual needs or circumstances. The VHA policy and practices for transition-related hormone therapy are informed by and generally consistent with, but independent of, the WPATH Standards of Care and the Endocrine Society guidelines. As noted earlier, VHA at this time does not conduct or pay for gender confirming surgeries.

In addition to readiness assessments, mental health professionals also provide gender counseling and gender-affirming psychotherapy, which can occur within the context of many different psychotherapy modalities. Whether a direct service provider, consultant, or advocate, mental health professionals are critical for fostering affirming, individualized, and equitable healthcare for transgender veterans in any healthcare system.

Gender affirming care best operates within an integrated health, patient-centered framework [34, 44]. It is important to note that there is no standard gender transition path. Each patient's transition is unique to their personal needs and goals, and these should be individually assessed with each patient. Some transgender veterans will seek all possible medical interventions for gender transitioning, including hormone therapy and gender confirmation surgeries (i.e., "top" [chest] and/or "bottom" [genital] surgery). Others will opt for hormone therapy alone without surgeries. Still others will pursue mainly social interventions, including changes in gender expression (e.g., clothes) and change in name and/or pronouns used. Transition-related goals may change over time in response to the individual's identity development, psychosocial factors, and social or medical transitioning.

Case Example
Lou is a 58-year-old Black Army veteran who was assigned male at birth. Lou identifies as pansexual and nonbinary and uses they/them pronouns. Lou has been referred for a Mental Health/Readiness Assessment before initiating feminizing hormone therapy. A complex and lengthy psychiatric history is revealed through a chart review.

At various times throughout their contacts with VA Psychiatry and Psychology departments, Lou has received diagnoses of major depressive disorder, severe with psychotic features; posttraumatic stress disorder; psychotic disorder NOS; bipolar disorder; cannabis use disorder; cocaine use disorder; substance-induced psychotic disorder; and borderline personality disorder. They currently take gabapentin daily, prescribed by their VA psychiatrist of 2 years. Lou reportedly has a history of cocaine dependence but has not used cocaine in 4 years; they currently endorse daily marijuana use.

When Lou arrives to their appointment, they enthusiastically and spontaneously share their political beliefs, cynicism toward the US military and government, and close relationships within a community of performers in the nearby city. Lou's mood is slightly expanded but denies any hallucinatory or delusional processes. They are quite verbose and at times difficult to redirect. Lou describes a long-standing sense (for the past 20 years) of not fully identifying as a man and having many negative opinions toward "compulsory masculinity." Lou states that they are seeking hormone therapy to "expand [their] horizons" and "unlock [their] femininity." They do not plan to seek transition-related procedures beyond feminizing hormones. Upon further inquiry, Lou expresses awareness of the anticipated effects of feminizing hormones, including physical changes that may be irreversible if they were to discontinue hormone therapy. Lou is excited by the opportunity to live "a box-free life" and to increase their potential of "seeing things from any gender angle."

> **Box 16.2 Resources Available for VHA Staff**
> - LGBT Veteran Care Coordinators
>   – Located at each VHA facility
>   – Roles include maintaining welcoming environment for SGM veterans, addressing gaps in clinical care, providing education and training for staff
> - Staff trainings
>   – Online trainings
>   - On-demand, outside VHA facilities (https://www.patientcare.va.gov/LGBT/LGBT_Veteran_Training.asp)
>   - Internal VA trainings through LGBT SharePoint
>   – Consultation on healthcare for transgender veterans through national e-consultation teams
>   – Interdisciplinary team training on transgender healthcare through Specialty Care Access Network - Extension for Community Healthcare Outcomes (SCAN-ECHO), multi-session, case-based videoconferencing
> - Interprofessional postdoctoral Psychology Fellowships in LGBT Health – 1 year positions at 9 VHA sites

In considering Lou's presentation and goals, several key points emerge in determining the best next steps:

- Lou has articulated their personalized transition-related goals (i.e., to take feminizing hormones but not pursue surgeries). An affirming, patient-centered approach includes supporting Lou's preferences, as long as health and safety risks are minimized.
- A discussion with Lou will facilitate their informed consent to receive hormone therapy. This discussion includes the anticipated physical effects of feminizing hormones, what changes are irreversible, and potential health risks.
- Lou's odd presentation and complex psychiatric history do not preclude their engagement in transition-related healthcare. Indeed, Lou's unstable emotionality may improve with treatment of their chronic gender dysphoria.
- Consistent use of Lou's identified name and gender pronoun will help create and maintain an affirming clinical environment.
- Lou might benefit from additional support:

- If Lou is at a VHA facility, the local LGBT Veteran Care Coordinator can be a helpful resource if Lou has negative experiences with other VHA providers regarding their gender identity, name, and pronouns.
- Psychotherapy services for untreated conditions or for ongoing support when initiating hormone therapy may be helpful.
- Referral to community transgender or LGBT support groups, if desired, may enhance social support.

Summary and Conclusion

SGM individuals are a key subgroup in the US military and veteran population. As visibility grows and cultural barriers diminish, it is likely that the SGM veteran population will continue to grow. For a variety of reasons, many SGM veterans will seek mental healthcare outside of the VHA. Therefore, it is critical that community mental health professionals are mindful of the intersecting health concerns of SGM veterans and able to provide culturally and clinically appropriate care.

Meyer's minority stress framework [1] provides a useful lens through which mental health professionals can better understand SGM health disparities. SGM veterans are disproportionately affected by psychiatric conditions, including depression and suicidal ideation, anxiety, problematic drinking and drug use and smoking, and posttraumatic stress. However, resilience mechanisms can serve as powerful counterbalances to minority stressors in the form of self-acceptance and LGBTQ pride, self-identity as an SGM, affirming and supportive relationships, and community engagement and activism.

Providing equitable and affirming care to SGM veterans has been embedded within VHA's treatment standards and guidelines. Mental health professionals in non-VHA healthcare systems can foster a welcoming clinical environment for SGM veterans by providing culturally attuned, affirming, and thoughtful approaches to clinical assessment and treatment. Mental health professionals can also play a powerful role as SGM consultants and advocates within interdisciplinary treatment teams, especially for transgender veterans. The provision of affirming patient-centered mental healthcare for SGM veterans in a welcoming clinical environment has the potential to reduce chronic minority stress, minimize maladaptive coping strategies, bolster adaptive coping skills, and foster personal growth and well-being. Ultimately, SGM veterans should be able to receive culturally responsive and appropriate mental healthcare wherever they get care.

References

1. Meyer I. Prejudice, social stress, and mental health in lesbian, gay, and bisexual populations: conceptual issues and research evidence. Psychol Bull. 2003;129(5):674–97.
2. Kauth MR, Shipherd JC, editors. Adult transgender care: an interdisciplinary approach for training mental health professionals. New York: Routledge; 2018.

3. Gates GJ. *How many people are lesbian, gay, bisexual, and transgender?* Los Angeles: Williams Institute, UCLA School of Law; 2011.
4. Gates GJ, Herman JL. *Transgender Military Service in the United States.* Los Angeles: Williams Institute, UCLA School of Law; 2014.
5. Gates GJ. *Lesbian, gay, and bisexual men and women in the US military: updated estimates.* Los Angeles: Williams Institute, UCLA School of Law; 2010.
6. Hoover KW, Tao KL, Peters PJ. Nationally representative prevalence estimates of gay, bisexual, and other men who have sex with men who have served in the US military. PLoS One. 2017;12(8):E01822222.
7. Brown GR. Transsexuals in the military: flight into hypermasculinity. Arch Sex Behav. 1988;17(6):527–37.
8. Kauth MR, Shipherd JC. Transforming a system: improving patient-centered care for sexual and gender minority veterans. LGBT Health. 2016;3(3):177–9.
9. National LGBT Health Education Center. Glossary of LGBT terms for health care teams. www.lgbthealtheducation.org/wp-content/uploads/LGBT-Glossary_March2016.pdf. Updated March 2016. Accessed 14 Nov 2017.
10. Bostwick WB, Boyd CJ, Hughes TL, McCabe SE. Dimensions of sexual orientation and the prevalence of mood and anxiety disorders in the United States. Am J Public Health. 2010;100(3):468–75.
11. McCabe SE, Hughes TL, Bostwick WB, West BT, Boyd CJ. Sexual orientation, substance use behaviors and substance dependence in the United States. Addiction. 2009;104(8):1333–45.
12. Department of Veterans Affairs. Provision of health care for veterans who identify as lesbian, gay or bisexual (VHA Directive 1340). https://www.va.gov/vhapublications/publications.cfm?pub=1. Accessed 14 Oct 2017.
13. Practitioners Disagree on NHS Recommendation to Ask Patients About Sexual Orientation. Psychiatry advisor https://www.psychiatryadvisor.com/practice-management/section/4032/. Published 30 Jan 2018. Accessed 8 April 2018.
14. Fletcher JB, Reback CJ. Mental health disorders among homeless, substance-dependent men who have sex with men. Drug Alcohol Rev. 2017;36(4):555–9.
15. Balsam KF, Rothblum ED, Beauchaine TP. Victimization over the life span: a comparison of lesbian, gay, bisexual, and heterosexual siblings. J Consult Clin Psychol. 2005;73(3):477–87.
16. Testa RJ, Habarth J, Peta J, Balsam K, Bockting W. Development of the gender minority stress and resilience measure. Psychol Sex Orientat Gend Divers. 2015;2(1):65–77.
17. Crenshaw K. Demarginalizing the intersection of race and sex: a black feminist critique of antidiscrimination doctrine, feminist theory and antiracist politics. Univ Chic Leg Forum. 1989;1989(1):139–67.
18. Cochran BN, Balsam KF, Flentje A, Malte CA, Simpson T. Mental health characteristics of sexual minority veterans. J Homosex. 2013;60:419–35.
19. Blosnich J, Foynes MM, Shipherd JC. Health disparities among sexual minority women. J Women's Health. 2013;22(7):631–6.
20. Lehavot K, Williams EC, Millard SP, Bradley KA, Simpson TL. Association of alcohol misuse with sexual identity and sexual behavior in women veterans. Subst Use Misuse. 2016;51(2):216–29.
21. Lehavot K, Simpson TL. Trauma, posttraumatic stress disorder, and depression among sexual minority and heterosexual women veterans. J Couns Psychol. 2014;61(3):392–403.
22. Mattocks KM, Sadler A, Yano EM, et al. Sexual victimization, health status, and VA healthcare utilization among lesbian and bisexual OEF/OIF veterans. J Gen Intern Med. 2013;28(Suppl 2):S604–8.
23. Brown GR, Jones KT. Mental health and medical health disparities in 5135 transgender veterans receiving healthcare in the veterans health administration: a case-control study. LGBT Health. 2016;3(2):122–31.
24. Blosnich JR, Brown GR, Shipherd JC, Kauth M, Piegari RI, Bossarte RM. Prevalence of gender identity disorder and suicide risk among transgender veterans utilizing veterans health administration care. Am J Public Health. 2013;103(10):e27–32.

25. Harrison-Quintana J, Herman JL. Still serving in silence: transgender service members and veterans in the National Transgender Discrimination Survey. LGBTQ Policy J. 2012;13:1–13.
26. Hatzenbuehler ML, Keyes KM, Hasin DS. State-level policies and psychiatric morbidity in lesbian, gay, and bisexual populations. Am J Public Health. 2009;99(12):2275–81.
27. Hatzenbuehler ML, McLaughlin KA, Keyes KM, Hasin DS. (2010). The impact of institutional discrimination on psychiatric disorders in lesbian, gay, and bisexual populations: a prospective study. Am J Public Health. 2010;100(3):452–9. https://doi.org/10.2105/AJPH.2009.168815
28. Blosnich JR, Marsiglio MC, Gao S, et al. Mental health of transgender veterans in US states with and without discrimination and hate crime legal protection. Am J Public Health. 2016;106(3):534–40.
29. Department of Veterans Affairs. Providing health care for transgender and intersex veterans (VHA Directive 2013–003). Retrieved from http://www.va.gov/vhapublications/ViewPublication.asp?pub_ID=2863. Accessed 14 Oct 2017.
30. Institute of Medicine. The health of lesbian, gay, bisexual, and transgender people: building a foundation for better understanding. Washington, DC: The National Academies Press; 2011.
31. James SE, Herman JL, Rankin S, Keisling M, Mottet L, Anafi M. The report of the 2015 U.S. transgender survey. Washington, DC: National Center for Transgender Equality; 2016.
32. Sherman MD, Kauth MR, Ridener L, Shipherd JC, Bratkovich K, Beaulieu G. An empirical investigation of challenges and recommendations for welcoming sexual and gender minority veterans into VA care. Prof Psychol Res Pract. 2014;45(6):433–42. https://doi.org/10.1037/a0034826.
33. Sherman MD, Kauth MR, Shipherd JC, Street RL. Communication between VA providers and sexual and gender minority veterans: a pilot study. Psychol Serv. 2014;11(2):235–42. https://doi.org/10.1037/a0035840.
34. Johnson L, Shipherd J, Walton HW. The psychologist's role in transgender-specific care with U.S. veterans. Psychol Serv. 2016;13(1):69–76.
35. Simpson TL, Balsam KF, Cochran BN, Lehavot K, Gold SD. Veterans administration health care utilization among sexual minority veterans. Psychol Serv. 2013;10(2):223–32.
36. Kauth MR, Barrera TL, Latini DM. Lesbian, gay, and transgender veterans' experiences in the veterans health administration: positive signs and room for improvement. Psychol Serv. 2018;01:25.
37. Fredriksen-Goldsen KI. The future of LGBT+ aging: a blueprint for action in services, policies, and research. J Am Soc Aging. 2016;40(2):6–15.
38. Monin JK, Mota N, Levy B, Pachankis J, Pietrzak RH. Older age associated with mental health resiliency in sexual minority US veterans. Am J Geriatr Psychiatry. 2017;25(1):81–90.
39. Hoy-Ellis CP, Shiu C, Sullivan KM, Kim HJ, Sturges AM, Fredriksen-Goldsen KI. Prior military service, identity stigma, and mental health among transgender older adults. The Gerontologist. 2017;57(suppl 1):S63–71. https://doi.org/10.1093/geront/gnw173.
40. Brown GR, Jones KT. Racial health disparities in a cohort of 5,135 transgender veterans. J Racial Ethn Health Disparities. 2014;1:257–66.
41. Balsam KF, Molina Y, Blayney JA, Dillworth T, Zimmerman L, Kaysen D. Racial/ethnic differences in identity and mental health outcomes among young sexual minority women. Cult Divers Ethn Minor Psychol. 2015;21(3):380–90.
42. Spoont MR, Sayer NA, Kehle-Forbes SM, Meis LA, Nelson DB. A prospective study of racial and ethnic variation in VA psychotherapy services for PTSD. Psychiatr Serv. 2017;68(3):231–7.
43. Dovidio JF, Fiske ST. Under the radar: how unexamined biases in decision-making processes in clinical interactions can contribute to health care disparities. Am J Public Health. 2012;102(5):945–52.
44. Chang SC, Singh AA. Affirming psychological practice with transgender and gender nonconforming people of color. Psychol Sex Orientat Gend Divers. 2016;3(2):140–7.
45. Zimmerman L, Darnell DA, Rhew IC, Lee CM, Kaysen D. Resilience in community: a social ecological development model for young adult sexual minority women. Am J Community Psychol. 2015;55:179–90.

46. Kauth MR, Barrera TL, Denton FN, Latini DM. Health differences among lesbian, gay, and transgender veterans by rural/small town and suburban/urban setting. LGBT Health. 2017;4(3):194–201.
47. Bukowski LA, Blosnich J, Shipherd JC, Kauth MR, Brown GR, Gordon AJ. Exploring rural disparities in medical diagnoses among veterans with transgender-related diagnoses utilizing veterans health administration care. Med Care. 2017;55(9):S97–S103.
48. Van Gilder BJ. Coping with sexual identity stigma in the U.S. military: an examination of identity management practices prior to and after the repeal of "Don't Ask, Don't Tell". Identity. 2017;17(3):156–75.
49. Chen JA, Granato H, Shipherd JC, Simpson T, Lehavot K. A qualitative analysis of transgender veterans' lived experiences. Psychol Sex Orientat Gend Divers. 2017;4(1):63–74.
50. Colpitts E, Gahagan J. The utility of resilience as a conceptual framework for understanding and measuring LGBTQ health. Int J Equity Health. 2016;15(1):60.
51. Rostosky SS, Riggle EDB. Same-sex couple relationship strengths: a review and synthesis of the empirical literature (2000-2016). Psychol Sex Orientat Gend Divers. 2017;4(3):1–13.
52. Maragh-Bass AC, Torain M, Adler R, et al. Is it okay to ask: transgender patient perspectives on sexual orientation and gender identity collection in healthcare. Acad Emerg Med. 2017;24(6):655–67.
53. Centers for Disease Control and Prevention. A guide to taking a sexual history. Accessed at https://www.cdc.gov/std/treatment/sexualhistory.pdf. 2011.
54. Hays PA. Addressing cultural complexities in practice: assessment, diagnosis, and therapy. 3rd ed. Washington, DC: American Psychological Association; 2016.
55. Brown TNT, Herman JL. Intimate partner violence and sexual abuse among LGBT people: a review of existing research. Los Angeles: The Williams Institute, UCLA School of Law; 2015.
56. Dichter ME, Cerulli C, Bossarte BM. Intimate partner violence victimization among women veterans and associated heart risks. Womens Health Issues. 2011;21(4):S190–4.
57. Dardis CM, Shipherd JC, Iverson KM. Intimate partner violence among women veterans by sexual orientation. Women Health. 2017;57(7):775–91.
58. Coolhart D, Provancher N, Hager A, Wang M. Recommending transsexual clients for gender transition: a therapeutic tool for assessing readiness. J GLBT Fam Stud. 2008;4(3):310–24.
59. World Professional Association for Transgender Health. Standards of care for the health of transsexual, transgender, and gender nonconforming people. Accessed at https://s3.amazonaws.com/amo_hub_content/Association140/files/Standards%20of%20Care%20V7%20-%202011%20WPATH%20(2)(1).pdf.2012.
60. Hembree WC, Cohen-Kettenis PT, Gooren L, Hannema SE, Meyer WJ, Murad MH, Rosenthal SM, et al. Endocrine treatment of gender-dysphoric/gender-incongruent persons: an Endocrine Society Endocrine Society clinical practice guideline. J Clin Endocrinol Metab. 2017;102(11):3869–903.

Older Veterans

17

John T. Little, Bryan A. Llorente, and Maria D. Llorente

Background and Demographics

Older veterans (typically those aged 65 years and above) have served in multiple conflicts, including World War II, the Korean War, the Vietnam War, and even the Persian Gulf War. In 2015, approximately 43% of men aged 65 or older were veterans (compared with only 5% of those under age 45 [1]. This higher proportion of veterans among older men is primarily due to the draft that was implemented from 1940 to 1973. The median age of draft-era veterans is 72 years, with the largest (median age 68 years) being those who served during the Vietnam era. Most of these veterans are white or non-Hispanic and have at least a high-school education. As veterans age, they move West and South, particularly to California, Texas, and Florida [2].

Veterans are living longer. Currently, approximately 2 million veterans are older than 80 years. Veterans who reach 100 years are predominantly male (94%) and white (82%) and served during World War II (92.5%) [3]. As a group, centenarian veterans were found to have a lower incidence of chronic illnesses after age 80 when compared with veteran octogenarians and nonagenarians. Interestingly, this cohort

---

J. T. Little (✉)
Departments of Psychiatry and Neurology, Georgetown University School of Medicine, Washington, DC, USA

Geriatric Mental Health Services, Department of Veterans Affairs Medical Center, Department of Psychiatry, Washington, DC, USA
e-mail: john.little5@va.gov

B. A. Llorente
College of Health Professions and Sciences, University of Central Florida, Orlando, FL, USA

M. D. Llorente
Georgetown University School of Medicine, Washington DC VA Medical Center, Department of Psychiatry, Washington, DC, USA

of veterans displayed similar compression of morbidity and extension of health span observed in nonveteran cohorts of centenarians, which are predominantly female.

Mental Health Considerations Among Older Veterans

Older veterans are at increased risk for mental health disorders for several reasons. First, older veterans, particularly men, have been found to be vulnerable to isolation and loneliness which are risk factors for depression [4, 5]. Second, older veterans are more likely to have been exposed to combat. Veterans also are more likely to enter occupations, such as police officers, firemen, and emergency medical personnel, with increased risk for traumatic exposures and associated stress-related conditions. As a result, veterans may experience chronic symptoms of PTSD and associated poorer outcomes [7–9], including a higher risk for suicide.

Third, older veterans have been found to have a higher prevalence of substance use disorders [10, 11]. Lastly, Vietnam veterans were exposed to Agent Orange. While this occupational exposure in and of itself is not known to cause mental health concerns, it is associated with several chronic medical conditions and cancer, which are significant stressors that add to the psychological burden of the older veteran.

Several recent studies have found that the Veterans Health Administration efforts to increase both detection of mental conditions through routine system-wide screening and access have increased mental health service utilization [12]. The increased detection and access have been reported to be contributory to the higher prevalence of some mental disorders in veteran populations utilizing the VA.

Serious Mental Illness

A recent meta-analysis reported that the pooled prevalence of schizophrenia among older veterans was 11.2% [11]. This rate is higher than that found in the general population and likely reflects the higher access and mental health service utilization of veterans who are engaged with VA services. Similarly, and for similar reasons, the prevalence rate of bipolar disorder is higher than that seen in the general population and averaged 3.9%.

Substance Use Disorders

Among older veterans, the pooled prevalence rates of substance use disorders were 5.7% and that of alcohol use disorders was 5.4% [11]. These rates are higher (more than double) than prevalence rates in the US older adult population. This finding could be due to the VA routinely screening for these disorders and thus identifying more cases than occurs in civilian groups. Conversely, this may also reflect the high proportion of substance and alcohol use found in Vietnam veterans, particularly those with PTSD, who are also more likely to receive their care in the VA.

Military-/Combat-Related PTSD

For some individuals, PTSD can be a chronic, life-long struggle, with periods of improved coping, alternating with periods of acute worsening, triggered by life stressors. A community sample found that 70% of older men and 41% of older women were exposed to at least one lifetime trauma [13]. The primary traumatic exposure to explain this gender difference was combat among the men. Among older male combat veterans, the prevalence of current PTSD was 29% [14], and more than half reported lifetime prevalence of PTSD. Among a large community primary care sample of older veterans, 12% endorsed PTSD symptoms [6]. These veterans reported poorer general health, little to no social support, and a higher prevalence of mental distress, death wishes, and suicidal ideation when compared with veterans who had no trauma exposure or who reported no PTSD symptoms. The data from this sample were further analyzed [7]. PTSD symptoms were found to have a chronic and fluctuating course and were associated with lower mental health quality of life. At least one large epidemiologic study has found that Vietnam veterans with PTSD may be at increased risk of death from multiple causes [9]. While the reasons for this finding are unknown, it is likely due to a combination of biopsychosocial factors. Further, veterans who have greater degrees of distress or whose symptoms significantly interfere with functioning, such as those who receive residential treatment, are likely to have behavioral causes of death, such as accidents (29.4%), chronic substance abuse (14.7%), and intentional death by suicide, homicide, or the police (13.8%) [15].

Assessment of PTSD

Older veterans may not spontaneously report trauma exposure or symptoms of PTSD. Initial visits should include routine inquiry regarding these experiences, even if the military service occurred many years ago. Older adults, including veterans, are more likely to endorse physical symptoms, such as insomnia or pain, rather than psychological concerns, such as anxiety or depression. Additionally, veterans may report irritability, difficulty getting along with supervisors or coworkers, or family conflicts as the primary concern. Additional questions can often identify an association with PTSD symptoms and trauma exposure. While normative studies for older adults are not yet available for the DSM-5 version of the Clinician-Administered PTSD Scale [16] or the PTSD Checklist [17], both of these instruments' older versions have been validated for use with older adults.

Course of PTSD

The symptoms of PTSD can continue into older age or at times may recur or worsen. There are several reasons for this. First, older veterans may have been coping with these symptoms through the use of illicit substances and/or alcohol. As they age and develop chronic medical conditions or experience adverse consequences of these behaviors, they stop using and then need to address their symptoms directly.

Second, many veterans may spend long hours in the workplace as a way to distract themselves and avoid their symptoms. After retirement, however, they no longer have this means to avoid and, with more free time, may experience increased introspection and recollection of traumatic events. Third, life-threatening diagnoses, such as cancer, can trigger similar feelings that were experienced when their life was threatened in combat. Veterans may note heightened anxiety, hypervigilance, and insomnia, but not make the connection with their previous combat experience.

Lastly, veterans may have been able to cope with their trauma exposure through repression of memories, but with the onset of neurocognitive disorders, they may become unable to continue to use this coping mechanism, and PTSD symptoms may recur. A recently described process, known as late-onset stress symptomatology (LOSS) refers to the development of increasing recollections and emotional responses to combat experiences. This can often occur in the context of physical limitations, health problems, or deaths of family and friends and may even develop in veterans who have led productive and functional lives [18, 19]. LOSS, when compared with PTSD, may be related to a search for meaning and growth in later life, rather than clinically significant distress [20].

Treatment of PTSD

There are very few randomized large clinical trials of psychotherapy efficacy to treat PTSD in older adults. The National Center for PTSD does report a pilot study that demonstrated that prolonged exposure was both efficacious and feasible with older veterans [21]. VA/DOD Clinical Practice Guidelines for PTSD reported a clinical trial of imaginal exposure in older persons following a cardiovascular event, and no adverse outcomes resulted [22]. The Guidelines report that trauma-focused psychotherapy is more effective than medications in the treatment of PTSD. However, if there are co-occurring depressive or other anxiety disorders, the use of selective serotonin reuptake inhibitors can be used. Only sertraline and paroxetine have FDA approval to treat PTSD. Prazosin has also been reported to be effective for combat-related PTSD with nightmares in both veterans and active-duty soldiers [23, 24]. However, more recently, a large multicenter randomized clinical trial has questioned this finding [25]. The patients in this larger trial were more psychosocially stable, and long period of placebo treatment (6 months) could have precluded patients who were more symptomatic from participation. There are patients, however, who do benefit from prazosin particularly for the nightmares.

While no randomized clinical trials have been specifically conducted among older veterans, a recent meta-analysis of meditation and yoga for PTSD was published [26], indicating a role for these two modalities in the management of PTSD. The American Heart Association has published a scientific statement that meditation may benefit cardiovascular risk and should be considered an adjunctive intervention. Both yoga and meditation are relatively low-cost and low-risk strategies and should be feasible to use with older veterans, experiencing PTSD symptoms.

Social Connectedness and Older Veterans

Social Connectedness and Health

With expanding research into social networks and their impact on human health, a correlation between social connectedness and overall mental and physical health has been reported, especially among older adults. Individuals who identify themselves as socially isolated face a higher risk of poorer general health, depression, and death from several infectious, neoplastic, and cardiovascular diseases, as well as suicide [27]. While social isolation, at any age, is a risk factor for morbidity and mortality, older adults are particularly vulnerable. Stress-related hormones, such as adrenaline and cortisol, normally regulate [28] blood pressure, blood sugar levels, and metabolism and assist with memory formulation. The overproduction of these hormones, which can occur when an individual experiences high levels of stress and lack of social connectedness, could lead to heart problems, high blood pressure, increased tobacco and alcohol use, and reduced health behaviors [29] and are particularly problematic among older adults who already have these comorbidities.

Military Cohesion

The military has a unique culture, which becomes embedded within the service member. Just because someone separates from the military, this cultural identity is not easily, nor typically, abandoned. A national poll taken in 2014 by *The Washington Post* and *The Keiser Family Foundation* found that 87% of Iraq and Afghanistan veterans were proud of their military service, despite 92% of that sample coming back with severe injuries [30].

Joining the military is unlike any other job. One's life is dependent on fellow service members and vice versa. Teamwork is a critical component of military culture. Unit cohesion has been defined as the "bonding together of soldiers in such a way as to sustain their will and commitment to each other, the unit, and mission accomplishment, despite combat or mission stress" [31].

Training is focused on developing horizontal cohesion (that with fellow service members) and vertical cohesion (allegiance to the commander). Therefore, social cohesion is integral to military service and military culture. Service members endure long periods of separation from family and civilian friends and endure significant stresses and hardships. They are exposed to traumatic and life-threatening events during combat. These unique shared experiences create bonds that are often stronger than family ties. Civilians do not fully understand these experiences and often have difficulty empathizing or relating.

A basic human need is to feel understood and to have like-minded people around you. The following social experiment illustrates this point. Simply engage in a conversation with someone, and after each time they voice an opinion, say "what?" as if you don't understand. The longer one does this, the angrier and more frustrated the other person will become. That frustration of not being understood is similar to what many isolated persons experience. Veterans who do not feel understood will experience increasing frustration and anger and often isolate socially.

A recent VA study of 800 National Guard and Reserve troops found that soldiers who reported higher levels of unit cohesion were more resilient to mental health problems, including PTSD. The researchers hypothesized that strong unit cohesion serves as a "natural intervention." Soldiers can discuss their problems with fellow service members who know what they may be trying to deal with and may help them learn strategies to cope with stressors [32]. This suggests that group therapy offers a treatment modality that may be particularly acceptable to veterans and effective in enhancing resilience.

Use of Group Therapy to Enhance Social Cohesion Among Veterans

Group therapy is an effective strategy that can be used either alone or as part of a comprehensive treatment plan in the management of PTSD, depression, and suicide prevention [33]. Yalom outlined the main principles of group therapy as follows [34]:

1. Instillation of hope: enables members to see people who are coping with similar problems and are in recovery.
2. Universality: members share similar experiences, which enables people to see that they are not alone.
3. Imparting information: members share resources and other information.
4. Altruism: members share coping strategies and help each other.
5. Development of socialization: members can practice new behaviors with others who are supportive.
6. Imitative behavior: members can model the behavior of each other or the facilitator.
7. Group cohesion: members gain sense of belonging and acceptance.
8. Catharsis: members share feelings with people who understand and can relieve guilt and distress.

Group therapy can promote cohesion and a sense of social connectedness among veterans who have the shared experience of combat and may only feel comfortable discussing these events with other combat veterans. These groups enable sharing of resources and information, as well as coping strategies.

Narrative Medicine and Film

An additional modality that can be used in the group format is narrative medicine [35]. This is an approach that aims to validate the experience of the patient by attending to the story of illness, not just the symptoms. Part of the value in telling the story is having the opportunity to have others serve as witness to the experience of the individual. At the same time, the individual has the opportunity to verbalize their thoughts and feelings about the experience and to have others validate these feelings and offer emotional support to promote healing.

In order to facilitate the telling of the story, different forms of stimuli can be used, including poetry, short stories, and film. There are several advantages for the use of film. First, many people are visual learners. Second, film serves as a therapeutic strategy by first showing the individual that they are not alone in experiencing the target symptoms and facilitates a sense of connectedness. Third, the person can utilize similar coping mechanisms to those depicted in the film and make adjustments based on their own experiences. Lastly, films demonstrate concepts of self-disclosure, making it easier for the individual to develop trust and share their personal story.

The utilization of film in treating veterans with mental health disorders is a relatively new concept, and more research is needed to determine effectiveness rates. However, in a pilot program, 96% of Vietnam combat veterans in a support group who were exposed to a documentary film about Vietnam veteran experiences reported that the film made them remember their experiences, 100% agreed they enjoyed talking about the experience with other veterans, and 94% agreed that watching the movie and discussing it afterward was helpful to their recovery [36].

Using film as part of a group modality enables veterans to process the film together in a safe and nonjudgmental setting. Because veterans may be in various stages of recovery, informing them at the onset that if at any time during the film they feel uncomfortable, they can leave the room increases sense of control. After the film, an open discussion is conducted. Utilizing open-ended questions throughout the discussion will allow the veterans to discuss and process the film together.

The selection of the film is also an important consideration. The intent is to facilitate discussion and social connectedness. Films that depict highly emotionally charged battle scenes, contain gore or shock footage, or deliver political sentiments are typically unsuitable. Films that are documentaries of specific events that occurred during the war, primarily told by veterans, are preferred. A final component of this type of session is to obtain feedback from the veterans to assess their preferences, the impact of the film on symptoms, and satisfaction with the therapeutic modality.

Dementia

In the Diagnostic and Statistical Manual of Mental Disorders, 5th Edition [37], *dementia* is subsumed under the newly named entity *major neurocognitive disorder*. Major neurocognitive disorder is defined in DSM-5 [37] as (a) a significant cognitive decline in one or more cognitive domains (complex attention, executive function, learning and memory, language, perceptual motor, or social cognition) and (b) interferes with independence in everyday activities and (c) does not occur exclusively in the context of delirium and (d) is not better explained by another mental disorder such as schizophrenia. The cause of major neurocognitive disorder in DSM-5 is specified (e.g., due to Alzheimer's disease). However, if cognitive decline and impairment are modest and do not interfere with independence in everyday activities and meet criteria (c) and (d) above, *mild neurocognitive disorder* is diagnosed according to DSM-5, and the cause of the mild neurocognitive disorder is also specified. Approximately one third of individuals with mild neurocognitive disorder develop dementia within 5 years [38].

Alzheimer's disease is the most common cause of dementia in the United States and accounts for 60–80% of cases [38]. According to the Alzheimer's Association, 11% of individuals age 65 or older have Alzheimer's disease versus 32% of individuals age 85 or older. The neuropathology in about half of these cases is due solely to Alzheimer's disease and in the remaining half of cases is due to Alzheimer's disease plus other dementias (mixed dementias). In 2013, death certificates indicated that Alzheimer's disease is the 6th leading cause of death in the United States and the 5th leading cause of death for Americans age 65 or older. The prevalence of Mixed Vascular-Alzheimer's disease in the elderly was found in a meta-analysis to be about 22% [39]. The percentage of dementia cases due to cerebrovascular disease, or stroke, alone is estimated at 10% [38].

Dementia with Lewy bodies (DLB) and Parkinson's disease (PD) are other common causes of dementia. The prevalence of DLB has been estimated at 1–2% of individuals over age 65 and about 5% of individuals over age 75 [40]. The prevalence of Parkinson's disease dementia (PDD) for individuals over age 65 has been estimated at 0.3–0.5%, accounting for about 3–4% of dementia cases in the general population [41]. The cumulative prevalence of PDD is 75% of PD patients surviving for 10 or more years [42]. Despite considerable clinical overlap, the key distinction between DLB and PDD is that cognitive impairment occurs first in DLB before motor symptoms, while the motor symptoms of parkinsonism occur (at least by a year) before the onset of cognitive impairment in PDD [40]. Clinical features of DLB and PDD include cognitive impairment, parkinsonism, visual hallucinations, and fluctuating attention. Neuropathological features of DLB and PDD include widespread cortical and subcortical alpha-synuclein/Lewy body plus Beta-amyloid and tau pathologies [40].

Frontotemporal dementia (FTD), or according to DSM-5 major neurocognitive disorder due to frontotemporal lobar degeneration, accounts for about 5% of dementia cases. FTD describes a cluster of syndromes characterized by executive dysfunction, behavioral changes, and a decrease in language functioning and is the second most common form of dementia in individuals younger than 65 years [43]. Approximately 25% of FTD cases are late onset [44]. The *behavioral variant* of FTD, accounting for approximately 60% of FTD cases, consists of impulsiveness, indifference, impatience, distractibility, carelessness, and stereotyped behaviors and compulsions. The *language variant* of FTD involves progressive fluent or dysfluent language dysfunction. Corticobasilar degeneration and progressive supranuclear palsy are conditions also included in the FDT family of illnesses [44].

Other causes of dementia, or major neurocognitive disorder, as outlined in DSM-5, may include human immunodeficiency virus (HIV) infection [45], Huntington's disease, prion disease such as Creutzfeldt-Jakob disease, substance use such as alcohol, other medical and neurological conditions such as brain tumors or normal pressure hydrocephalus, or multiple etiologies. Traumatic brain injury may also cause or contribute to the development of dementia and is of special concern to veterans.

In a large retrospective study utilizing the electronic medical records of 188,764 US veterans age 55 or older, traumatic brain injury (TBI) was associated with a 60% increase in risk of developing dementia over a 9-year follow-up period even after accounting for confounding influences [46]. In addition, in the same study, the risk of dementia increased in an additive manner when TBI was combined with other comorbidities including depression, posttraumatic stress disorder, and cerebrovascular disease. On the average, veterans with TBI developed dementia 2.1 years earlier than those without TBI. The risk for development of dementia after TBI was elevated for all dementia subtypes except there were an insufficient number of cases to examine for association between TBI and frontotemporal dementia. In the same study, the magnitude of the increased risk for dementia was similar for all types of TBI diagnoses and severity.

The pathologic entity associated with repetitive head trauma is known as chronic traumatic encephalopathy (CTE) [47]. The clinical presentation of CTE involves cognitive and behavioral impairments and may include chronic headaches, poor impulse control, aggression, depression, suicidal ideation, cognitive impairment, and dementia [48]. Pathologic studies on athletes with history of repetitive head injuries have indicated neuronal loss and tau-positive protein deposition in neurons [49, 50]. The frequent association of CTE with other neurodegenerative disorders suggests that repetitive brain trauma and hyperphosphorylated tau protein deposition promote the accumulation of other abnormally aggregated proteins such as amyloid beta protein and alpha-synuclein [50]. Age of initial exposure, duration of exposure, genetic predisposition, and other environmental factors have been implicated in contributing to the development of CTE [47]. In a recent neuropathological case series of 202 deceased football players, CTE was diagnosed in 87% of cases with a mean age of death at 67 years [51]. Among 84 cases with severe CTE pathology, 89% had behavioral or mood symptoms, 95% had cognitive symptoms, and 85% had signs of dementia based on interviews with informants. In the same study, among 27 cases with mild CTE pathology, 96% had behavioral or mood symptoms, 85% had cognitive symptoms, and 33% had signs of dementia based on informant interviews. Given that traumatic brain injuries may occur in different forms including from blast exposures, it is a serious health concern for veterans [48].

Both posttraumatic stress disorder (PTSD) and depression have been shown to increase the risk of dementia among older veterans [46]. In another large retrospective cohort study (238,532 patients, 97% male, with a mean age of 68.8 years at baseline), utilizing the Department of Veterans Affairs National Patient Care Database, veterans with posttraumatic stress disorder were found to have a 7-year cumulative incident dementia rate of 10.6%, whereas those without PTSD had a rate of 6.6% [52]. The authors concluded that patients with PTSD were nearly twice as likely to develop dementia as compared to those without PTSD. Utilizing similar methods, another study examined depression status and dementia among 281,540 veterans ages 55 years and older at baseline and found that the 7-year incident dementia cumulative rate was nearly twice as likely for veterans with depression or dysthymia at baseline compared to those without depression or dysthymia after adjusting for demographics and comorbidities [53].

Assessment of Cognitive Impairment

Assessment of cognitive impairment first involves obtaining an accurate history of cognitive decline which optimally involves corroborating history from a family member or informant. Neurological exam, mental status exam, and laboratory studies (e.g., thyroid level, B12, RPR, metabolic panel, structural brain scan) will help identify illnesses that can cause dementia syndromes. The Mini-Mental State Exam (MMSE) and Montreal Cognitive Assessment (MOCA) are commonly utilized brief-structured cognitive screening tools that help to quantify severity of cognitive impairment.

Formal neuropsychological testing helps to clarify cognitive strengths and weaknesses in different cognitive domains, can assist in clarifying diagnosis, and thus can be very useful in helping to guide clinical management. Fluorodeoxyglucose (FDG) positron emission tomography (PET) brain scan can help distinguish Alzheimer's versus frontotemporal dementia based on regional metabolic patterns [54].

Decision-Making Capacity

Assessment of decision-making capacity is an important clinical issue with older patients. There can be a potential ethical tension between the clinician's duty to respect the individual's autonomous decision-making and the clinician's duty to protect the individual with diminished capacity for autonomous decision-making [55]. Capacity for health care decision-making is generally defined in four dimensions: (a) understanding, (b) appreciation, (c) reasoning, and (d) expression of choice.

Understanding denotes the ability to comprehend the clinical information presented as well as the nature and potential risks and benefits of the proposed treatment and alternatives. *Appreciation* involves the application of the relevant information to one's own situation. *Reasoning* refers to the ability to rationally manipulate the information. *Expression of choice* indicates the ability to communicate a clear and consistent decision.

Among the different structured or semi-structured capacity instruments available, the MacArthur Competence Assessment Tool for Treatment [56] appears to be the most widely used in studies of health care decision-making capacity [55].

Treatment of Neurocognitive Disorders

Recommended treatment of mild cognitive impairment includes observation and the use of nonpharmacological therapies such as controlling vascular risk factors (exercise, healthy diet, and smoking cessation) and cognitive rehabilitation such as using memory cues and organizational aids [57]. For patients with Alzheimer's dementia, several FDA-approved medications may provide modest symptomatic benefits. There are three cholinesterase inhibitors approved for Alzheimer's disease: *donepezil* (all stages of dementia), *galantamine* (mild to moderate dementia), and *rivastigmine* (all stages of dementia). Rivastigmine is also approved for mild to moderate Parkinson's disease dementia. Additionally, *memantine*, thought to prevent the excitotoxicity effects of glutamate in the brain, is approved for moderate to severe Alzheimer's disease and may be administered alone or in combination with a cholinesterase inhibitor.

Recently, Dysken et al. demonstrated that vitamin E, when compared with placebo, slowed the progression of Alzheimer's disease by almost 20% per year [58]. Brain-healthy lifestyles such as maintaining physical exercise, mental stimulation, stress reduction, and good nutrition are also recommended for individuals with dementia [54]. In 2017, there were 105 agents in the Alzheimer's disease treatment development pipeline, divided among phases I, II, and III, with 70% considered as potential disease-modifying therapies [59]. Many of these trials employ biomarkers (e.g., amyloid detected by imaging) to identify trial participants and as outcome measures.

Management of behavioral symptoms of dementia is an important clinical issue that may affect, for example, whether an individual can be maintained in a home setting or would require a specialized care placement in an assisted living residence or nursing home. At the same time, no pharmacotherapy has FDA approval for neuropsychiatric symptoms due to dementia, except for pimavanserin which has been approved recently for psychosis in Parkinson's disease [60].

Nonpharmacological approaches are employed first for behavioral disturbances in dementia and may be very helpful. Such nonpharmacological interventions, for example, may include ensuring adequate supervision, addressing hearing or visual deficits, implementing good sleep hygiene, using memory aids, providing education to the caregiver, improving communication between caregiver and patient, simplifying the environment, and minimizing alcohol intake [57].

For agitation in Alzheimer's disease, a range of medications including selective serotonin antidepressants (SSRIs), anticonvulsants, cholinesterase inhibitors, memantine, benzodiazepines, and antipsychotics have been used but have shown minimal efficacy and/or substantial side effects [60]. For psychotic symptoms in Alzheimer's disease, antipsychotic medications have minimal efficacy and are associated with many side effects. For example, antipsychotic medication use in dementia is associated with a higher risk of cerebrovascular or cardiovascular events and mortality, and the FDA has issued black box warnings for use of antipsychotics for dementia-related psychosis [57].

For apathy in mild Alzheimer's disease, methylphenidate has provided improvement in community-dwelling veterans [61]. For depression in Alzheimer's disease, only small to null effect sizes have been found with SSRIs and serotonin-norepinephrine reuptake inhibitor (SNRI) treatment trials, while there is some evidence that psychosocial interventions such as increasing social contacts or exercise can be helpful [60].

In frontotemporal dementia, a small number of studies have reported improvement of behavioral symptoms with the use of SSRIs [43]. Some studies have suggested that donepezil provides benefit for behavioral symptoms such as hallucinations in Lewy body dementia [62]. Despite their limitations in dementia, pharmacological approaches have been suggested as first-line interventions in certain conditions: major depression with or without suicidal ideation, psychosis causing harm or potential for harm, and aggression with risk to self or others [63].

Specialty Geriatrics Care in VHA

Geriatrics and extended care (GEC) services are provided by the Veterans Health Administration (VHA) in home and community-based settings as well as skilled nursing homes and residential settings [64]. Home- and community-based services assist chronically ill or disabled veterans who remain in their homes and may include adult day health care, home health aide care, home-based primary care, hospice care, palliative care, skilled home health care, telehealth care, and respite care. Residential settings and nursing home care provided by VHA include medical foster homes, community and VA nursing homes, and state veteran homes. Some of the listed home- and community-based services, such as hospice care and palliative care, can also be provided in residential settings and nursing homes. An important goal of all GEC services is to provide veteran-centric care that addresses veteran's requirements and preferences for sites, systems, providers, and styles of care [65].

Conclusions

Veterans 65 years and older have unique military occupational exposures, many of which have long-lasting consequences. As time goes on, additional conditions are being identified as being associated with both toxic exposures, such as Agent Orange, and psychological traumatic exposures. PTSD can recur in later life for multiple reasons. Principles of supportive therapy and narrative medicine are helpful in combatting social isolation among older combat veterans. Dementia of varying causes is more prevalent among older veterans. Comprehensive team-based geriatric services are important in the management of this group of veterans, and VA medical centers offer a continuum of these models of care.

References

1. https://www.census.gov/newsroom/blogs/random-samplings/2016/11/who_are_veterans.html.
2. VA DATA. https://www.va.gov/vetdata/docs/Demographics/New_Vetpop_Model/Vetpop_Infographic_Final31.pdf.
3. Kheirbek RE, Fokar A, Shara N, Bell-Wilson LK, Moore HJ, Olsen E, Blackman MR, Llorente MD. Characteristics and incidence of chronic illness in community-dwelling predominantly male U.S. veteran centenarians. J Am Geriatr Soc. 2017;65:2100–6. https://doi.org/10.1111/jgs.14900.
4. Royal British Legion: a UK household survey of the ex-service community. http://media.britishlegion.org.uk/Media/2273/2014householdsurvey_execsummary.pdf. Accessed 11 Mar 2018.
5. Kuwert P, Knaevelsrud C, Pietrzak RH. Loneliness among older veterans in the United States: results from the National Health and Resilience in Veterans Study. Am J Geriatr Psychiatry. 2014;22:564–9.
6. Durai UN, Chopra MP, Coakley E, Llorente MD, Kirchner JA, Cook JM, Levkoff SE. Exposure to trauma and PTSD symptoms in older veterans attending primary care: comorbid conditions and self-rated health status. AJGP. 2011;59(6):1087–92.
7. Chopra M, Zhang H, Kaiser AP, Moye JA, Llorente MD, Oslin DW, Spiro A III. PTSD is a chronic, fluctuating disorder affecting the mental quality of life in older adults. AJGP. 2014;22(1):86–97.
8. Bullamn TA, Kang HK. Posttraumatic-stress-disorder and the risk of traumatic deaths among Vietnam veterans. J Nerv Ment Dis. 1994;182:604–10.
9. Boscarino J. Posttraumatic-stress-disorder and mortality among U.S. Army veterans 30 years after military service. Ann Epidemiol. 2006;16:248–56.
10. Colliver JD, Compton WM, Gfroerer JC, et al. Projecting drug use among aging baby boomers in 2020. Ann Epidemiol. 2006;16:257–65.
11. Williamson V, Stevelink SAM, Greenberg K, Greenberg N. Prevalence of mental health disorders in elderly US military veterans: a meta-analysis and sytematic review. AJGP 2018. Available online at http://www.ajgponline.org/article/S1064-7481(17)30523-7/pdf. Accessed 11 Mar 2018.
12. Wiechers IR, Karel MJ, Hoff R, et al. Growing use of mental and general health care services among older veterans with mental illness. Psychiatr Serv. 2015;66:1242–4.
13. Creamer MC, Parslow RA. Trauma exposure and posttraumatic stress disorder in the elderly. a community prevalence study. Am J Geriatr Psychiatr. 2008;16:853–6.
14. Engdahl B, Dikel TN, Eberly R, Blank A Jr. Posttraumatic stress disorder in a community group of former prisoners of war: a normative response to severe trauma. Am J Psychiatr. 1997;154:1576–81.
15. Drescher K, Rosen C, Burling T, et al. Causes of death among male veterans who received residential treatment for PTSD. J Trauma Stress. 2003;16:535–43.
16. National Center for PTSD. Clinician-Administered PTSD Scale for DSM-IV. 1998. Available at: http://www.clintools.com/victims/resources/assessment/ptsd/protected/CAPSIV.pdf. Accessed 11 Mar 2018.
17. Weathers FW, Huska JA, Keane TM. PCL-C for DSM-IV. Boston: National Center for PTSD Behavioral Science Division; 1991.
18. Davison EH, Pless AP, Gugliucci MR, King LA, King DW, Salgado DM, Spiro A III, Bachrach P. Late-life emergence of early-life trauma: the phenomenon of late-onset stress symptomatology among aging combat veterans. Res Aging. 2006;28:84–114.
19. King LA, King DW, Vickers K, Davison EH, Spiro A III. Assessing late-onset stress symptomatology among aging male combat veterans. Aging Ment Health. 2007;11:175–91.
20. Potter CM, Pless Kaiser A, King LA, King DW, Davison EH, Seligowski AV, Brady C, Spiro A III. Distinguishing late-onset stress symptomatology from posttraumatic stress disorder in older combat veterans. Aging Ment Health. 2012.

21. National Center for PTSD. PTSD Assessment and Treatment in Older Adults. 2017. Available at: https://www.ptsd.va.gov/professional/treatment. Accessed 11 Mar 2018.
22. Department of Veterans Affairs and Department of Defense. (2017). VA/DOD clinical practice guideline for the Management of Posttraumatic Stress Disorder and Acute Stress Disorder. Washington, DC. Available at: https://www.healthquality.va.gov/guidelines/MH/ptsd/.
23. Raskind MA, Peskind ER, Kanter ED, Petrie EC, Radant A, Thompson CE, Dobie DJ, Hoff D, Rein RJ, Straits-Tröster K, et al. Reduction of nightmares and other PTSD symptoms in combat veterans by prazosin: a placebo-controlled study. Am J Psychiatry. 2003;160(2):371–3.
24. Raskind MA, Peterson K, Williams T, Hoff DJ, et al. A trial of prazosin for combat trauma PTSD with nightmares in active-duty soldiers returned from Iraq and Afghanistan. Am J Psychiatry. 2013;170(9):1003–10.
25. Raskind MA, Peskind ER, Chow B, Harris C, Davis-Karim A, Holmes HA, Hart KL, McFall M, Mellman TA, Reist C, et al. Trial of prazosin for PTSD in military veterans. N Engl J Med. 2018;378(6):507–17.
26. Gallegos AM, Crean HF, Heffner KL. Meditation and yoga for posttraumatic stress disorder: a meta-analytic review of randomized controlled trials. Clin Psychol Rev. 2017;58:115–24.
27. Cacioppo J, Hawkley L. Social isolation and health, with an emphasis on underlying mechanisms. Perspect Biol Med. 2003;46(3 Suppl):S39–52.
28. Qualls SH. (2014, March 6). What social relationships can do for health. Retrieved November 01, 2017, from http://www.asaging.org/blog/what-social-relationships-can-do-health.
29. Institute of Medicine Committee on Health and Behavior. Health and behavior: the interplay of biological, behavioral, and societal influences. Washington, DC: National Academy Press; 2001.
30. Clement, S. (2014, April 08). Few regrets: 89% of Iraq and Afghanistan vets would do it all over again. Retrieved November 01, 2017, from https://www.washingtonpost.com/news/post-nation/wp/2014/04/08/few-regrets-89-of-iraq-and-afghanistan-vets-would-do-it-all-over-again/?utm_term=.eec9be3dee8a.
31. Manning F. Morale and Cohesion in Military Psychiatry. *Military Psychiatry: Preparing in Peace for War* 1982;82(February):1–9.
32. Dept of Veterans affairs Office of Research & Development. Unit Cohesion could be key to PTSD resiliency. 2014. Available at: https://www.research.va.gov/currents/summer2014/summer2014-27.cfm Accessed 12 Mar 2018.
33. Kanas N. Group therapy for patients with chronic trauma-related stress disorders. Int J Group Psychother. 2005;55(1):161–6.
34. Yalom ID, Lesczc M. The theory and practice of group psychotherapy. New York: Basic Books; 2005.
35. Charon R. Narrative medicine: a model for empathy, reflection, profession and trust. JAMA. 2001;286(15):1897–902.
36. Llorente MD, Mehta R. Use of video as a stimulus for trauma narratives in Vietnam combat veterans with PTSD. 2017 Presented at the American Psychiatric Association annual meeting, San Diego.
37. American Psychiatric Association, diagnostic and statistical manual of mental disorders, 5th ed. American Psychiatric Publishing, Washington, DC, 2013, pp 591–643.
38. Alzheimer's association: Alzheimer's & dementia 2016, 12:459–509.
39. Custodio N, Montesinos R, Lira D, et al. Mixed dementia: a review of the evidence. Dement Neuropsychol. 2017;11(4):364–70.
40. Jellinger KA. (2017). Dementia with Lewy bodies and Parkinson's disease-dementia: current concepts and controversies. J Neural Transm; published online 08 December, 2017.
41. Aarsland D, Kurz MW. The epidemiology of dementia associated with Parkinson's disease. Brain Pathol. 2010;10:633–9.
42. Aarsland D, Kurz MW. The epidemiology of dementia associated with Parkinson's disease. J Neurol Sci. 2010;289:18–22.
43. Young JJ, Lavakumar M, Tampi D, et al. Frontotemporal dementia: latest evidence and clinical implications. Ther Adv Psychopharmacol. 2018;8(1):33–48.

44. Onyike CU, Diehl-Schmid J. The epidemiology of frontotemporal dementia. Int Rev Psychiatry. 2013;25(2):130–7.
45. Farhadian S, Patel P, Spudich S. Neurological complications of HIV infection. Curr Infect Dis Rep. 2017;19(50):1–7.
46. Barnes DE, Kaup A, Kirby KA, et al. Traumatic brain injury and risk of dementia in older veterans. Neurology. 2014;83:312–9.
47. Savica R. Head trauma and neurodegeneration in veterans: an additional piece of the puzzle. Neurology. 2014;83:298–9.
48. Hasoon J. Blast-associated traumatic brain injury in the military as a potential trigger for dementia and chronic traumatic encephalopathy. The Army Medical Department Journal 2017, (Jan-Jun) 102–105.
49. McKee AC, Cantu RC, Nowinski CK, et al. Chronic traumatic encephalopathy in athletes: progressive tauopathy following repetitive head injury. J Neuropathol Exp Neurol. 2009;68(7):709–35.
50. McKee AC, Stein TD, Nowinski CJ, et al. The spectrum of disease in chronic traumatic encephalopathy. Brain. 2013;136:43–64.
51. Mez J, Daneshvar DH, Kiernan PT, et al. Clinicopathological evaluation of chronic traumatic encephalopathy in players of American football. JAMA. 2017;318(4):360–70.
52. Yaffe K, Vittinghoff E, Lindquist K, et al. Posttraumatic stress disorder and risk of dementia among US veterans. Arch Gen Psychiatry. 2010;67(6):608–13.
53. Byers AL, Covinsky KE, Barnes DE, Yaffe K. Dysthymia and depression increase risk of dementia and mortality among older veterans. Am J Geriatr Psychiatry. 2012;20:664–72.
54. Small FW. Detection and prevention of cognitive decline. Am J Geriatr Psychiatry. 2016;24:1142–50.
55. Palmer BW, Harmell AL. Assessment of healthcare decision-making capacity. Arch Clin Neuropsychol. 2016;31:530–40.
56. Grisso T, Appelbaum PS, Hill-Fotouhi C. The MacCAT-T: a clinical tool to assess patients' capacities to make treatment decisions. Psychiatr Serv. 1997;48:1415–9.
57. Kimchi EZ, Lyketsos CG. Dementia and mild neurocognitive disorders. In: The textbook of geriatric psychiatry. 5th ed: Washington, D.C.: The American Psychiatric Publishing. 2015; p. 177–242.
58. Dysken MW, Sano M, Asthana S, Vertrees JE, Pallaki M, Llorente M. et.alEffect of vitamin E and memantine on functional decline in Alzheimer disease: the TEAM-AD VA cooperative randomized trial. JAMA. 2014;311(1):33–44.
59. Cummings J, Lee G, Mortsdorf T, et al. Alzheimer's disease drug development pipeline: 2017. Alzheimer's & dementia: translational research & clinical. Interventions. 2017;3:367–84.
60. Lanctot KL, Amatniek J. Ancoli-Israel, et al: neuropsychiatric signs and symptoms of Alzheimer's disease: new treatment paradigms. Alzheimer's & dementia: translational research & clinical. Interventions. 2017;3:440–9.
61. Padala PR, Padala KP, Lensing SY, et al. Methylphenidate for apathy in community-dwelling older veterans with mild Alzheimer's disease: a double-blind, randomized, placebo-controlled trial. Am J Psychiatry. 2018;175:159–68.
62. Cummings J, Lai T, Hemrungrojn S, et al. Role of donepezil in the management of neuropsychiatric symptoms in Alzheimer's disease and dementia with Lewy bodies. CNS Neurosci Ther. 2016;22:159–66.
63. Gerlach LB, Kales HC. Managing behavioral and psychological symptoms of dementia. Psychiatr Clin N Am. 2018;41:127–39.
64. US Dept. of Veterans Affairs. Geriatrics & Extended Care Available at: https://www.va.gov/geriatrics. Accessed 13 Mar 2018.
65. Shay K, Hyduke B, Burris JF. Strategic plan for geriatrics and extended care in the veterans health administration: background, plan, and progress to date. J Am Geriatr Soc. 2013;61:632–8.

Women Veterans

18

Kasey M. Llorente, Keelan K. O'Connell, Margaret Valverde, and Elspeth Cameron Ritchie

Introduction

Sybil Ludington warned colonial militiamen that "the British were coming" to Danbury, Connecticut. She rode on horseback 40 miles, which was longer than Paul Revere's ride. She was a 16-year-old teenager. Margaret Corbin is the first American woman to receive a lifetime pension for wounds suffered in battle. She defended Fort Washington in New York during the Revolutionary War, during a battle in which her husband was killed, and she took over the cannon when the gunner was killed. She was wounded and left for dead, treated by a local doctor and survived. Women have served honorably in the US military since the Revolutionary War, in a wide range of capacities and roles. These roles have changed over time, and with each change, American women have responded admirably and achieved the mission.

K. M. Llorente (✉)
Creighton University, Omaha, NE, USA
e-mail: kll46560@creighton.edu

K. K. O'Connell
Walter Reed National Military Medical Center, Department of Behavioral Health, Bethesda, MD, USA

M. Valverde
George Washington University Hospital, Psychiatry and Behavioral Sciences, Washington, DC, USA

E. C. Ritchie
Department of Psychiatry, MedStar Washington Hospital Center, Washington, DC, USA

Georgetown University School of Medicine, Washington, DC, USA

George Washington University School of Medicine, Washington, DC, USA

Uniformed Services University of the Health Sciences, Silver Spring, MD, USA

Mental Health Community Based Outpatient, Washington, DC, USA

© Springer Nature Switzerland AG 2019
E. C. Ritchie, M. D. Llorente (eds.), *Veteran Psychiatry in the US*,
https://doi.org/10.1007/978-3-030-05384-0_18

Today, U.S. women veterans number approximately two million. The proportion of women veterans is expected to increase at an average rate of about 18,000 per year for the next 10 years, and by 2043, women are projected to make up 16.3% of all living veterans [1]. As with all veterans, there is a continuum of service, with many female veterans alternating between active duty, and reserve and veteran status. A thorough and extensive review may be found in *Women at War* by the senior author [2]. Unlike their male counterparts, who are predominantly older, approximately 37% of women veterans are of reproductive age—between 18 and 45 years old. Nearly 44% of female veterans are now enrolled in and use services provided by the Veterans Health Administration (VHA), allowing healthcare providers to learn about the effects of military service on women's health. Understanding the unique healthcare needs of women veterans affected by an array of experiences, including combat exposure, military sexual trauma, toxic occupational exposures, and mental health and medical consequences, is paramount to providing exceptionally high-quality care for these women when they return home.

Women veterans differ from men in several significant ways, including the prevalence and presentation of certain mental health disorders, as well as in their response to behavioral health treatment modalities. These differences are attributed to a number of different factors, including biological sex differences and social and cultural influences. The Office of Research on Women's Health within the National Institutes of Health has identified "further understanding of sex/gender differences in fundamental mechanisms and patterns of behavioral and social functioning relevant to health and well-being" as an important goal for 2020 [1]. Identification of these differences is an initial and crucial step in knowing how to best meet women's mental and general healthcare needs.

Demographics of US Women Veterans

Who are our women veterans? US servicewomen and veterans come from diverse backgrounds and differ in many ways from their civilian counterparts who never served in the military. Data from the 2015 American Community Survey (ACS) provide an in-depth profile of the nearly two million women veterans living in the United States. and Puerto Rico today [1]. The largest percentage (33.2%) of women veterans living today have served during the post-9/11 period (September 2001–present), and many were deployed as part of Operation Enduring Freedom/Operation Iraqi Freedom/Operation New Dawn (OEF/OIF/OND). The remaining women veterans by period of military service include peacetime only (24.9%), pre-9/11 (23.3%), Vietnam era (13.1%), Korean War (3.0%), and World War II (2.5%).

Compared with nonveteran women, women veterans, on average, are older, with a median age of 50 years, versus 46 years for nonveteran women. A total of 62.4% of women veterans are between the ages of 35 and 64 years compared to 49% of women nonveterans [1]. In 2015, 19% of women veterans were African Americans, compared with 12% of nonveteran women [1]. In contrast, the percentage of women veterans who were Hispanic was almost half that of nonveterans (9% compared with 16%). As the percentage of Hispanics in the general population rises, their representation in the military is expected to increase as well. Currently, the percentage of Asian women veterans is less than half of nonveterans (2% compared with 5.5%).

Due to military enlistment requirements that stipulate that recruits must have a high school diploma or a GED, veterans have higher overall educational attainment at all educational levels than nonveterans [1]. Further, working-age women veterans (17–64 years) have a slightly higher labor force participation rate (71.5%) than nonveteran women (70.1%), although they differ somewhat in the specific kinds of work they perform [1]. Almost half of employed women veterans (49%) worked in management, professional, or other related occupations, compared with 41% of nonveteran women. A higher percentage of employed women veterans work in the government sector (34%) than nonveteran women (16%).

In part related to the higher educational attainment, women veterans are less likely than nonveteran women to be living in poverty in every age group [1]. Despite this, about 10% of women veterans have incomes below the poverty threshold, with highest rates (17.5%) found among the youngest women (17–24 years) [1]. Young women veterans (ages 17–24) were more likely to be married than similar age civilian women counterparts (30% vs 8%, respectively), but they were also more likely to be divorced (8% vs 1%, respectively). A higher percentage of women veterans in all age groups are currently divorced.

Identifying Women Veterans' Mental Healthcare Needs

Research consistently shows that female veterans are more likely than male veterans to be diagnosed with a mental health condition [3]. Further, women veterans are twice as likely to have experienced past-year severe psychological distress in comparison to their male counterparts [3]. In addition, relative to male veterans, women veterans have been found to have higher rates of both mental health and medical comorbidities [3, 4], indicating the potential need for intensive care coordination, more frequent follow-up visits, and higher utilization. These findings are consistent with currently observed patterns of VA mental healthcare utilization, in that women veterans with mental illness are more frequent users of VA mental health services relative to their male counterparts [5].

Now that the ban on women serving in combat has been lifted, it is also likely that combat exposure will have a significant effect on the incidence and prevalence of combat-related consequences, both positive [6] and negative [7]. As a result, it is crucial that mental healthcare providers inquire about military service and are aware of veteran deployment histories in order to better understand the veteran's perspective and possible contributory factors for psychological stress and mental health conditions. In addition, the interaction between deployment and family relationships has a significant impact on reintegration into civilian life.

Post-Traumatic Stress and Major Depressive Disorders

Post-traumatic stress disorder (PTSD) and major depressive disorder are the two most prevalent primary service-connected conditions among women veterans, with prevalence rates of 11.8% and 6.5%, respectively. In 2015, nearly 48,000 women veterans received VA compensation for PTSD, while roughly 26,500 did so for major depressive disorder [9].

Causes of deployment-related stress include actual combat trauma exposure, sexual harassment and assault in the military and family separations, conflicts, and interpersonal difficulties. These stressors are also associated with reduced postmilitary quality of life and can adversely affect work, romantic relationships, and parenting [9].

Experiences of being wounded or injured during deployment may be more strongly associated with PTSD symptoms for women than men [9], an important consideration due to the changing nature of warfare and the recent lift on the ban restricting women from some combat roles, including positions in the infantry, armor, and special operations. Women not directly in combat do experience associated trauma through support activities, such as medical support or the handling of human remains [9]. Repeated traumatic exposure increases the likelihood of PTSD [9].

Women veterans report the highest rates of lifetime and past-year post-traumatic stress disorder compared with female civilians, male veterans, and civilians. Encouragingly, men and women veterans are more likely than civilians to utilize a variety of treatment sources (i.e., psychotropic medications, psychotherapy, other). Women veterans are also more likely to seek help for PTSD symptoms than their male veteran counterparts [1].

A study [7] found that among women veterans, major depression follows the onset of other comorbid disorders. Anxiety and eating disorders co-occurred more commonly among women veterans compared to male veterans, and nicotine and alcohol use disorders were found less often. Among women veterans in mid-life and older, those with depression had a 60% greater chance of having coronary artery disease than those without depression, regardless of nicotine history [8]. For each additional co-occurring mental health condition, the risk increases by an additional 40%. Early identification and treatment of depressive disorders, in conjunction with an assessment of whole health and recommendations for health lifestyle choices, including physical activity, are thus crucially important and possibly lifesaving for women veterans.

Military Sexual Trauma

Military sexual trauma (MST) is the term used by the VA and defined in federal law to refer to "Psychological trauma which resulted from a physical assault of a sexual nature, battery of a sexual nature or sexual harassment which occurred while the veteran was serving on active duty, active duty for training, or inactive duty training" [2]. The sexual activity was against the veteran's will. The veteran may report feeling pressured into the activity. Examples include threats of negative consequences for refusal to be sexually cooperative, implied faster promotions, or better treatment in exchange for sex. At times, the activity occurs when the veteran may have been unable to consent (when intoxicated). Other examples of activities that are included as MST are unwanted sexual touching or grabbing; threatening, offensive remarks about a person's body; unwelcome sexual advances; and repeated, unsolicited verbal or physical contacts of a sexual nature that are threatening in character.

Exposure to MST is a significant risk factor for subsequent development of PTSD, as well as a contributory factor for homelessness among women veterans. While both women and men do experience MST and sexual harassment, women are 20 times more likely than men to be assaulted during military service. Among OEF/OIF/OND women veterans, nearly one third (31%) diagnosed with PTSD also reported a history of MST, compared to only 1% of male OEF/OIF veterans diagnosed with PTSD [9]. Psychiatric symptoms and morbidity were notable after all military-associated traumas, although those seeking care for MST-related events demonstrated more severe PTSD, depressive, and dissociative symptoms and were more likely to meet criteria for non-PTSD anxiety and psychotic disorders [10, 12].

While still on active duty, service members report fearing retaliation and adverse repercussions for reporting MST. Often, they feel that nothing will be done to address the report and the behavior and therefore will not submit a report. MST survivors also report a loss of professional and personal identity. Despite the increased attention, a recent Department of Defense (DoD) report indicated that MST survivors may experience retraumatization through being questioned about the validity of the experience and being blamed [11].

The perpetrator of MST is often a coworker or a commanding officer. Service members may also experience intimate partner violence (IPV) which also can lead to mental health conditions, including anxiety, depression, unhealthy substance use, and suicidal thinking. One third of women veterans report experiencing IPV, compared with less than a quarter of civilian women [13]. Women who have experienced IPV may experience physical injuries as well, such as stab wounds or broken bones or sexually transmitted infections. Additionally, they may experience long-term adverse health effects such as obesity; problems with their heart, stomach, or digestive systems; difficulties with pregnancies; chronic pain; and other stress-related difficulties such as headaches. Over half of women veterans (53.3%) who have ever experienced IPV had a mental health diagnosis and have significantly higher odds of each type of mental health morbidity except psychoses. Similar findings were noted when adjusting for military sexual trauma [13, 14]. These findings highlight the mental health burden associated with past-year IPV among women veterans and underscore the need to address psychological and sexual trauma.

Substance Use Disorders

Recent studies of women veterans in outpatient substance abuse treatment programs have found a high prevalence of comorbid mental disorders such as PTSD, major depressive disorder, and other serious mental illnesses [15, 16]. OIF/OEF/OND women veterans who used large quantities of alcohol and drugs were more likely to screen positive for PTSD than those not using substances [14, 16]. Further, women veterans who present for treatment for PTSD were more likely to be prescribed benzodiazepine (38.3%) than men presenting to the same clinic (29.8%) [17]. Benzodiazepines have high potential for abuse and dependence and may complicate the management of PTSD, such that they should only be used in the lowest effective doses and for brief periods of time in this population.

Suicide

While a great deal of attention has been directed to the high rate of suicide among veterans, a disproportionately high prevalence of completed suicides has been found among women veterans. The suicide rate among women veterans is nearly three times higher than that of women in the general population (9.8 per 100,000 vs 3.4 per 100,000) [18]. Men and women veterans in younger age groups (18–34 years) have the highest suicide rate of all veterans. Although it is unclear why younger age is a factor in completed suicides, this trend may represent a cohort effect related to particular conflicts or experiences shortly after returning from conflict. Factors that have been identified that contribute to increased suicidality in women veterans include high comorbidity with substance use disorders, combat exposure/deployment, and mental health disorders [19]. Some women veterans may self-medicate with substances to relieve psychological symptoms [15], which can then lead to increased impulsivity and suicidal action.

A challenge in suicide prevention is identifying subgroups of individuals who are likely to benefit from suicide-related intervention [20]. Women veterans with substance use disorders and/or comorbid depression or PTSD are such a subgroup [21]. Further, women veterans who report poor mental health are also more likely to endorse multiple health problems, suggesting a need for integrated primary care and mental health strategies to simultaneously address medical and mental health problems. Alternatively, screening for depression, PTSD, MST, and substance use disorders in primary care settings is likely to identify these individuals earlier to then offer treatment services as soon as possible. These patients should also be routinely screened for suicidal thinking [22]. More research will need to be done to more fully understand the interrelationship between substance use, mental illness, and suicidality to be able to develop more effective interventions.

Biological Considerations

Hormonal changes during the life cycle can have an effect on mental health. Currently, among women veterans seeking VA healthcare, 42% are in their reproductive years (ages 18–44) and 29% are in the perimenopausal period (ages 45–55) [5]. Ovarian hormones, particularly estrogen and progesterone, undergo major fluctuations during specific transition periods, such as the transition from pregnancy to postpartum, as well as the transition into menopause. These transitions are associated with elevated susceptibility to depression [23].

Reproductive mental health issues can also affect treatment decisions. Up to 20% of pregnant women in the general population experience mood or anxiety disorders during pregnancy, and 10–15% experience postpartum depression [23]. In reproductive aged women, it is imperative that providers discuss contraception counseling, pregnancy testing, and risk/benefit counseling prior to prescribing medications that are potentially teratogenic. While there are risks to psychotropic medication use during pregnancy, untreated mental health disorders can also adversely affect the patient, her baby, and her family. The risks and benefits of each treatment option should be carefully discussed with patients to ensure understanding and informed decision-making.

Management of Biological Functions in Deployment

One particular challenge faced by deployed women is the management of menstruation in resource-limited areas. Menstrual suppression with oral contraceptives (OCPs) has become increasingly commonplace, although the unpredictability of a combat zone poses a challenge to adherence [24]. With limited access to sanitation products, deployed women are at a heightened risk for urogenital infections [25, 26]. Often during deployment, women resort to suppressing urination or limiting fluid intake in order to avoid urinating while being surrounded by their male counterparts or stepping off the path to find privacy behind a bush and risking an encounter with an improvised explosive device (IED). These same barriers push women to maintain tampons and pads in place for longer than the recommended time frame. Each of these practices poses a risk for women to develop urinary tract infections (UTIs), bacterial vaginosis (BV), and toxic shock syndrome (TSS) [25]. Further, limited access to healthcare in often austere environments can leave these infectious diseases undiagnosed and untreated. Without antibiotic therapy, persistent BV can increase the risk of recurrent vaginitis along with an increased rate of other sexually transmitted infections (STIs) [27]. BV further appears to prolong the course of human papillomavirus (HPV) infection [28]. In fact, an association was found between cervical intraepithelial neoplasia/squamous intraepithelial lesions (CIN/SIL) and women with a history of BV [29]. Women deployed to combat zones during the Gulf War were found to have a higher occurrence of abnormal pap smears and breast cysts compared to the general population [30]. Upon return from deployment, women veterans should receive prompt evaluation, screening, and close follow-up for all STIs, cervical cancer, and breast masses.

Pregnancy

Pregnancy places a great deal of physiologic and emotional stress on the body. Coupled with the chronic stress of war exposure and its lingering psychological effects, this places women veterans at high risk for pregnancy-associated complications. Moreover, pregnancy can exacerbate or even precipitate underlying mental health conditions [31]. Antepartum complications, prolonged postpartum hospital stays, and rehospitalizations after delivery have all been observed to occur at a higher frequency among women who served in OEF/OIF/OND compared to the general population [30].

Active duty women face pregnancy challenges that are similar to those seen in the general population, in addition to having many other unique challenges specific to military employment. Service women in certain fields, however, such as fuel handlers and those in combat environments, may be occupationally exposed to a number of toxic elements, such as petroleum, during pregnancy or postpartum, which may jeopardize the health of the service member or her fetus/newborn [2].

Pregnant active duty service members may not be deployed to combat theaters and are protected from deployment for at least 6 months postpartum (depending on her branch of service). However, most postpartum guidelines recommend breastfeeding an infant for at least the first year after giving birth, which may be impossible if a woman is deployed to the field or war zone during that time [2].

During pregnancy, limitations may be placed on the service member to ensure her safety, as well as that of the unborn fetus. These limitations can affect various categories of job functions and include physical (exemption from the physical readiness program), ergonomic (exemptions from standing at parade rest for >15 min, lying in the prone position for a prolonged period, lifting greater than 25 pounds, performing work at heights, exposure to excessive heat or vibration), and environmental (restricting exposure to chemicals, toxins, or radiation).

Pregnant servicewomen are afforded the opportunity for counseling by an occupational healthcare provider. Commanding officers, supervisory personnel, and healthcare professionals "are responsible for providing for the health and safety of the servicewoman and her unborn child while maintaining optimum job and career performance" [32]. Per DoD instructions, pregnancy status is not to "adversely affect the career patterns of naval servicewomen," although many women voice concerns about discrimination and job advancement should they become pregnant.

If a service member desires an abortion, this procedure is illegal in many countries where female service members are stationed. A woman who requests an abortion who is stationed in a country where abortion is prohibited must go on leave to a country that provides legal abortion (usually the United States) or risk an illegal abortion. The military health system and TRICARE do not pay for abortions, except in the case of rape and incest [4].

Among pregnant veterans with PTSD, while the full mechanism remains unknown, PTSD appears to dysregulate hormones controlled by the hypothalamic-pituitary axis (HPA) [33]. Chronic stress blunts the release of cortisol, disinhibiting corticotropin-releasing hormone (CRH) and norepinephrine (NE). PTSD amplifies the stress reaction in pregnancy without allowing the compensatory mechanisms to cope with that added stress. This bolstered anxiety increases the risk of developing pregnancy-related complications that can lead to adverse maternal and neonatal outcomes.

Two particularly common antepartum conditions, gestational diabetes and preeclampsia, occur at a higher prevalence among women diagnosed with PTSD compared with other populations [34, 35]. Further alterations in the levels of thyroid hormones similarly result from neurobiological changes in PTSD [33]. The skewed levels of thyroid hormone lead to menstrual irregularities; hyperemesis gravidarum; increased anxiety, which can be transferred to the fetus; and elevated heart rate and blood pressure, which can lead to cardiovascular complications.

The higher prevalence of mental health conditions among pregnant veterans can lead to risky behaviors, such as drug and alcohol abuse, and reduced adherence with prenatal checkups [36]. Alcohol abuse in pregnancy can lead to fetal structural abnormalities and poor neurologic development. Illicit drug abuse can result in a variety of complications ranging from neonatal withdrawal symptoms to antepartum placental abruption. Poor adherence with prenatal care can have a further wide range of effects, including neural tube defects, vertically transmitted infections, and overall poor maternal health.

Caring for pregnant patients requires a great deal of collaboration and trust between the patient and doctor. Veteran status intensifies this requirement. Civilian providers should ask their patients if they have served in the military. Once identified as a veteran, those planning to become pregnant should undergo thorough mental health screening prior to and following conception. Those identified with mental health conditions should receive appropriate therapy and close follow-up for signs of worsening moods or behaviors. Physicians aware of these heightened risks for antepartum, postpartum, and neonatal complications among women veterans will be better prepared to act accordingly to prevent negative outcomes.

Breastfeeding

Long duty hours, inflexible work schedules, and frequent separations from baby and family can make it difficult for active duty mothers who wish to breastfeed to continue breastfeeding after returning to work. The Department of Defense (DoD) has endorsed Healthy People 2020 target goals for health promotion and disease prevention, but a DoD-wide lactation policy does not exist [37]. However, each branch of service has implemented lactation policies or support recommendations for their respective service members in an effort to support breastfeeding and optimize the health of military members and their families [2].

In a recent survey of female active duty service members who have given birth within the past 2 years, a majority of respondents stated that the lack of time and space for pumping was the primary obstacle to continue breastfeeding [37]. Even in garrison, places to pump milk in a hygienic manner may be limited [2]. Many active duty mothers stated that despite lactation policies in place, the lack of support from coworkers and supervisors had a negative influence on their decision to continue breastfeeding: minorities, younger age, less maternal education, and lower income levels are all characteristics associated with lower breastfeeding prevalence [37].

Infertility

Nearly 16% of women veterans self-reported struggling with impaired fertility compared to 12% of women in the general population [38]. Higher rates of infertility have been observed among veterans with mental health conditions compared to those without such a diagnosis [38]. Further risk factors include younger age, obesity, black or Latina ethnicities, physical trauma, and military sexual trauma (MST) [39, 40]. However, only a small number of OEF/OIF/OND women veterans received an infertility diagnosis from the VA. Until very recently, few veterans received full workups and treatments, which included controlled ovarian hyperstimulation, reverse tubal ligation surgery, or artificial insemination/intrauterine insemination [40, 41]. In 2017, the VA began to include in vitro fertilization as a treatment option for specific service-connected conditions that cause infertility in both male and female veterans with those conditions [42].

Amputations, Prosthetic Devices, and Women

Of those receiving services within the VA, female veterans with amputations are seen more frequently for rehabilitative and prosthetic services than their male counterparts. Furthermore, of women with amputation who are domiciled, 57% live alone compared to 36% of males with amputations [43]. While learning to live with an amputation is challenging, women face numerous additional challenges that are often overlooked or underappreciated in the use of their prostheses as compared to their male counterparts. For instance, women generally require smaller prosthetic components compared to men because of their smaller bone structure and muscle mass. Collectively, poor cosmesis, few female-specific components, heavy prosthetic weight, combined with socket fitting challenges can lead to poor prosthetic fit and appearance, skin integrity concerns, pistoning, and unwanted noise [43].

Pregnancy is another concern for women veterans with amputations of traumatic etiology. Pregnancy-related fluid retention and weight fluctuations of the residual limb may cause abnormal wear on prosthetic components (e.g., prosthetic feet) requiring more frequent monitoring. Further, these changes can affect the fit of the prosthetic socket and may necessitate a category change in selected components [43]. Lastly, pregnancy alters the woman's center of mass throughout the pregnancy, which can adversely affect balance and prosthetic alignment and can lead to an increased risk of falls for the prosthetic user.

There are also a few relevant medical differences among women veterans with amputations when compared with male counterparts. Although there does not appear to be a gender difference for frequency of residual limb pain or phantom limb pain, women with amputations tend to report greater pain and pain that interferes with the function and activities of daily living to a greater extent than males [43]. Similarly, all individuals living with lower limb loss are at an increased risk of associated comorbidities such as osteoporosis and osteoarthritis in proximal and contralateral joints. However, the risk of osteoarthritis among women with amputation is significantly elevated [43]. Providers should work closely with female amputees to develop strategies for weight management, lower extremity strengthening, and activity modification to ensure optimal health and prevent disease.

Social and Cultural Considerations

Marriage

Social and cultural factors can have an impact on women's mental health. Gender differences in social resources and socioeconomic status (SES) are known, and research indicates that SES is a key factor in determining the psychological health of women [1].

As a group, military women marry at earlier ages, likely related to access to the larger ratio of men in the military and financial incentives related to military benefits for married couples (housing and supplemental food allowances).

Most military marriages (93%) are between a male service member and a female civilian spouse. Records from more than six million service members between 1996 and 2005 were utilized to assess patterns and trends in marriage and marital dissolution among military personnel [44]. Study findings indicated that active duty females had higher rates of marital dissolution than their male counterparts, and these findings were consistent across time and branch of service [44].

During 2005, divorce rates among women service members were more than double those of men serving on active duty (6.60% vs. 2.60%). Differences in rates of dissolution were most pronounced for enlisted women married to civilian men [44]. An increase in the number of months deployed increased military couples' chances of marital dissolution, with stronger effects for dual-military couples and female service members. More importantly, even in the absence of deployment, the risk of divorce for nondeployed women married for 3 years was double that of nondeployed men married for the same period. Based on women's higher risks for marital dissolution, women are also more likely than men to enter single-parent and stepparent families [44].

Spouses of all active duty service members face the challenges of coping with their spouse's long and irregular work schedules, experiencing concern for their spouses' safety during deployment and being susceptible to the effects of their spouses' military service on their mental health which can lead to depression, anxiety, and PTSD [44]. Husbands of active duty female service members find themselves facing the additional challenge of performing nontraditional gender roles such as housekeeping and childcare.

While military activities and support resources are available to support military spouses of both genders, there is a stigma attached to males' utilization of resources leading to a common perception among male spouses that activities and support resources were not designed to meet their needs. This perception can lead to increased feelings of isolation and exclusion from the military and civilian community. Furthermore, husbands reported susceptibility to the effects of their spouses' military service on their own mental health and can lead to depression, anxiety, and PTSD in the husband [44].

Despite the challenges of military lifestyle, husbands married to military wives describe many positive aspects as well, including a stable income and military family benefits such as healthcare and tuition assistance. Husbands perceived their wives' service as honorable. Many felt that the couples' ability to overcome challenges, such as separation and relocations, strengthened the marriage by fostering communication with their wives and children. Such findings highlight both potential risk and protective factors associated with wives' military service [44].

Homelessness

Homelessness among veterans has been steadily decreasing over the past decade. In spite of this, homelessness among women veterans remains a significant societal problem. Among women, military service is associated with a 2–4 times increased likelihood of experiencing homelessness [1]. Factors found to be associated with the experience of homelessness in women veterans include unemployment, disability with low income, history of MST, fair to poor health, tobacco use, and a positive screen for an anxiety disorder or PTSD [45].

Compared to homeless male veterans, homeless women veterans are younger and have higher rates of unemployment and mental illness [45]. These women are often of childbearing age. Gender-based violence (i.e., domestic and sexual violence) is a leading cause of homelessness for women in the general population, and this also holds true among women veterans. Among homeless veterans who receive VA health services, nearly 40% of the women reported having experienced MST [46]. Homeless women veterans are more likely than male veterans to have young children in their custody, suggesting that there may be different origins for homelessness but certainly indicating a need for different solutions (e.g., housing for women and children) to mitigate the risk for homelessness and to facilitate the establishment of permanent housing [4].

In 2009, the VA, together with the Department of Labor, introduced the Trauma-Informed Care for Women Veterans Experiencing Homelessness guide. Approximately $8.6 million in reintegration grants were released for homeless women veterans and veterans with children [1]. Additional resources include emergency shelters, transitional housing programs, and permanent housing. However, resources that are female gender-specific or that include options in housing for families with young children have lagged and not been able to keep up with the demand for those services.

Best Practices for Gender-Sensitive Mental Healthcare

Women in general tend to be nurturers and caregivers, prioritizing the needs of others and often putting their own self-care on the back burner. Providing care for others can make for a stressful life. Prolonged stress affects mental well-being and, ultimately, physical well-being. To overcome these adverse outcomes, women veterans must have access to medical and mental health services that are comprehensive, integrated, and collaborative.

The 2015 Study of Barriers for Women Veterans to VA Health Care [47] surveyed more than 8400 women veterans who currently use or do not use VA services and identified 9 barriers to accessing care: (1) comprehension of eligibility requirements and scope of services, (2) effectiveness of outreach about women's health services, (3) effect of driving distance on access to care, (4) location and hours, (5) child care, (6) acceptability of integrated care, (7) gender sensitivity, (8) mental health stigma, and (9) safety and comfort. Although this study focused on barriers specific to acquiring VA healthcare, the findings are likely generalizable to other healthcare settings.

Comprehension of Eligibility Requirement and Scope of Services The VA is a large and often bureaucratic agency that despite offering a wide variety of healthcare services is often difficult to navigate. As a result, women veterans who are unfamiliar with this system often have an inadequate or incomplete understanding of resources that are available to them and on how to access these services.

Effectiveness of Outreach According to findings from the VA study, brochures are the most preferred source of information in VA users and non-users alike, perhaps due to the permanence and trustworthiness that brochures provide. Respondents also indicated a preference for postal mail (46%) and email (26%) for future communications. Notably, as disability level increases, the preference for telephone use also increases [47]. Further, women veterans indicated they would like to receive information "early and often," both before they separate from service and repeatedly after separation [47].

Effect of Driving Distance on Access to Care Women who are able to make transportation arrangements use healthcare services more frequently. Women veterans of all ages prefer to drive themselves (80%), followed by having family or friends drive them (14%). Of women with a 70–100% disability rating, 12% indicate having a very hard or somewhat hard time finding appropriate transportation [47]. These veterans would benefit from information regarding transportation benefits. Some veterans are eligible to be picked up at home and transported to and from visits. Some are eligible for travel benefits that provide mileage reimbursement. Some programs can provide public transportation vouchers. Social work staff are often able to provide information regarding community resources that provide transportation.

Location and Hours Women veterans rank quality of providers and availability of needed services as the dominant reasons for selecting one healthcare facility over another, even if it is farther away. Furthermore, healthcare facilities with convenient appointment times are used more frequently by women veterans. Among employed and unemployed women veterans, morning appointments are the most preferred time slots because afternoon appointments may run behind schedule.

Respondents prefer to schedule their own appointment times and dates rather than being assigned one without their consent, to ensure availability and ability to attend appointments [47].

Childcare Young, unmarried women who live in urban settings report the most difficulty in obtaining childcare. The majority of women surveyed indicated that on-site childcare would be very helpful and might influence their decision to use a particular healthcare facility [47].

Acceptability of Integrated Care Comprehensive care is defined as having one provider who can deliver all general medical care, as well as all routine women's health care, such as pap smears, contraception, and menopause care. Comprehensive care is becoming more common throughout the healthcare industry as it often results in better coordination, communication, and control of costs, as well as improved outcomes and higher levels of patient satisfaction. Seventy-five percent of female veterans rated having a single provider for all care as very or somewhat important, while 65% indicate having a female provider for their women's services as very or somewhat important [47]. Women throughout all demographic categories show a preference for women-only settings, but women who previously experienced unwanted sexual attention, threat, or force of sex are particularly sensitive to mixed-gender settings. As a result, an increasing number of VA hospitals now have women-specific clinics. All VA hospitals are also required to have providers who are certified to provide gender-specific care.

Mental Health Stigma More than half of women veterans (52%) indicate they have needed mental health care [47]. Unfortunately, 24% of women veterans indicated they were hesitant to seek care for mental health issues, citing concerns about the medications used (62%), concerns about potential negative impacts on their job (54%), concerns that others would think less of them (47%), preference for spiritual/religious counseling (40%), uncertainty that treatment would be helpful (36%), thinking less of oneself (32%), and concern for negative effects on relationships with family/spouse (37%).

When clinicians recognize that stigma is a significant barrier to care, they can often broach the subject directly to begin to address the stigma. An alternate strategy is to integrate mental health services directly into primary care settings. This is an initiative that has been implemented throughout the VA system and has served to increase access to mental health services.

Conclusion

This chapter provides information for clinical practice, with the goal of identifying and serving the unique mental healthcare needs of women veterans. The demographics of women veterans were reviewed, and how military service can affect a woman veteran's postmilitary life was discussed. Known gender differences between male and female veterans in the prevalence of certain mental health conditions were summarized. Gender differences in biological, social, and cultural factors that influence mental health, such as reproductive health needs and gender disparities in economic resources, as well as the importance of gender-sensitive mental health care to address the unique healthcare needs of women veterans, were also discussed. Although much progress has been made to provide and improve gender-sensitive care for women veterans, there is still much work to be done. Future collaborative efforts among researchers, clinicians, administrators, policy makers, and the veterans consumers themselves will continue to optimize treatment outcomes for this very important emerging population.

References

1. Women veteran's report: the past, present and future of women veterans. Department of Veterans Affairs. National Center for Veterans Analysis and Statistics. February 2017. Available at https://www.va.gov/vetdata/docs/SpecialReports/Women_Veterans_2015_Final.pdf. Accessed January 2018.
2. Ritchie EC, Naclerio A, editors. Women at war. Oxford: Oxford University Press; 2015.
3. Runnals JJ, Garavoy N, McCutcheon SJ, Robbins AT, Mann-Wroel M, Ventimiglia A, Strauss JL, Mid-Atlantic Mental Illness Research Education and Clinical Center Women Veterans Workgroup. Systematic review of gender differences in mental health and unique needs of women veterans. Womens Health Issues. 2014;24(5):485–502.
4. Ross ID, Garavoy ND, McCutcheon SJ. The woman veteran experience. In: Ritchie EC, Naclerio AL, editors. Women at war. New York/Oxford: Oxford University Press; 2015.
5. Frayne SM, Phibbs CS, Saechaeo F, Maisel NC, Friedman SA, Finaly A, Haskell S. Sourcebook: women veterans in the Veterans Health Administration. Volume 3. Sociodemographics, utilization, costs of care, and health profile. Washington, DC: Women's Health Evaluation Initiative, Women's Health Services, Veterans Health Administration, Department of Veterans Affairs; 2014.
6. Lahav Y, Kanat-Maymon Y, Solomon Z. Posttraumatic growth and dyadic adjustment among war veterans and their wives. Front Psychol. 2017;30(8):1102.
7. Curry JF, Aubuchon-Endsley N, Brancu M, Runnals JJ, VA Mid-Atlantic MIRECC Women Veterans Research Workgroup, et al. Lifetime major depression and comorbid disorders among current-era women veterans. J Affect Disord. 2013;152:434–40.
8. Gerber MR, King MW, Iverson KM, Pineles SL, Haskell SG. Association between mental health burden and coronary artery disease in U.S. women veterans over 45: a national cross-sectional study. J Womens Health (Larchmt). 2018;27(3):238–44.
9. Smith BN, Taverna EC, Fox AB, Schnurr PP, Matteo RA, Vogt D. The role of PTSD, depression and alcohol misuse symptom severity in linking deployment stressor exposure and post-military work and family. Clin Psychol Sci. 2017;5(4):664–82.
10. Hoge CW, Terhakopian CA, Castro CA, et al. Association of posttraumatic stress disorder with somatic symptoms, health care visits, and absenteeism among Iraq war veterans. Am J Psychiatry. 2007;164:150–3.
11. Department of Defense annual report on sexual assault in the military fiscal year 2015 (2016). Retrieved from http://www.sapr.mil/public/docs/reports/FY15_Annual/FY15_Annual_Report_on_Sexual_Assault_in_the_Military.pdf. Accessed June 16, 2018.
12. Cloitre M, Stolbach BC, Herman JL, van der Kolk B, Pynoos BL, Wang J, Petkova E. A developmental approach to complex PTSD: childhood and adult cumulative trauma as predictors of symptom complexity. J Trauma Stress. 2009;22:399–408.
13. Dichter ME, Sorrentino A, Bellamy S, Medvedeva E, Roberts CB, Iverson KM. Disproportionate mental health burden associated with past-year intimate partner violence among women receiving care in the Veterans Health Administration. J Trauma Stress. 2017;30(6):555–63.

14. Scoglio AA, Shirk SD, Hoff RA, et al. Gender-specific risk factors for psychopathology and reduced functioning in post-9/11 veteran sample. J Interpers Violence. 2017; https://doi.org/10.1177/0886260517746182.
15. Leeies M, Pagura J, Sareen J, Bolton JM. The use of alcohol and drugs to self-medicate symptoms of posttraumatic stress disorder. Depress Anxiety. 2010;27:731–6.
16. Gifford E, Tavakol R, Wang K, et al. Female veterans in outpatient substance use disorder specialty care. Palo Alto: Center for Health Care Evaluation; 2011.
17. Bernardy NC, Lund BC, Alexander B, Jenkyn AB, Schnurr PP, Friedman MJ. Gender differences in prescribing among veterans diagnosed with posttraumatic stress disorder. J Gen Intern Med. 2012;28:542–8.
18. Kaplan MS, McFarland N. Firearm suicide among veterans in the general population: findings from the National Violent Death Reporting System. J Trauma. 2009;67:503–7.
19. Gibbons RD, Brown CH, Hur K. Is the rate of suicide among veterans elevated? Am J Public Health. 2012;102:17–9.
20. Ilegen MA, Bohnert AS, Ignacio RV, et al. Psychiatric diagnoses and risk of suicide in veterans. Arch Gen Psychiaty. 2010;67:1152–8.
21. Seal CH, Cohen G, Waldrop A, et al. Substance use disorders in Iraq and Afghanistan veterans in VA health care, 2001–2010: implications for screening diagnosis and treatment. Drug Alcohol Depend. 2011;116:93–101.
22. Kimerling R, Makin-Byrd K, Louzon S, Ignaocio RV, McCarthy JF. Military sexual trauma and suicide mortality. Am J Prev Med. 2016;50(6):684–91.
23. Zsido RG, Villringer A, Sacher J. Using position emission tomography to investigate hormone-mediated neurochemical changes across the female lifespan: implications for depression. Int Rev Psychiatry. 2017;29(6):589–96.
24. Powell-Dunford NC, Coda AS, Moore JL, Crago MS, Kelly AM, Deuster PA. Menstrual suppression for combat operations: advantages of oral contraceptive pills. Womens Health Issues. 2011;21(1):86–91.
25. Trego LL. Prevention is the key to maintaining gynecologic health during deployment. J Obstet Gynecol Neonatal Nurs. 2012;41:283–92.
26. Lowe NK, Ryan-Wegner NA. Military women's risk factors for and symptoms of genitourinary infections during deployment. Mil Med. 2003;168(7):569–74.
27. Bautista CT, Wurapa E, Sateren WB, Morris S, Hollingsworth B, Sanchez JL. Bacterial vaginosis: a synthesis of the literature on etiology, prevalence, risk factors, and relationship with chlamydia and gonorrhea infections. Mil Med Res. 2016;3:4.
28. Guo YL, You K, Qiao J, Zhao YM, Geng L. Bacterial vaginosis is conducive to the persistence of HPV infection. Int J STDs AIDS. 2012;23(8):581.
29. Gillet E, Meys JF, Verstraelen H, Verhelst R, De Sutter P, Temmerman M, Vanden Broeck D. Association between bacterial vaginosis and cervical intraepithelial neoplasia: systematic review and meta-analysis. PLoS One. 2012;7:e45201.
30. Coughlin SS, Krengel M, Sullivan K, Pierce PF, Heboyan V, Wilson LCC. A review of epidemiologic studies of the health of Gulf War women veterans. J Environ Health Sci. 2017;3(2) https://doi.org/10.15436/2378-6841.17.1551.
31. Miller LJ, Gladioli NY. Gender-specific mental health care needs of women veterans treated for psychiatric disorders in a Veterans Administration Women's Health Clinic. Med Care. 2015;53(4;1):93–6.
32. Department of the Navy. OPNAV Instruction 6000.1C. Available at: www.jag.navy.mil/distrib/instructions/OPNAV6000.1CPregnancyandParenthood.pdf. Accessed 17 June 2018.
33. Sherin JE. Post-traumatic stress disorder: the neurobiological impact of psychological trauma. Dialogues Clin Neurosci. 2011;13(3):263–78.
34. Katon J, Mattocks K, Zephyrin L, Reiber G, Yano EM, Callegari L, Schwarz EB, Brandt C, Haskell S. Gestational diabetes and hypertensive disorders of pregnancy among women veterans deployed in service of operations in Afghanistan and Iraq. J Women's Health. 2013;23(10):792–800.

35. Shaw JG, Asch SM, Katon JG, Shaw KA, Kimerling R, Frayne SM, Phibbs CS. Post-traumatic stress disorder and antepartum complications: a novel risk factor for gestational diabetes and preeclampsia. Pediatr Perinat Epidemiol. 2017;31(3):185–94.
36. Boyd MA, Bradshaw W, Robinson M. Mental health issues of women deployed to Iraq and Afghanistan. Arch Psychiatr Nurs. 2013;27(1):10–22.
37. Martin SE, Drake E, Yoder L, et al. Active duty Women's perceptions of breast-feeding support in the military setting. Mil Med. 2015;180(11):1154–60.
38. Katon J, Cypel Y, Raza M, Zephyrin L, Reibar G, Yano EM, Barth S. Self-reported infertility among male and female veterans serving during operation enduring freedom/operation Iraqi freedom. J Women's Health. 2014;23(2):175–83.
39. Centers for Disease Control and Prevention. Frequently asked questions about infertility. 2017. Available from: https://www.cdc.gov/reproductivehealth/infertility/index.htm. Accessed 17 June 2018.
40. Mattocks K, Kroll-Desrosiers A, Zephyrin L, Katon J, Weitlauf J, Bastion L, Haskell S, Brandt C. Infertility care among OEF/OIF/OND women veterans in the Department of Veterans Affairs. Med Care. 2015;53(4):68–75.
41. Ryan GL, Mengeling MA, Booth BM, Torner JC, Syrop CH, Sadler AG. Voluntary and involuntary childlessness in female veterans: associations with sexual assault. Fertil Steril. 2014;102(2):539–47.
42. Department of Veterans Affairs Office of Community Care. 2018. Available at: https://www.va.gov/COMMUNITYCARE/programs/veterans/ivf.asp. Accessed 17 June 2018.
43. Randolph BJ, Nelson LM, Highsmith JM. A review of unique considerations for female veterans with amputation. Mil Med. 2016;181(4):66–8.
44. Southwell KH, Shelley M, McDermid-Wadsworth M. The many faces of military families: unique features of the lives of female service members. Mil Med. 2016;181(1):70–9.
45. Metraux S, Cusack M, Byrne TH, et al. Pathways into homelessness among post-9/11-era veterans. Psychol Serv. 2017;14(2):229–37.
46. Pavao J, Turchik JA, Hyun JK, Karpenko J, Saweikis M, McCutcheon S, Kane V, Kimerling R. Military sexual trauma among homeless veterans. J Gen Intern Med. 2014;28(2):536–41.
47. Study of barriers for women veterans to VA Health Care: final report. Department of Veterans Affairs. April 2015. https://www.womenshealth.va.gov/WOMENSHEALTH/docs/Womens%20Health%20Services_Barriers%20to%20Care%20Final%20Report_April2015.pdf. Accessed Jan 2018.

Military Environmental Exposures and Mental Health

19

Matthew J. Reinhard, Michelle Kennedy Prisco, Nicholas G. Lezama, and Elspeth Cameron Ritchie

Introduction

Many years ago, Paracelsus (1493–1541) made this observation about the toxicity of chemicals [1]. This rings true today, as the risk for environmental exposure health effects depends on many factors, to include the exposed substance, corresponding dose and the health of the exposed individual.

DoD and VA mental health-care providers see numerous Veterans who have deployed to combat, humanitarian missions, or other locations where environmental toxins exist. To date, approximately 1,965,534 service members from the recent conflicts in Iraq and Afghanistan have separated from service [2]. Veterans from earlier combat deployments like the Korean War, Vietnam War, and the Gulf War

M. J. Reinhard (✉)
War Related Illness and Injury Study Center, Washington DC Veterans Affairs Medical Center, Washington, DC, USA

Department of Psychiatry, Georgetown University Medical School, Washington DC Veterans Affairs Medical Center, Washington, DC, USA

Uniformed Services University of the Health Sciences, Silver Spring, MD, USA
e-mail: matthew.reinhard@va.gov

M. K. Prisco · N. G. Lezama
War Related Illness and Injury Study Center, Washington DC Veterans Affairs Medical Center, Washington, DC, USA

E. C. Ritchie
Department of Psychiatry, Georgetown University Medical School, Washington DC Veterans Affairs Medical Center, Washington, DC, USA

Department of Psychiatry, MedStar Washington Hospital Center, Washington, DC, USA

George Washington University School of Medicine, Washington, DC, USA

Uniformed Services University of the Health Sciences, Silver Spring, MD, USA

Mental Health Community Based Outpatient, Washington, DC, USA

© Springer Nature Switzerland AG 2019
E. C. Ritchie, M. D. Llorente (eds.), *Veteran Psychiatry in the US*,
https://doi.org/10.1007/978-3-030-05384-0_19

(GW) also seek health care from DoD/VA. Even peacetime Veterans may be subject to possible exposure events.

Some of these service members and Veterans report environmental exposure concerns they believe are associated with certain health conditions. These service members and their families also have concerns about reproductive health effects that environmental exposures may have on their offspring. Women of childbearing age who are pregnant or lactating may be concerned about transmitting toxins to their offspring [3, 4].

For these reasons, it is important that VA, DoD, and civilian providers who interact with Veterans and service members have a basic understanding of military exposure concerns and the potential impact these exposures may have on physical, mental, and overall health. Given the target audience of this book, the purpose of this chapter is to provide an overview of occupational and environmental exposures in the military population to mental health providers who may see these service members and Veterans in their clinical practice.

Military Environmental Exposures

Military service members encounter a range of occupational and/or environmental exposures during military service that may cause acute and/or long-term health effects. Military exposures typically are categorized as garrison exposures, which are exposures occurring in military nonwar settings, or combat exposures, which are exposures occurring during combat operations.

Garrison occupational exposures may include occupational exposures found in civilian workplace settings like petroleum, metals, noise, solvents, or asbestos [5]. Combat environmental exposures include military unique exposures like chemical and biological warfare agents, burn pit smoke, and deployment health prophylactics like anthrax vaccinations and pyridostigmide bromide tablets [6].

Historical Military Exposures

From the Civil War to recent conflicts in Iraq and Afghanistan, different environmental exposures place military personnel at risk for adverse health effects [7–9]. Some historical military environmental exposure concerns include (1) Agent Orange herbicides used during Vietnam War [10]; (2) burning oil well fires [11]; (3) chemical and biological warfare agent concerns [6]; (4) depleted uranium [11]; (5) use of health prophylactics like vaccinations and pyridostigmide bromide during the Gulf War (GW) 1990–1991 [6]; (6) burn pits, sulfur fires [7], and sodium dichromate; (7) antimalarial regimens like mefloquine used during more recent wars in Iraq and Afghanistan [12]; and (8) environmental exposure concerns at military garrison sites like Camp Lejeune (past water contamination) [13] and Fort McClellan (radioactive compounds, chemical warfare agents, airborne polychlorinated biphenyls) [14].

The Department of Veterans Affairs (VA) now presumes that certain chronic, unexplained symptoms existing for 6 months or more may be related to GW service [15]. A variety of different environmental exposures (i.e., infections, airborne exposures, vaccines, neurotoxins, combat stress) have been investigated as to potential causes for these medically unexplained symptoms [16–18]. To date, the etiology of these poorly understood combat syndromes remains elusive [16].

In addition to military historical exposures, there are many ubiquitous environmental exposures present in deployment environments. Examples include harsh climates, austere living conditions, industrial pollution, incoming fire and explosive events, threat or experience of combat, noise hazards, infectious diseases, and carrying heavy equipment [19, 20].

Prevalence

After recent conflicts, service members were asked if they had environmental exposure concerns they wished to discuss with a health-care provider following a deployment [21]. This was done primarily through the Post Deployment Health Assessment, which is completed when service members return from deployment, and then again through a Re-Assessment survey 3–6 months later.

Approximately 12–45% of Operation Enduring Freedom/Operation Iraqi Freedom (OEF/OIF) Veterans reported a military environmental exposure concern they believe impacted their health [21]. The frequency of these environmental exposure concerns often rose 3–6 months after a deployment [21], with deployed Veterans reporting a mean of 2.7 environmental exposure concerns [20].

Research also shows that many Veterans from prior wars (e.g., Gulf War and Vietnam Veterans) still have environmental exposure concerns they wish to discuss. Approximately 20% of GW Veterans report persistent medically unexplained symptoms they attribute to deployment environmental exposure (s) [22]. Research studies and news reports also illustrate that many Vietnam Veterans still have questions about Agent Orange, the herbicide used during the Vietnam conflict [23, 24].

Significance

Given the prevalence of military environmental exposures and the impact these exposures may have on health, health-care providers must be familiar with these concerns. If service members and Veterans encounter health-care providers not familiar with these exposures, perceptions of mistrust may arise that make it difficult for these individuals to engage in recommended treatments. If people believe their environmental exposure concerns are not adequately addressed by a trusted and credible authority [25], they may view these informational sources as untrustworthy. They also may be at greater risk for holding beliefs that are incongruous with their actual risk for developing exposure-related disease [26].

Service members and Veterans who report military environmental exposure concerns they believe are not addressed in a timely and accurate manner also may be at risk for higher rates of chronic health conditions and higher health-care utilization, seek more disability benefits, and rate VA care as less satisfactory compared to Veterans who do not have these concerns [27–30]. They also may be less adherent and receptive to recommended treatments if they believe the cause of their health symptoms is tied to an unaddressed military environmental exposure concern [31, 32].

Occupational and Environmental Medicine Overview

Occupational and environmental medicine is a complex field that is constantly evolving. When speaking to service members or Veterans about military occupational or environmental exposure concerns, it is important to remember basic occupational and medicine concepts. An environmental exposure is typically defined as an event (s) in which a potentially toxic environmental substance enters the body [33]. Depending on the makeup of the exposure, some exposures are more hazardous and toxic than others.

Protective Mechanisms

The body has many protective mechanisms (i.e., skin barriers, respiratory and gastrointestinal linings) to protect itself from harmful exposures [34]. Many service members also receive training and guidance about protective measures (i.e., use of personal protective measures, health prophylactic measures, ventilation systems) to minimize potential exposure health effects.

Service members (particularly those deployed) frequently operate in austere environments, with limited resources, that may affect their ability to engage in self-protective exposure measures. This is complicated by the increased number of combat deployments in recent years. All of these factors may put service members at increased risk for potential military occupational and/or environmental exposure health effects.

Occupational and Environmental Hazards

Occupational Safety and Health Administration (OSHA) classifies occupational and environmental exposures into hazard categories for identification purposes [35] (see Table 19.1). Contributing risk factors for exposure disease like characteristics of the exposure and individual host factors [1, 36] also are listed in Table 19.1.

Table 19.1 Occupational and environmental hazards [35]

Category	Definition	Examples
Physical	Exposures that may cause health effects without touching the body	Radiation (ionizing radiation and nonionizing radiation), exposure to ultraviolet radiation from the sun, hot and cold temperature extremes, loud noises
Chemical	Exposure to chemicals in any form (solid, liquid, gas)	Solvents, paints, gasolines, pesticides, and gases like carbon monoxide, propane
Biological	Exposures that occur through contact with people, animals, plants, or other organisms	Blood or bodily fluids, bacteria/viruses, mold/fungi, insect/animal bites, animal droppings, contact with infectious plants
Ergonomic	Types of work, body positions, or work conditions that place strain on the body	Repetitive movements, poor posture, frequent lifting
Safety factors	Unsafe conditions that lead to falls, injury, and/or illness	Spills on floors or tripping over obstacles, frayed electrical cords, unsafe machinery, working from heights
Work organization factors	Spills on floors or tripping over obstacles, frayed electrical cords, unsafe machinery, working from heights	Workload demands, lack of respect, workplace violence, sexual harassment

Contributing factors [1, 36]: Exposure dose, frequency of exposure, other exposures an individual may have encountered, and underlying individual health factors to include genetics, presence of chronic health conditions, and social habits

Exposure Routes

When assessing for health effects related to environmental exposures, occupational and environmental medicine physicians also ask about exposure routes as this can provide a clearer understanding about the potential health effects that may arise. Depending on the exposure route, certain health effects may occur (see Table 19.2) [1, 34, 36–38].

Challenges and Pitfalls

Given the complexities associated with occupational and environmental exposure disease, it is sometimes difficult for health-care providers to determine who may be at risk for environmental exposure disease and which health condition (s) may be related to an environmental exposure (s). It is not always easy to determine which health effects are associated with an environmental exposure, [11] particularly if there is conflicting science [39]. Some of the challenges and pitfalls associated with conducting these exposure assessments are outlined below:

Table 19.2 Exposure routes

Exposure Route	Effects [1, 34, 36–38]
Skin or eye	Dermal exposure may cause mild effects like transient redness or mild dermatitis. More severe effects may include destruction of skin tissue or other significant skin conditions Ocular exposures may cause mild to severe health effects ranging from mild redness and irritation to more severe conditions like corneal abrasions, burns, blindness, and other health effects depending on injury and absorption rates
Inhalation	Exposures that are inhaled are either exhaled or deposited in the respiratory tract. If deposited in the respiratory tract, respiratory irritation or disease may occur. Once a substance is systemically absorbed, other health effects may occur depending on the substance absorbed and the affected target organs
Ingestion	Chemicals that are ingested may not cause harm to the gastrointestinal tract unless they are irritating or corrosive. Chemicals that are insoluble in the gut may get excreted. Chemicals that are soluble may be absorbed through the gastrointestinal tract lining and transported to other parts of the body where they may cause damage
Injection	This includes intravenous, intramuscular, intradermal, intraperitoneal, and/or subcutaneous injections with a contaminated or hazardous substance. Health effects depend on the injection exposure route, dose, and properties of the substance injected

Image: http://www.riley.army.mil/News/Photos/igphoto/2001326834/
Source—U.S. Army
Description—Soldiers conducting MOPP gear exchange during training at the National Training Center at Fort Irwin, California

- It can be difficult to determine what environmental exposures a service member encountered due to lack of individual exposure data [40, 41]. In many instances, service members are deployed to remote or primitive environments where environmental monitoring is not available, and service members do not have individual exposure monitoring devices. Given the limitations associated with environmental sampling and collecting individual samples [42], there seldom is a simple biomarker that can definitively answer an environmental exposure question.
- Many disease etiologies are multifactorial (i.e., genetics, social habits, underlying health conditions, environmental exposures). For this reason, it may

not be easy to determine whether an exposure is associated with a certain disease.
- These uncertainties can be frustrating for service members/Veterans. This is particularly the case when disability benefits are requested.
- There are many examples of social media posts and web blogs attributing military environmental exposures to a variety of medical conditions to include some that are medically ill-defined. The impact of these media reports may increase perceptions that an association exists between an environmental exposure and a health condition even when there is no definitive scientific information supporting this.
- There have been past controversies in how occupational and environmental exposures have been addressed. There have been reports of governments/companies improperly handling or disposing of chemicals and reports of inadequate responses to environmental exposure concerns.
- Given this history, some people are skeptical or harbor suspicions about how occupational and environmental exposure concerns are addressed currently. This skepticism and suspicion also may make it more difficult for health-care providers to address the underlying exposure concern.

Clinical Exposure Evaluations

When conducting occupational and environmental exposure evaluations, accurate diagnosis requires a thorough clinical and exposure history, physical examination, relevant laboratory and diagnostic testing, and specialty consultation as indicated [43]. If neurological, neuropsychiatric, or psychiatric sequelae are suspected, relevant specialty consultation is indicated. Results of the exposure evaluation will guide medical treatment, and emphasis should be placed on avoiding repeated exposures to hazardous exposures [43].

Potential Neuropsychiatric and Behavioral Symptoms

Occupational exposure to metals, solvents, pesticides, or other toxins can cause neurological or behavioral sequelae, especially if the exposure is above recommended thresholds. The immediate effects of toxic exposures may involve all regions of the nervous system, whereas delayed effects are likely related to focal deficits. Diffuse damage to the central nervous system may cause alterations in thinking, consciousness, or attention, sometimes in combination with abnormalities of movement. Focal dysfunction can cause a myriad of syndromes, depending on which area of the brain is involved and the extent and severity of damage [24].

Unique Military Exposures and Associated Neuropsychiatric Symptoms

Agent Orange Herbicides

The US military sprayed herbicides over Vietnam from 1962 to 1971 [24]. The herbicide mixtures used were named from the colors of storage drum identification bands. The main chemical mixture sprayed was Agent Orange, a 50:50 mixture of 2,4-D and 2,4,5-T [24]. The most toxic form of dioxin, 2,3,7,8-tetrachlorodibenzo-*p*-dioxin (TCDD), was an unintended contaminant generated during the production of 2,4,5-T, which was present in Agent Orange as well as some other formulations sprayed in Vietnam [24].

In response to Vietnam Veteran health concerns and uncertainty about long-term effects from sprayed herbicides, Congress passed the Agent Orange Act of 1991. This act directed the VA to ask the National Academy of Sciences (NAS) to evaluate the scientific and medical information regarding the health effects of exposure to Agent Orange, other herbicides used in Vietnam, and the various components of those herbicides, including TCDD. The NAS reviews new literature and publishes updates every 2 years.

Currently, the VA recognizes certain diseases as presumptive diseases associated with Agent Orange exposure. Veterans who were exposed to Agent Orange or other herbicides during military service are eligible for an Agent Orange Registry health exam for possible long-term health problems related to herbicide exposure [24, 44].

The National Academies of Science Veterans and Agent Orange committee concluded there is inadequate or insufficient evidence to determine whether there is an association between herbicide exposure and cognitive or neuropsychiatric disorders [24]. The committee distinguished behavioral health conditions such as posttraumatic stress disorder (PTSD), depression, and anxiety from neurologic conditions. "First, military service alone, including deployment and service in Vietnam, confers a range of potentially traumatic psychological exposures that may be expected to increase the risk of developing PTSD and related psychological comorbidities. To illustrate this point, compelling evidence has established that the prevalence of PTSD is more than twice as high for operational infantry units exposed to direct combat than in the general population [45]. Given the known relationship between combat exposure and an increased risk of mental health conditions, a synthesis of the literature would not provide the opportunity to disentangle any potential adverse effects from exposure to the chemicals of interest (COIs) on mental health outcomes [24]. Second, a review of the vast toxicology literature that relates to the COIs reveals that there is a dearth of reports that address the potential associations that may influence the risk of developing mental health conditions [24]."

Gulf War Illness

The 1991 Gulf War (GW) was conducted by a multinational coalition in response to the Iraqi invasion of Kuwait. A troop buildup (Operation Desert Shield) was followed by a 6-week air campaign and 4 days of ground combat (Operation Desert Storm). GW Veterans may have been exposed to a variety of environmental and chemical hazards that carried potential health risks. GW exposures include chemical warfare agents released by the destruction of Iraqi facilities, extensive spraying and use of pesticides, pyridostigmine bromide (PB) pills given prophylactically to protect troops against nerve agent exposure, and smoke from oil well fires set by the Iraqi troops as they withdrew from Kuwait [16, 17].

Operation Desert Shield and Desert Storm Veterans have experienced multiple health complaints and disorders. Approximately 25% of these Veterans have Gulf War Illness (GWI), a condition characterized by medically unexplained chronic symptoms that can include fatigue, headaches, joint pain, indigestion, insomnia, dizziness, respiratory disorders, and memory problems [46]. VA refers to these illnesses as chronic multi-symptom illness and undiagnosed illnesses.

Some research has raised the concern of pesticide and PB exposures to GWI [46], while exposures to low-level nerve gas agents, contaminants from oil well fires, multiple vaccinations, and combinations of these exposures cannot be ruled out [16, 17]. Other research also has suggested that Gulf War Veterans have higher rates of neurological disorders such as ALS, brain cancer, stroke, migraine headaches, neuritis, and neuralgia, alone or in combination with medically unexplained illnesses [46].

According to the last report issued by the Committee on Gulf War and Health, ALS was the only neurological condition for which the committee found limited/suggestive evidence for an association related to GW deployment [16]. It is important to note that higher rates of ALS is not specific to GW Veterans as the VA established ALS as a presumptive compensable illness for all Veterans, based on a 2006 Institute of Medicine report [47].

Psychiatric conditions were studied in Operation Desert Shield and Desert Storm Veterans after their multiple health concerns became known. Posttraumatic stress disorder (PTSD) occurs in approximately 3–6% of Gulf War Veterans [46]. Research on PTSD and other psychiatric disorders among Gulf War Veterans shows lower rates of these conditions than in Veterans of other wars and far lower than the prevalence of GWI [46]. Combat stressors, self-reported stress reactions, and exposure to other stressful events do not explain or predict GWI. The 2010 Institute of Medicine report concluded that "the excess of unexplained medical symptoms reported by deployed Gulf War veterans cannot be reliably ascribed to any psychiatric disorder [17]."

Environmental Exposures and Neuropsychiatric Conditions

In addition to the above unique military exposures, environmental exposures may cause neuropsychiatric effects in several different ways. First, some toxins may have primary psychiatric and neuropsychiatric effects on the central nervous system, such as organophosphates (chemical warfare agents, pesticides) and many solvents [48]. In addition, acute and perhaps continued long-term effects have been reported by some taking prophylaxis medications (e.g., mefloquine) [49].

Second, even in the absence of primary neuropsychiatric effects, anxiety and depression may occur as a result of coping with chronic disease related to military environmental exposure (s) (i.e., Agent Orange-related cancer, burn pit related respiratory disease). Third, psychiatric symptoms such as anxiety may occur when there is a vaccuum of accurate information, or accurate information is not provided in a timely manner as to whether symptoms may be related to a harmful toxin exposure. Imagine a Gulf War service member hearing chemical alarms related to possible missile attacks along with orders to quickly put on Mission Oriented Protective Posture Gear (MOPP) in extreme heat situations, and how this may lead to increased levels of anxiety especially when one is concerned about a potential exposure to a lethal, colorless, and odorless chemical warfare agent. It is reasonable for service members/Veterans to connect or question whether possible toxic exposures may contribute to their current health symptoms in some way. Veterans also may present for care without specific recall of potential exposure events. Rather, they may present with exposure concerns that are broad and nonspecific in nature (i.e., deployed to the Gulf War).

Given these examples, it is easy to understand why some service members and Veterans may not trust DoD and VA officials and, by extension, the health-care providers that work for those agencies who may be viewed as purveyors of government misinformation. In cases like this, employing risk communication methods is essential to address these exposure concerns.

Risk Communication

Experts recommend using risk communication techniques when discussing military environmental exposure concerns with Veterans. Risk communication is defined as "an interactive process of exchange of information and opinions among individuals, groups, and institutions, concerning a risk or potential risk to human health or the environment" [50].

In the clinical context, risk communication is characterized as a two-way exchange of information between a patient and clinician about the nature, magnitude, significance, and/or control of a risk [51] in order to put an environmental exposure concern into context. An important element of risk communication is to make sure the patient is an active participant in the discussion and his/her concerns are elicited and acknowledged.

To be effective, risk communication needs to be responsive to the concerns of the target patient or audience. This is especially critical when the topic is controversial in nature or there are a number of unknown factors as is the case with military environmental exposure education [52]. Good risk communication may not always address the underlying concern or change perceptions, but poor risk communication may result in an increased perception of risk and, more importantly, a decrease in trust toward the information source [52].

Principles of Risk Communication

When conducting risk communication, health-care providers must remember the following principles [53]:

- Engage the service member and Veteran as an active partner. The goal is to have an informed discussion, not diffuse or dismiss the concern.
- Listen carefully to the service members' and Veterans' specific concerns. People often care more about trust, credibility, competence, fairness, and empathy than statistics and details.
- Be honest, frank, and open. Trust and credibility are difficult to obtain. If lost, they are difficult to regain.
- Work with other credible sources. If you do not know an answer, seek help from other credible sources.
- Recognize the role of media on people's perceptions of military environmental exposure concerns. Sometimes, media reports focus more on politics than risk, simplicity over complexity, and danger over safety.
- Speak clearly and with compassion. If a tragic event like an illness, injury, or death occurred, acknowledge it—whether it may or may not be related to an environmental exposure event.
- Recognize that service members and Veterans may understand risk information, but may not agree with information conveyed. In these cases, people may not be satisfied with the information provided.

Health-care providers may not be able to answer the underlying specifics of Veteran's military environmental exposure concern, but they can engage the service member/Veteran in the conversation and provide them with referral resources that better address the concern and follow-up to determine that the concern was addressed.

Summary

Given the complexities and controversies surrounding military environmental exposure concerns in the deployed population, some people may feel as if their military exposure concerns are not taken seriously and dismissed as "all in the head." This can cause resentment and mistrust. These feelings of resentment and mistrust can be further exacerbated if these service members and Veterans perceive that their health-care providers do not fully understand the complexities of environmental exposures and dismiss the exposure concerns as psychological in nature.

Understanding that your patient has exposure concerns and the context from which these exposure concerns may arise, having a basic working knowledge of the most common toxins, utilizing risk communication principles, and knowing where to refer for more information are essential. These concepts should be part of the whole health model of care that includes asking how military environmental exposure concerns may impact quality of life and financial, occupational, social, community, and spiritual factors.

For More Information

There are a number of occupational and environmental exposure and deployment health resources available:

- *Department of Veterans Affairs Post-Deployment Health Services*: conducts epidemiological studies on Veterans' health and develops and provides information on military exposure (s) and related health effects, deployment health research, environmental exposure fact sheets, and VA post-deployment resources. https://www.publichealth.va.gov/index.asp
- *Department of Veterans Affairs' War Related Illness and Injury Study Center (WRIISC)*: VA's national post-deployment health resource that seeks to advance post-deployment health care through clinical, education, and research programs. https://www.warrelatedillness.va.gov/
- *DoD's Deployment Health Branch*: provides product development and deployment health execution guidance. https://health.mil/Military-Health-Topics/Health-Readiness/Public-Health/Deployment-Health
- *Army Public Health Center*: Identifies and assesses current and emerging health threats for military populations and develops and communicates public health solutions. Issues Periodic Occupational and Environmental Monitoring Summaries (POEMS) for specific military sites. Issues periodic publications and surveillance reports. https://phc.amedd.army.mil/Pages/default.aspx
- *National Institute for Occupational Safety and Health (NIOSH)*: research programs, data and statistics, and publications and products on a variety of occupational health topics. https://www.cdc.gov/niosh/index.htm
- *Centers for Disease Control and Prevention (CDC)—National Center for Environmental Health*: provides resources on a variety of environmental health topics. https://www.cdc.gov/nceh/
- *Agency for Toxic Substances and Disease Registry*: facts sheets, training, and resources for questions about toxic substances. https://www.atsdr.cdc.gov/
- *Environmental Protection Agency*: Resources for environmental exposure topics. https://www.epa.gov/
- *Occupational Safety and Health Administration (OSHA)*: Provides resources on safe and healthful working conditions for working men and women. https://www.osha.gov/about.html

References

1. University of Nebraska- Lincoln. Toxicology and Exposure Guidelines (revised 1/03). [On-line]. {cited 7 March 2018}. Accessed https://ehs.unl.edu/documents/tox_exposure_guidelines.pdf
2. Analysis of VA health care utilization among Operation Enduring Freedom, Operation Iraqi Freedom, and Operation New Dawn Veterans: Cumulative from 1st Qtr FY 2002 through 3rd Qtr FY 2015 [online] (October 1, 2001 – June 30, 2015) {cited 5 March 2018}. Accessed

https://www.publichealth.va.gov/docs/epidemiology/healthcare-utilization-report-fy2015-tr3.pdf
3. Bell MR, Ritchie EC. Breastfeeding in the military. Part I: information and resources provided to servicewomen. Mil Med. 2003;8(10):807–12.
4. Bell MR, Ritchie EC. Breastfeeding in the military. Part II: resource and policy considerations. Mil Med. 2003;8(10):813–6.
5. Veterans Health Administration, Office of Patient Care Services, Post-Deployment Health Services. Public Health: Military Exposures-Occupational Hazards [online]. (2018) {cited 2018 Mar 19} https://www.publichealth.va.gov/exposures/categories/occupational-hazards.asp
6. Teichman R. Health hazards of exposures during deployment to war. J Occup Environ Med. 2012;54(6):655–8.
7. Morris MJ, Rawlins FA, Forbes DA, et al. Deployment-related respiratory issues. US Army Med Dep J. 2016;2-16:173–8.
8. Hyams KC, Wignall FS, Roswell R. War syndromes and their evaluation: from the U.S. Civil War to the Persian Gulf War. Ann Intern Med. 1996;125:398–405.
9. Hyams KC, Riddle J, Trump DH, et al. Protecting the health of United States military forces in Afghanistan: applying lessons learned since the Gulf War. Clin Infect Dis. 2002;34(supp 5):S208–14.
10. DeFraites RF, Richards EE. Assessing potentially hazardous environmental exposures among military populations: 2010 symposium and workshop: summary and conclusions. Mil Med. 2011;176:17–21.
11. Richards EE. Responses to occupational and environmental exposures in the U.S. military-World War II to the present. Mil Med. 2011;176:22–8.
12. Nevi RL. Mefloquine prescriptions in the presence of contraindications: prevalence among US military personnel deployed to Afghanistan, 2007. Pharmacoepidemiol Drug Saf. 2010;19(2):206–10.
13. Veterns Health Administration, Office of Patient Care Services, Post-Deployment Health Services. Public Health: Military Exposures-Camp Lejeune Past Water Contamination [online]. (2018) {cited 2018 Mar 19} https://www.publichealth.va.gov/exposures/camp-lejeune/
14. Veterans Health Administration, Office of Patient Care Services, Post-Deployment Health Services. Public Health: Military Exposures-Potential Exposure at Fort McClellan [online]. (2018) {cited 2018 Mar 19} https://www.publichealth.va.gov/exposures/fort-mcclellan/index.asp
15. Murphy FM, Mather SH, Brown MA. Innovation in Veterans' health care and assistance: the Department of Veterans Affairs 10 years after the Gulf War. Mil Med. 2002;167(3):191–5.
16. Committee on Gulf War and Health: Institute of Medicine. Gulf War and health, volume 10, update on health effects of serving in the Gulf War. Washington, DC: National Academies Press; 2016.
17. Committee on Gulf War and Health: Institute of Medicine. Gulf War and health, volume 8: update of health effects of serving in the Gulf War. Washington, DC: National Academies Press; 2010.
18. Nettleman M. Gulf War illness: challenges persist. Trans Am Clin Climatol Assoc. 2015;126:237–47.
19. Spelman JF, Hunt SC, Seal KH, et al. Post deployment care for returning combat Veterans. J Gen Intern Med. 2012;27(9):1200–9.
20. Helmer D, Rossignol M, Blatt M, et al. Health and exposure concerns of Veterans deployed to Iraq and Afghanistan. J Occup Environ Med. 2007;49(5):475–80.
21. Armed Forces Health Surveillance Center. Update: deployment health assessments, U.S. armed forces, December 2010. MSMR. 2010;17(12):14–5.
22. Veterans Health Initiative: Guide to Gulf War Veterans' Health. DVA-EES. March 2002.
23. Veterans Health Initiative: Vietnam Veterans and Agent Orange. DVA-EES. First released March 2002. Updated June 2008.

24. National Academies of Sciences, Engineering, and Medicine. Veterans and agent orange: update 2014. Washington, DC: The National Academies Press; 2016.
25. Peters R, Covello V, McCallum D. The determinants of trust and credibility in environmental risk communication: an empirical study. Risk Anal. 17(1):43–54.
26. Zikmund-Fisher BJ, Turkelson A, Franzblau A, et al. The effect of misunderstanding the chemical properties of environmental contaminants on exposure beliefs: a case involving dioxins. Sci Total Environ. 2013;1(447):293–300.
27. Landrigan PJ. Illnesses in Gulf War veterans: causes and consequences. JAMA. 1997;277(3):259–61.
28. Dursa EK, Barth SK, Schneiderman AI, et al. Physical and mental health status of Gulf War and Gulf era Veterans: results from a large population-based epidemiological study. J Occup Environ Med. 2016;8(1):41–6.
29. Tsai J, Rosenheck RA. US Veterans' use of VA mental health services and disability compensation increased from 2001 to 2010. Health Aff (Millwood). 2016;35(6):966–73.
30. Committee on Gulf War and Health: Institute of Medicine. Gulf War and health: treatment for chronic multi-symptom illness. Washington, DC: National Academies Press; 2013.
31. McAndrew LM, Teichman RF, Osinubi OY, et al. Environmental exposure and health of Operation Enduring Freedom/Operation Iraqi Freedom veterans. J Occup Environ Med. 2012;54(6):665–9.
32. McAndrew LM, Helmer DA, Phillips LA, et al. Iraq and Afghanistan Veterans report symptoms consistent with chronic multisymptom illness one year after deployment. J Rehabil Res Dev. 2016;53(1):59–70.
33. Links MJ. Principles of Exposure, Dose, and Response. Johns Hopkins Bloomberg School of Public Health [online]. (2006) {cited 2017 Oct 25}. Accessed http://ocw.jhsph.edu/courses/environmentalhealth/pdfs/lecture1.pdf
34. Agency for Toxic Substances and Disease Registry. Toxicology Curriculum for Communities Trainer's Manual. Module Two: Routes of Exposure. [online]. (2018) {cited 2018 Mar 19} https://www.atsdr.cdc.gov/training/toxmanual/pdf/module-2.pdf
35. Occupational Safety and Health Administration [online]. Safety Hazards/Biological Hazards/Physical Hazards/Ergonomic Hazards/Chemical Hazards/Work Organization Hazards. (2018) {cited 2018 Mar 19} https://www.osha.gov/dte/grant_materials/fy10/sh-20839-10/circle_chart.pdf
36. Occupational Safety and Health Administration [online]. Understanding Chemical Hazards: Factsheet A. {cited 2018 Mar 25} https://www.osha.gov/dte/grant_materials/fy11/sh-22240-11/ChemicalHazards.pdf
37. Blackburn J, Levitan EB, MacLennan PA, et al. A case-crossover study of risk factors for occupational eye injuries. J Occup Environ Med. 2012;54(1):42–7.
38. Zakrzewski H, Chung H, Sander E, et al. Evaluation of occupational ocular trauma: are we doing enough to promote eye safety in the workplace? Can J Ophthalmol. 2017;54(4):338–42.
39. Gaydos JC. Military occupational and environmental health: challenges for the 21st century. Mil Med. 2011;176(7 Suppl):5–8.
40. Baird C. Deployment exposure and long-term health risks: the shadow of war. US Army Med Dep J. 2016;2-16:167–71.
41. May LM, Weese C, Ashley DL, et al. The recommended role of exposure biomarkers for the surveillance of environmental and occupational chemical exposures in military deployments: policy considerations. Mil Med. 2004;169(10):761–7.
42. Mallon TM. Progress in implementing recommendations in the National Academy of Sciences reports: Protecting those who serve: strategies to protect the health of deployed U.S. forces. Mil Med. 2011;176(7):9–16.
43. Dembert ML. Occupational Chemical Exposures and Psychiatric Disorders. Jefferson J Psychiatry. 1991;9(1):57–69.
44. Veterans Health Administration, Office of Patient Care Services, Post-Deployment Health Services: Benefits Overview for Agent Orange Exposure. Accessed Apr 4, 2018 at https://www.publichealth.va.gov/exposures/agentorange/benefits/index.asp

45. Kok BC, Herrell RK, Thomas JL, et al. Post-traumatic stress disorder associated with combat service in Iraq or Afghanistan: teconciling prevalence differences between studies. J Nerv Ment Dis. 2012;200:444–50.
46. White RF, Steele L, O'Callaghan J, et al. Recent research on Gulf War Illness and other health problems in veterans of the 1991 Gulf War: effect of toxicant exposures during deployment. Cortex. 2016;74:449–75.
47. Institute of Medicine. Amyotrophic lateral sclerosis in veterans: review of the scientific literature. Washington, DC: The National Academies Press; 2006.
48. Albers J, Berent S. Neurobehavioral toxicology: neurological and neuropsychological perspectives, Volume III. New York: Taylor & Francis; 2009.
49. Food and Drug Administration [online]. FDA Drug Safety Communication: FDA approves changes for antimalarial drug mefloquine hydrochloride due to risk of serious psychiatric and nerve side effects. https://www.fda.gov/Drugs/DrugSafety/ucm362227.htm.
50. National Research Council. Improving risk communication: National Research Council. Washington, DC: DC National Academy Press; 1989.
51. Covello VT. Risk communication: an emerging area of health communication research. In: Deetz SA, editor. Communication yearbook 15. Newbury Park: Sage; 1992. p. 359.
52. Santos SL, Helmer D, Teichman R. Risk communication in deployment-related exposure concerns. J Occup Environ Med. 2012;54(6):752–9.
53. Raab C, Harkins DK, Prisco MK, et al. Chapter 23: risk communication: an essential element of effective care. Airborne hazards related to deployment. Texas: Borden Institute, US Army Medical Department Center and School Fort Sam Houston; 2015. p. 231–8.

Neuropsychiatric Quinism: Chronic Encephalopathy Caused by Poisoning by Mefloquine and Related Quinoline Drugs

20

Remington L. Nevin

Background

Quinolines are a class of neurotoxic drug that have been widely used against parasitic febrile disease, particularly malaria, for hundreds of years since the Western discovery in the seventeenth century of the curative powers of the bark of the cinchona tree [1]. Quinine, a naturally occurring derivative first isolated from cinchona bark in the nineteenth century, is the prototypical quinoline drug from which the class derives its name. Quinine and its naturally occurring stereoisomer quinidine, and the related cinchona derivatives cinchonine, and its stereoisomer cinchonidine, are known as the cinchona alkaloids [2].

The cinchona alkaloids have a narrow therapeutic index in clinical use [3], and poisoning by the drugs, due to overdose or idiosyncratically, can occur either in treatment or prevention of parasitic disease. Use of the drugs is associated with a condition traditionally known as cinchonism, marked by a range of neuropsychiatric symptoms, including dizziness, vertigo, visual disturbances, and tinnitus, which are often attributed to peripheral neurotoxicity [4, 5], but which may be equally attributable to central neurotoxicity. Cinchonism is often accompanied by gastrointestinal symptoms such as abdominal pain, nausea, emesis, and diarrhea [4]. Cinchonism is also recognized as having psychiatric manifestations including cognitive impairment consistent with a limbic encephalopathy [6]. However, other psychiatric effects of the cinchona alkaloids, including depression, anxiety, mania, irritability, paranoia, personality change, and psychosis, have historically been attributed to the effects of cerebral malaria. As cerebral malaria is a disease for which the cinchona alkaloids were previously the only effective treatment, the drugs were a ubiquitous confounding exposure [7].

R. L. Nevin (✉)
The Quinism Foundation, White River Junction, VT, USA
e-mail: rnevin@quinism.org

Synthetic quinoline drugs were first manufactured in the early twentieth century as substitutes for the cinchona alkaloids in the treatment and prevention of malaria [8]. Similar symptoms of limbic encephalopathy were noted during early use of the synthetic drug quinacrine, including the same symptoms of depression, anxiety, mania, irritability, paranoia, personality change, psychosis, and cognitive impairment seen with the cinchona alkaloids. These more serious symptoms were frequently predicted by the development of prodromal symptoms including abnormal dreams and insomnia, which often developed idiosyncratically during early use of quinacrine [7].

Similar symptoms of limbic encephalopathy, and a similar propensity to neurologic and gastrointestinal effects as seen from the cinchona alkaloids, were subsequently reported following the more recent synthesis of related quinoline antimalarial drugs, including chloroquine, mefloquine, and tafenoquine [7]. These and other quinolines have also been demonstrated to be neurotoxic, both in vitro and in vivo, with neurohistopathological findings marked by neuronal loss in focal areas of the brain and brainstem [9].

The common signs and symptoms produced by the quinolines, and their common underlying neurotoxicity, suggest the existence of a unique medical disorder caused by a poisoning of the central nervous system by this class of drug. In this chapter, the term *neuropsychiatric quinism* is presented as a common term for the limbic encephalopathy and corresponding brain and brainstem dysfunction produced by quinoline poisoning. The term quinism, previously an obsolete synonym for cinchonism, is repurposed in this context to describe the broader family of medical disorders caused by quinoline poisoning.

This chapter will briefly review the likely pathophysiology of neuropsychiatric quinism and its corresponding clinical features and what is known of its epidemiology, with a particular focus on neuropsychiatric quinism from exposure to mefloquine. As this chapter will demonstrate, chronic symptoms consistent with those of neuropsychiatric quinism are likely to affect considerably greater than 1% of those exposed to this drug.

The chapter will then provide a brief history of the use of the quinoline drugs in military settings and illustrate some historical examples where the effects of the drugs may have been misattributed. The chapter will then describe how the clinical features of neuropsychiatric quinism may serve to mimic several common neuropsychiatric conditions now prevalent among veterans, particularly traumatic brain injury (TBI) and posttraumatic stress disorder (PTSD).

The chapter will next discuss considerations in the diagnosis and management of the condition. It will conclude with a discussion of the implications of neuropsychiatric quinism in the clinical care of veterans and the provision of disability compensation, and how research into several conditions, including PTSD and TBI, is likely to have been confounded by unmeasured exposure to the quinolines.

Pathophysiology

While the quinolines have diverse acute pharmacological and toxicological targets in the central nervous system too numerous to mention, several quinolines have been demonstrated to be neurotoxic in vitro and to induce a remarkable pattern of focal neuronal injury in various regions of the brain and brainstem in vivo, suggesting a common neurotoxic class effect across the quinolines.

Quinoline poisoning has been found in humans to induce injury to the hippocampus in cells of the pyramidal layer near the hilus of the dentate gyrus, accompanied by injury to the globus pallidus and basilar pons; and specifically to the oculomotor, trochlear, abducent, and vestibular nuclei [10], as well as the dorsal columns, inferior olive, and red nucleus [11]. Quinoline poisoning in humans has also been found to induce injury to the roots of the trigeminal, vestibulocochlear, and vagus nerves [12], and the nucleus gracilis [13].

In monkey studies, a similar but much broader pattern of neurotoxic injury has been observed, with various quinolines causing highly focal and cell-specific injury across a wide range of brain and brainstem structures. These include the oculomotor, Edinger–Westphal, trochlear, and abducent nuclei; the vestibular, cochlear, facial, and superior olivary nuclei and the inferior colliculus; the inferior olivary, red, and lateral reticular nuclei; the lateral cuneate nuclei; the paraventricular and supraoptic, anterior hypothalamic, and habenular nuclei; the pulvinar nuclei; the medial dorsal nucleus; the substantia nigra; the ambiguous and hypoglossal nuclei [14, 15]; and the dorsal motor nucleus of the vagus [16]. In other animal studies, related neurotoxic injury has been observed in the cuneate and gracile nuclei and in the solitary tract [17], and in cells in the entorhinal areas of the piriform cortex [18].

It is unclear why the quinolines cause this particular and highly focal pattern of neurotoxicity, which is suggestive of a cell-type-specific susceptibility. The specific molecular mechanisms of this neurotoxicity are also unclear.

Clinical Features

The clinical features of neuropsychiatric quinism reflect the localization of observed neurotoxic injury across the quinolines, with chronic dysfunction in affected areas of the brain and brainstem providing the most parsimonious explanation for the pattern of observed signs and symptoms from the disorder [9].

Auditory disturbances associated with neuropsychiatric quinism, including hyperacusis and tinnitus [19, 20], are consistent with dysfunction of the cochlear, superior olivary, and facial nuclei, and of the inferior colliculus. Visual disturbances including photophobia, binocular dysfunction, and difficulties in focusing, convergence, and accommodation [10, 21–23], are similarly consistent with dysfunction in the oculogyric and Edinger–Westphal nuclei. Similarly, symptoms of nystagmus, dizziness, and vertigo [24–26] are consistent with dysfunction in the vestibular nuclei. Related complaints of disequilibrium and unsteady gait [27, 28] can reflect these effects possibly worsened by loss of distal proprioception, consistent with dysfunction in the dorsal columns and gracile and cuneate nuclei. Paresthesias and dysesthesias, frequently attributed to peripheral causes, are similarly consistent with dysfunction in these areas and in other sensory nuclei. Movement disorders, such as ataxia and extrapyramidal syndrome [29–31], are also consistent with such dysfunction, and with related dysfunction in the globus pallidus, inferior olivary, red, and lateral reticular nuclei. Similarly, a propensity toward seizures in neuropsychiatric quinism [32–35] is consistent with a broader dysfunction and the creation of seizure foci, while headaches and migraine, a common finding in various neurotoxicity syndromes, are also reported.

Dysautonomia has also been reported in neuropsychiatric quinism, marked by lasting orthostatic hypotension, and sexual dysfunction including erectile and ejaculatory dysfunction [36]. These and other complaints, such as altered thermal regulation, are broadly consistent with dysfunction in various areas of the brainstem, including the paraventricular, supraoptic, and anterior hypothalamic nuclei, while related complaints of neuroendocrine abnormalities are consistent with dysfunction in adjacent areas.

An interesting manifestation of neuropsychiatric quinism is its effects on the gastrointestinal system. In human cases, lasting gastrointestinal complaints, including often severe abdominal pain and tenderness [8, 23, 37], often manifest only several days after dosing [36] and remain persistent, consistent with dysfunction of the dorsal motor horn of the vagus. Common related complaints, including nausea, emesis, and diarrhea, are consistent with such dysfunction, and to dysfunction in related brainstem chemoreceptor trigger areas.

Neuropsychiatric quinism is also associated with the interesting manifestation of both central and obstructive sleep apnea, the latter of which is consistent with impaired innervation of the genioglossal muscle from dysfunction of the hypoglossal nucleus [38–40]. Similarly, complaints of impaired swallowing [10] are consistent with such dysfunction, and with impaired innervation of the esophagus, resulting from dysfunction in the nucleus ambiguous and the dorsal motor horn of the vagus.

While less understood, the diverse psychiatric effects seen in neuropsychiatric quinism plausibly reflect dysfunction in the hippocampus, and in diverse other regions of the brain known to be affected by quinoline neurotoxicity, including the substantia nigra, habenular and pulvinar nuclei, and the medial dorsal nucleus. As with the association of neuropsychiatric quinism with seizure, these effects may also reflect to some degree the onset of an acquired temporal lobe epilepsy consistent with the creation of seizure foci [35].

Case reports of poisoning by quinoline drugs are consistent with encephalopathy of the limbic system, with symptoms of anxiety, depression, mania, irritability, paranoia, personality change, psychosis, and cognitive dysfunction [7]. Neuropsychiatric quinism is also associated with a risk of violent behavior [41–43], and consistent with its association with psychosis and other symptoms of mental illness, with a risk of self-injurious behavior, suicidal ideation, and completed suicide [43–45].

Symptoms of anxiety seen in cases of neuropsychiatric quinism can include a sense of apprehension, unease, or a sense of impending doom or death, panic, and fear and various phobias, including agoraphobia. Symptoms of depression can include tearfulness, sadness, fatigue, malaise and lethargy, and a sense of helplessness, pessimism, or hopelessness. Symptoms of mania can include emotional lability, euphoria, expansiveness, flight of ideas, inattention, disinhibition, inappropriate behavior, and hypersexuality and occasional paraphilia [7, 46, 47].

Neuropsychiatric quinism can also include symptoms of irritability, and in some cases can include symptoms of aggression, anger, and often extreme rage. Those suffering from neuropsychiatric quinism may also suffer from paranoia. Personality change, often with paranoid features, is a common feature of the disorder, with persecutory delusions, magical thinking, and hyperreligious thoughts not uncommonly reported. Other symptoms of psychosis can include auditory, olfactory, and visual hallucinations, often featuring zoopsia, and often with some degree of preserved insight. In certain cases, neuropsychiatric quinism may include delusional misidentification and dissociative symptoms, including derealization and depersonalization [7, 46, 47].

Symptoms of cognitive dysfunction in neuropsychiatric quinism are diverse and include temporospatial disorientation, disturbances in attention and concentration, including impairment of short-term and working memory, problems with word-finding, and impairment of explicit memory, including anterograde and retrograde amnesia. In acute cases, dysfunction can progress to delirium or can mimic delirium with consciousness preserved [7, 46, 47].

These diverse neuropsychiatric effects may be preceded by prodromal symptoms such as abnormal dreaming or restlessness and often severe insomnia, which herald an idiosyncratic susceptibility to quinoline toxicity at the lower doses used in prophylaxis of parasitic disease, such as the weekly use of mefloquine for prevention of malaria [7]. The vivid dreams associated with the prodrome of neuropsychiatric quinism are occasionally associated with parasomnias, such as sleep paralysis, and hypnopompic and hypnogogic hallucinations [7, 48], and have been described as "awakening dreams which at times were of a frightening and nightmare quality" [49], and "terrifying nightmares with often technicolor clarity—often remembered days later" [50].

As risk factors for susceptibility to idiosyncratic quinoline toxicity remain unknown, the risk minimization strategy adopted by drug regulators for mefloquine has long included a requirement that the drug be discontinued at the onset of certain prodromal symptoms [51], namely "anxiety, depression, restlessness or confusion." Some years later, drug regulators clarified that all "psychiatric symptoms" were prodromal [52]. However, the requirement to discontinue the drug at the onset of such symptoms has long been widely overlooked or misunderstood. Only recently did international drug regulators clarify mefloquine's labeling with boxed warnings, and add abnormal dreams, nightmares, and insomnia explicitly as symptoms requiring the drug's immediate discontinuation [53].

Epidemiology

Those suffering from neuropsychiatric quinism may appear to be suffering from various neurologic disorders, as well as from a wide range of psychiatric disorders listed in the Diagnostic and Statistical Manual of Mental Disorders, 5th Edition (DSM-5). These span the diagnostic nosology, particularly as various anxiety disorders, depressive disorders, manic and bipolar disorders, personality disorders, and conversion and factitious disorders.

As a newly described disorder, previously mistaken for other conditions, the epidemiology of neuropsychiatric quinism remains poorly defined. For example, although efforts have been made to ascertain the burden of various psychiatric and neurologic disorders to which symptoms of quinoline exposure have been attributed [54, 55], such effects have failed to define the epidemiology of neuropsychiatric quinism as a distinct disorder, and have themselves been hampered by methodological limitations including inadequate power, misclassification, and bias [56].

Based on limited studies, certain chronic effects consistent with those of neuropsychiatric quinism are likely to affect considerably greater than 1% of those exposed to mefloquine. For example, among those reporting nightmares with use of mefloquine, 21% report these continuing over 3 years after discontinuing use [48]. As abnormal dreams and nightmares are reported in at least 14% taking mefloquine [57], it is likely that 21% of these, or over 2% of those taking mefloquine, continue to experience nightmares chronically after use.

As the quinolines have been ubiquitous exposures among certain populations, including among military personnel, neuropsychiatric quinism is likely to be the cause of a significant burden of disease in these groups, but considerable additional study is needed to determine the absolute burden of disability attributable to quinoline poisoning versus other causes.

Neuropsychiatric Quinism in Recent Military History

Neuropsychiatric quinism has likely contributed to several notable incidents of neuropsychiatric illness, and to overall patterns of neuropsychiatric morbidity, associated with various events in recent military history. For example, quinine was widely used during the Macedonian campaign in World War I, where large numbers of psychiatric casualties, likely from quinine, appear to have been misattributed to the effects of malaria [58].

In the early years of World War II (WWII), British commander Orde Wingate survived a suicide attempt [59], likely resulting from the psychiatric effects of his use of quinacrine [60]. The US military's initial widespread use of quinacrine, beginning in the South Pacific campaign, was almost immediately associated with reports of a novel form of neurosis, described as "unique in medical history" [61]. Military researchers would subsequently observe an increased rate of psychosis in US military units administered quinacrine in the South Pacific theater [62]. Quinacrine was also administered to US troops during the early weeks of the Italian campaign [63]. This use suggests the possibility that the infamous incidents in which General Patton slapped two hospitalized soldiers, including one admitted for an "anxious breakdown," but accused by Patton of cowardice and thought to be malingering, may have involved unrecognized neuropsychiatric quinism. One soldier had recently contracted malaria [64], to which at least one of his contemporaries had likely misattributed his psychiatric symptoms [64], and the other would subsequently be diagnosed with malaria after being admitted for acute anxiety [65].

With the development of chloroquine [66] and primaquine resulting from a WWII-era drug development effort, these drugs would gradually replace quinacrine and the highly neurotoxic drug pamaquine [10], previously widely used for treatment, for use in treatment and prevention of malaria during the subsequent Korean war [67]. To what degree symptoms of neuropsychiatric quinism from these drugs contributed to patterns of morbidity and disability is not clear, although accounts of "persistent stress reaction" among veterans plausibly exposed to quinolines describe relatively common symptoms such as severe headache, dizziness, abdominal discomfort, diarrhea, difficulty swallowing, and concentration and memory impairment that are more consistent with neuropsychiatric quinism than with a purely trauma- or stress-related disorder [68].

Similarly, widespread use of chloroquine and primaquine during the war in Vietnam was accompanied by reports of a "toxic neurasthenia" syndrome, marked by symptoms of headache, rage, gastrointestinal complaints, and concentration and memory impairment, similarly inconsistent with a purely trauma- or stress-related disorder. While such cases were initially attributed to pesticide exposure [69], they may be equally attributable to neuropsychiatric quinism.

A more general "post-Vietnam syndrome," noted in the psychiatric literature from the era, and from which the diagnosis of PTSD would ultimately evolve [70], was notable for initial reports that differed significantly from this subsequent diagnosis, including headaches, and prominent features of rage and psychosis [71], and gastrointestinal symptoms including diarrhea [72]. Vietnam veterans subsequently diagnosed with PTSD have been found to have prominent symptoms of anger, rage, and memory and concentration impairment, not fully accounted for by this diagnosis [73]. Perhaps most intriguingly, Vietnam veterans treated for cerebral malaria, almost certainly with quinolines, have been found to have prominent symptoms of psychosis, rage, and memory and concentration impairment. Certain of these symptoms have been previously attributed to the sequelae of cerebral malaria [74, 75], but with improved understanding of the more limited symptomatology of this disorder [7], these findings may be considered more consistent with unrecognized neuropsychiatric quinism.

With the development of mefloquine to counter rising resistance of the malaria parasite to chloroquine [76], and the drug's subsequent widespread use in various military settings beginning in the early 1990s, reports would emerge of unusual behavior and extreme acts of violence associated with mefloquine use during various operations, including in Somalia, Afghanistan, and Iraq. Although eventually replaced by safer and non-neurotoxic alternatives by policy in the militaries of most English-speaking Western nations by early- to mid-2010s, mefloquine was a ubiquitous exposure on deployments throughout much of past quarter century [77], including in the US, Canadian, Irish, and UK militaries, and particularly during the period of sustained deployments associated with the recent epidemics in PTSD and TBI. In contrast, exposure to quinolines in the Australian military, where mefloquine use has traditionally been deprioritized, has been mostly limited to a series of controversial trials of mefloquine and tafenoquine [78].

Neuropsychiatric Quinism, TBI, and PTSD

One factor previously limiting recognition of neuropsychiatric quinism as a distinct disorder is that, particularly in recent military settings where confounding exposures such as traumatic stressors and blast are common, the symptoms of neuropsychiatric quinism are likely to have been misattributed to TBI and to PTSD [79].

As a chronic encephalopathy, and therefore, an acquired form of brain injury, many of the neurological symptoms of neuropsychiatric quinism may seem indistinguishable from those of TBI, particularly tinnitus, dizziness, vertigo, visual disturbance, and headache. Similarly, psychiatric symptoms such as cognitive dysfunction, irritability, personality change, and insomnia, are common to both TBI and to neuropsychiatric quinism. More specific combinations of psychiatric symptoms of neuropsychiatric quinism, including nightmares, insomnia, anxiety, depression, irritability, aggression, panic, and dissociation, may similarly readily mimic those of PTSD.

Although a strict application of DSM-5 PTSD diagnostic criterion H—which requires the condition not be due to the physiological effects of a substance or medication—will formally exclude the diagnosis of PTSD in cases of neuropsychiatric quinism, this diagnostic exclusion did not apply to earlier diagnostic criteria [79]. US military authors have cautioned that mefloquine use may "confound the diagnosis" of PTSD [80], and that "the significant overlap in symptoms associated with mefloquine toxicity and PTSD obscures the distinction between these diagnoses" [28]. There is evidence that this has resulted in PTSD being diagnosed disproportionately in those exposed to mefloquine. For example, in one military study of non-combat-deployed personnel, exposure to mefloquine resulted in a near-doubling of the rate of PTSD diagnosis as compared to those who lacked such exposure [54].

Diagnosis

Although occasionally associated with pathognomonic signs, the diagnosis of neuropsychiatric quinism should typically be made clinically, on the basis of reported history, after reasonably excluding other causes of persistent symptoms. Frequently, key to the diagnosis of neuropsychiatric quinism is establishing a history of symptomatic exposure to the quinolines and establishing the temporal onset of one or more persistent symptoms to such symptomatic exposure [81], rather than to other postulated causes, such as blast or traumatic stressors. In other cases, where multiple potentially confounding exposures exist, the clinician may need to attempt to disentangle the effects of blast or traumatic stressors from the effects of quinoline exposure, by considering the pattern of symptoms, and identifying characteristic features of neuropsychiatric quinism. In certain cases where attribution to other disorders, including psychiatric illness, has been made, the clinician may need to assess the patient's response to conventional therapies for these, and reexamine existing diagnoses in light of additional evidence of neurologic signs or symptoms of neuropsychiatric quinism.

Given the ubiquity of use of quinolines in military settings, particularly among veterans of recent wars presenting with chronic neuropsychiatric symptoms that have proven unresponsive to traditional therapies, clinicians should assess for the possibility of neuropsychiatric quinism in their patients by screening for symptomatic quinoline exposure [81]. Such screening involves first determining the likelihood of exposure to one or more of the quinoline drugs that have been in use as antimalarial drugs during recent military conflicts, including the drugs chloroquine, primaquine, mefloquine, and tafenoquine, in contrast to non-quinoline antimalarial drugs.

Although certain of these quinoline drugs were previously used commonly in the treatment of malaria disease, in more recent years, exposure to such drugs will likely have been in the form of these drugs being administered during deployment for the prevention of malaria. Drugs administered weekly for such purpose include mefloquine, chloroquine, or tafenoquine. Occasionally, such exposure will have been in the form of these drugs being administered daily. Drugs administered daily for such purpose include primaquine, and occasionally, mefloquine and tafenoquine, during brief initial loading doses. As well, primaquine and tafenoquine may have been administered daily for a period upon return from deployment as presumptive anti-relapse therapy.

Although in certain cases, the veteran's medical records will document such exposure, quinoline drugs have frequently been issued or dispensed as a public health measure under command direction, occasionally without documentation. In such cases, the clinician may need to rely on the veteran reliably reporting or presenting other evidence of use of such drugs. The clinician may also need to rely on the veteran demonstrating evidence of deployment to areas where use of such drugs could be inferred by policy or procedure. In cases where the veteran's history or documentation is considered unreliable, consultation with those with expertise in travel medicine and military medicine may aid in establishing likely exposures.

With exposure to one or more quinoline drugs thus established, the clinician should identify evidence of the veteran experiencing one or more symptoms consistent with the prodrome of quinoline encephalopathy during or soon following exposure to these drugs. Although chronic effects have been reported from quinolines after only a single prophylactic dose [82], prodromal symptoms may not manifest until after several doses [83], reflecting population heterogeneity in idiosyncratic susceptibility. If the veteran reports experiencing symptoms consistent with a prodrome, whether attributed to use of the drug or not—and particularly if the veteran reports continued use despite the onset of such symptoms—this should be considered evidence of an increased risk of neuropsychiatric quinism.

With symptomatic quinoline exposure thus confirmed, the clinician should then determine whether the onset of one or more of persistent symptoms correlates temporally to such symptomatic exposure. When the prodromal symptoms themselves have become chronic, particularly insomnia, or abnormal dreams or nightmares, this can often aid in more confidently assigning the diagnosis as the cause if the quality, temporality, and severity of these symptoms are explored during a thorough history. For example, persistent abnormal dreams or nightmares featuring imagery unrelated to specific actual traumatic stressors, which clearly develop within the first few doses of mefloquine and prior to any subsequent traumatic stressors, should in fact be considered evidence of the development of neuropsychiatric quinism. The persistence of such abnormal dreams or nightmares following exposure to traumatic stressors may readily confound a subsequent diagnosis of PTSD unless such a thorough history is taken.

In certain settings, the development of an appropriate questionnaire will assist in the process of screening both for exposure to quinolines, and for such symptomatic exposure. Such a questionnaire may consider historical patterns of quinoline use specific to the population to whom it is administered, and inquire of other exposures, such as blast and traumatic stressors, that could confound subsequent diagnosis of the disorder.

When existing psychiatric diagnoses are being reconsidered following confirmation of symptomatic quinoline exposure, it is helpful to consider the known epidemiology of prodromal and other acute symptoms. While certain of the symptoms of neuropsychiatric quinism may have been attributed to other causes, such as coincidental or latent psychiatric illness, the very common incidence of such symptoms from quinoline exposure should be considered in the attribution of causation. For example, symptoms of abnormal dreams, nightmares, and insomnia are very common with use of mefloquine, occurring in greater than 10% of users. Similarly, symptoms of anxiety, depression, and confusion affect greater than 1% of users [57]. The onset of multiple such symptoms, in temporal association with each other, particularly over a brief period during early use of the medication, may, by the principle of parsimony, be considered most likely to represent adverse effects of the medication than a result of coincidental or latent psychiatric illness.

Although neuroimaging should be considered in the workup of a suspected case of neuropsychiatric quinism, and particularly in cases with worrisome neurologic features or in cases where the differential diagnosis includes acute or evolving processes, conventional neuroimaging should be expected to be normal in most cases [46, 47]. Similarly, although abnormal electroencephalography (EEG) in the absence of other more likely causes should be considered consistent with neuropsychiatric quinism, EEG is similarly expected to be normal in most cases [46, 47]. Although there is insufficient experience with novel forms of neuroimaging, functional imaging and very high resolution imaging, as well as quantitative EEG (QEEG), may hold promise [46, 47].

In several case reports featuring contested diagnoses, the demonstration of additional neurologic features of neuropsychiatric quinism, particularly through specialist referral, have been sufficient to establish the diagnosis with relative certainty. For example, following symptomatic exposure to mefloquine or another quinoline, the development of additional symptoms of dizziness and vertigo, together with objective evidence of central vestibulopathy on specialist examination, in the absence of another more likely cause for these findings [25, 28, 30], should be considered strongly suggestive of the diagnosis. Specialist referral should be considered particularly in cases where symptoms may have contributed to consideration of somatoform or factitious disorder [25]. Specialist referral should also be made in cases where there may be legal considerations to the diagnosis [79].

Management

As a newly defined disorder, there is little published evidence suggesting which therapies may be effective for neuropsychiatric quinism. Current recommendations for management of neuropsychiatric quinism rest on establishing the extent of the disorder through additional specialist referrals, with consideration of symptomatic treatment where appropriate. Proper management also rests on the discontinuation or avoidance of potentially unhelpful therapies, and the avoidance of settings or environments that may exacerbate the disorder [46].

For example, a common feature of neuropsychiatric quinism is pronounced anxiety, apprehension, agoraphobic avoidance, and panic, particularly in certain environments. While certain of these symptoms may reflect a true organic anxiety, the frequent association of these symptoms with additional symptoms of dizziness, disequilibrium, vertigo, and visual disturbances in many patients, suggests a potential contribution of clinical or even subclinical vestibulocular dysfunction to the etiology. Consistent with a "supermarket syndrome," those suffering from neuropsychiatric quinism may demonstrate avoidance of particular environments [84], such as those with bright or flickering lights, or where there may be complex visual stimuli where loss of a visual horizon or excessive movement may induce vestibular decompensation. A similar agoraphobic avoidance of certain activities or modes of transport may reflect a similar vestibular sensitivity [85]. In such cases, referral to an otorhinolaryngologist, neuro-otologist, or neuro-otologist, for rotary chair and other sensitive testing for central vestibular disorders, would be appropriate. Such testing may aid in identifying those for whom further management and vestibular rehabilitation would be appropriate.

Similarly, those suffering neuropsychiatric quinism may experience complex visual disturbances, including problems with accommodation, binocular dysfunction, and visual processing, which may elude cursory optometric or ophthalmologic examination. Referral to a neuro-optometric specialist may aid in identifying visual disturbances that could benefit from specific neuro-optometric rehabilitation.

In cases where temporal lobe seizure disorder or other forms of induced epilepsy are suspected due to neuropsychiatric quinism, referral to neurology for management is appropriate. There is little direct evidence to guide pharmacologic management specifically of neuropsychiatric quinism, but where evidence of these disorders exists, conventional management would seem appropriate.

In contrast, the use of other pharmacotherapies should be approached with caution [46, 86]. Although the psychiatric symptoms of neuropsychiatric quinism may mimic those of several conventional psychiatric disorders, including various anxiety, mood, depressive, attention, and psychotic disorders, pharmacologic therapies for these disorders have never been specifically tested for safety or efficacy in neuropsychiatric quinism. Similarly, there is no specific evidence that the psychiatric disorders, for which these medications have demonstrated efficacy, share an underlying etiology in common with neuropsychiatric quinism such that the drugs' action would be expected to be therapeutic. Properly designed clinical trials will be necessary to determine which pharmacologic therapies may be helpful in neuropsychiatric quinism.

Similarly, equally untested treatments, such stellate ganglion block, which has demonstrated efficacy in such conditions as PTSD [87], may hold promise, but must be similarly subjected to proper tests of efficacy and safety in cases of neuropsychiatric quinism. Lastly, neurofeedback, which has been employed in TBI [88] and which appears anecdotally to offer some improvement in neuropsychiatric quinism, must also be subjected to properly designed clinical trials.

In many cases, particularly among veterans who have suffered for many years through treatments that have proven unhelpful or even counterproductive, the diagnosis of neuropsychiatric quinism and the determination that the veteran is in fact suffering from the effects of a poisoning will provide significant therapeutic benefit in and of itself. In many cases, the veterans will themselves have long suspected that their chronic symptoms were attributable to such a poisoning. However, in the absence of medical recognition, these veterans may have experienced considerable frustration. The clinician should not underestimate the therapeutic benefit that comes from veterans simply having their suspicions confirmed. Nor should the clinician underestimate the change in prognosis that can occur from simply acknowledging the condition, which in some settings has long been denied by various authorities.

Implications and Conclusions

Particularly given the ubiquity of exposure to quinolines in military settings, and the likelihood of misdiagnosis, neuropsychiatric quinism is likely to emerge as a significant public health problem in veteran populations. Recognition of neuropsychiatric quinism as a diagnosis is also likely to have important legal and policy implications, including in the areas of veteran compensation, military research, and drug development. This final section briefly discusses certain of these implications.

In recent years, in jurisdictions such as the United States and Australia with statutory veteran compensation systems, several successful claims or administrative findings have linked quinoline exposure with the development of various chronic neuropsychiatric effects. While not yet formally acknowledging neuropsychiatric quinism, these jurisdictions have, through various formal decision-making processes, acknowledged a likely causal link between quinoline exposure and various psychiatric and neurologic disorders consistent with neuropsychiatric quinism [89, 90]. In these jurisdictions, in due course, particularly given inconsistencies in documentation of exposure to the quinolines, adoption of a formal process of presumption, similar to what has been established for Agent Orange, may prove most efficient in managing the burden of claims associated with neuropsychiatric quinism.

Similarly, in jurisdictions such as the United Kingdom and Ireland, which rely on litigation to award claims for service-connected neuropsychiatric disabilities, several cases have been successfully settled in favor of claimants alleging harm from their use of the quinolines [91, 92]. In the coming years, such claims are likely to increase in number, suggesting the utility of a similar statutory compensation scheme to increase efficiencies and to avoid duplicative and expensive litigation.

Particularly problematic for the military research community is the potential for a significant body of work to be invalidated by growing recognition of neuropsychiatric quinism. In particular, much military research on PTSD and TBI has been conducted among populations with ubiquitous exposure to the quinolines, yet only rarely has this exposure been measured or considered in analysis. Exposure to the quinolines is likely to be correlated both with exposure to blast and other sources of concussive injury, and with exposure to traumas. Similarly, exposure to quinolines provides a separate, independent causal pathway for the development of symptoms previously attributed to TBI and PTSD, and is thus an unmeasured, but critical, confounder. The effects of confounding from unmeasured quinoline exposure on the internal validity of much of the current body of military PTSD and TBI research has yet to be fully considered, but calls urgently for the inclusion of quinoline exposure, and preferably symptomatic quinoline exposure, as an essential covariate in future analysis [93–95].

Lastly, the fact that many of the quinolines in common use were initially developed by governments and militaries is itself worthy of some note. Militaries in several jurisdictions continue to invest and collaborate in the development of quinoline drugs, while acknowledging the inherent neurotoxicity of certain of these. With growing recognition of neuropsychiatric quinism as a class effect, these militaries may need to reconsider the utility of this class of drug. The history of the development and use of the quinolines in military settings teaches that several decades may pass before the particular dangers of a given drug are fully recognized [9].

Conflict of Interest Statement Dr. Nevin serves as consultant and expert witness in legal cases involving claims of adverse effects from antimalarial drugs.

References

1. Greenwood D. The quinine connection. J Antimicrob Chemother. 1992;30(4):417–27.
2. Sullivan DJ. Cinchona alkaloids: quinine and quinidine. In: Staines HM, Krishna S, editors. Treatment and prevention of malaria. Basel: Springer Basel; 2012. p. 45–68.
3. Hofheinz W, Merkli B. Quinine and quinine analogues. In: Peters W, Richards W, editors. Antimalarial drugs II: current antimalarials and new drug developments. Berlin: Springer; 1984. p. 61–81.
4. Bateman DN, Dyson EH. Quinine toxicity. Adverse Drug React Acute Poisoning Rev. 1986;5(4):215–33.
5. Balfour AJ. The bite of Jesuits' bark. Aviation, space, and environmental medicine. Aviat Space Environ Med. 1989;60(7 Pt 2):A4–5.
6. Summers WK, Allen RE, Pitts FN. Does physostigmine reverse quinidine delirium? West J Med. 1981;135(5):411–4.
7. Nevin RL, Croft AM. Psychiatric effects of malaria and anti-malarial drugs: historical and modern perspectives. Malar J. 2016;15:332.
8. Russell PF. Plasmochin, plasmochin with quinine salts and atabrine in malaria therapy. Arch Intern Med. 1934;53(2):309–20.
9. Nevin RL. Idiosyncratic quinoline central nervous system toxicity: historical insights into the chronic neurological sequelae of mefloquine. Int J Parasitol Drugs Drug Resist. 2014;4(2):118–25.

10. Loken AC, Haymaker W. Pamaquine poisoning in man, with a clinicopathologic study of one case. Am J Trop Med Hyg. 1949;29(3):341–52.
11. Kono R. Introductory review of subacute myeolo-optico-neuropathy (SMON) and its studies done by the SMON Research Commission. Jpn J Med Sci Biol. 1975;28 Suppl(4):1–21.
12. Shiraki H. Neuropathology of subacute myelo-optico-neuropathy, "SMON". Jpn J Med Sci Biol. 1971;24(4):217–43.
13. Ricoy JR, Ortega A, Cabello A. Subacute myelo-optic neuropathy (SMON). First neuropathological report outside Japan. J Neurol Sci. 1982;53(2):241–51.
14. Schmidt IG, Schmidt LH. Neurotoxicity of the 8-aminoquinolines. I. Lesions in the Central Nervous System of the Rhesus Monkey Induced by Administration of Plasmocid. J Neuropathol Exp Neurol. 1948;7(4):368–98.
15. Schmidt IG, Schmidt LH. Neurotoxicity of the 8-aminoquinolines. II. Reactions of various experimental animals to plasmocid. J Comp Neurol. 1949;91(3):337–67.
16. Schmidt IG, Schmidt LH. Neurotoxicity of the 8-aminoquinolines. III. The effects of pentaquine, isopentaquine, primaquine, and pamaquine on the central nervous system of the rhesus monkey. J Neuropathol Exp Neurol. 1951;10(3):231–56.
17. Dow G, Bauman R, Caridha D, Cabezas M, Du F, Gomez-Lobo R, et al. Mefloquine induces dose-related neurological effects in a rat model. Antimicrob Agents Chemother. 2006;50(3):1045–53.
18. Ismail T, Mauerhofer E, Slomianka L. The hippocampal region of rats and mice after a single i.p. dose of clioquinol: loss of synaptic zinc, cell death and c-Fos induction. Neuroscience. 2008;157(3):697–707.
19. Fusetti M, Eibenstein A, Corridore V, Hueck S, Chiti-Batelli S. Mefloquine and ototoxicity: a report of 3 cases. Clin Ter. 1999;150(5):379–82.
20. Bernard P. Alterations of auditory evoked potentials during the course of chloroquine treatment. Acta Otolaryngol. 1985;99(3–4):387–92.
21. Telgt DS, van der Ven AJ, Schimmer B, Droogleever-Fortuyn H. a, Sauerwein RW. Serious psychiatric symptoms after chloroquine treatment following experimental malaria infection. Ann Pharmacother. 2005;39(3):551–4.
22. Wittes R. Adverse reactions to chloroquine and amodiaquine as used for malaria prophylaxis: a review of the literature. Can Fam Physician. 1987;33(November):2644–9.
23. West JB, Henderson AB. Plasmochin intoxication. Bull US Army Med Dep. 1944;82(November):87–99.
24. Hardgrove M, Applebaum IL. Plasmochin toxicity; analysis of 258 cases. Ann Intern Med. 1946;25:103–12.
25. Nevin RL. Limbic encephalopathy and central vestibulopathy caused by mefloquine: a case report. Travel Med Infect Dis. 2012;10(3):144–51.
26. Hart CW, Naunton RF. The ototoxicity of chloroquine phosphate. Arch Otolaryngol. 1964;80:407–12.
27. De Oliveira JAA. Antimalarial drug - quinine. In: Audiovestibular toxicity of drugs. Boca Raton: CRC Press; 1989. p. 147–63.
28. Livezey J, Oliver T, Cantilena L. Prolonged neuropsychiatric symptoms in a military service member exposed to mefloquine. Drug Saf Case Rep. 2016;3(1):7.
29. Lysack JT, Lysack CL, Kvern BL. A severe adverse reaction to mefloquine and chloroquine prophylaxis. Aust Fam Physician. 1998;27(12):1119–20.
30. Chansky PB, Werth VP. Accidental hydroxychloroquine overdose resulting in neurotoxic vestibulopathy. BMJ Case Rep. 2017;2017 https://doi.org/10.1136/bcr-2016-218786.
31. Singhi S, Singhi P, Singh M. Extrapyramidal syndrome following chloroquine therapy. Indian J Pediatr. 1979;46(373):58–60.
32. Newell HW, Lidz T. The toxicity of atabrine to the central nervous system. Am J Psychiatry. 1946;102:805–18.
33. Patchen LC, Campbell CC, Williams SB. Neurologic reactions after a therapeutic dose of mefloquine. N Engl J Med. 1989;321(20):1415–6.

34. Martin AN, Tsekes D, White WJ, Rossouw D. Chloroquine-induced bilateral anterior shoulder dislocation: a unique aetiology for a rare clinical problem. BMJ Case Reports. 2016;2016 https://doi.org/10.1136/bcr-2015-214292.
35. Ferrier TM, Schwieger AC, Eadie MJ. Delayed onset of partial epilepsy of temporal lobe origin following acute clioquinol encephalopathy. J Neurol Neurosurg Psychiatry. 1987;50(1):93–5.
36. Craige B, Eichelberger L, Jones R, Alving A, Pullman TN, Whorton CM. The toxicity of large doses of pentaquine (SN-13,276), a new antimalarial drug. J Clin Invest. 1948;27(3 Pt 2):17–24.
37. Clayman CB, Arnold J, Hockwalk RS, Yount EH, Edgcomb JH, Alving AS. Toxicity of primaquine in Caucasians. J Am Med Assoc. 1952;149(17):1563–8.
38. Saboisky JP, Butler JE, McKenzie DK, Gorman RB, Trinder JA, White DP, et al. Neural drive to human genioglossus in obstructive sleep apnoea. J Physiol. 2007;585(Pt 1):135–46.
39. Fleury Curado T, Fishbein K, Pho H, Brennick M, Dergacheva O, Sennes LU, et al. Chemogenetic stimulation of the hypoglossal neurons improves upper airway patency. Sci Rep. 2017;7:44392.
40. Ramchandren S, Gruis KL, Chervin RD, Lisabeth LD, Concannon M, Wolfe J, et al. Hypoglossal nerve conduction findings in obstructive sleep apnea. Muscle Nerve. 2010;42(2):257–61.
41. Gebhart F. Some psychoactive prescription drugs associated with violence. Drug Topics. 2011;March:37.
42. Moore TJ, Glenmullen J, Furberg CD. Prescription drugs associated with reports of violence towards others. PLoS One. 2010;5(12):e15337.
43. Mohan D, Mohandas E, Rajat R. Chloroquine psychosis: a chemical psychosis. J Natl Med Assoc. 1981;73(11):1073–6.
44. Good MI, Shader RI. Lethality and behavioral side effects of chloroquine. J Clin Psychopharmacol. 1982;2(1):40–7.
45. Jousset N, Rougé-Maillart C, Turcant A, Guilleux M, Le Bouil A, Tracqui A. Suicide by skull stab wounds: a case of drug-induced psychosis. Am J Forensic Med Pathol. 2010;31(4):378–81.
46. Nevin RL, Ritchie EC. The mefloquine intoxication syndrome: a significant potential confounder in the diagnosis and management of PTSD and other chronic deployment-related neuropsychiatric disorders. In: Posttraumatic stress disorder and related diseases in Combat Veterans. Cham: Springer International Publishing; 2015. p. 257–78.
47. Ritchie EC, Block J, Nevin RL. psychiatric side effects of mefloquine: applications to forensic psychiatry. J Am Acad Psychiatry Law. 2013;41(June):224–35.
48. Ringqvist Å, Bech P, Glenthøj B, Petersen E. Acute and long-term psychiatric side effects of mefloquine: a follow-up on Danish adverse event reports. Travel Med Infect Dis. 2015;13(1):80–8.
49. Engel GL, Romeno J, Ferris EB, Schmidt LH. Malaria Report #212: the effect of atabrine on the central nervous system. In: Malaria Rreports Volume 2. Washington, DC: Board for the Coordination of Malarial Studies; 1944.
50. Boudreau E, Schuster B, Sanchez J, Novakowski W, Johnson R, Redmond D, et al. Tolerability of prophylactic Lariam regimens. Trop Med Parasitol. 1993;44(3):257–65.
51. Nevin RL. A serious nightmare: psychiatric and neurologic adverse reactions to mefloquine are serious adverse reactions. Pharmacol Res Perspect. 2017;5(4):e00328.
52. Nevin RL, Byrd AM. Neuropsychiatric adverse reactions to mefloquine: a systematic comparison of prescribing and patient safety guidance in the US, UK, Ireland, Australia, New Zealand, and Canada. Neurology Ther. 2016;5(1):69–83.
53. European Medicines Agency. Pharmacovigilance Risk Assessment Committee (PRAC). Minutes of the meeting on 23–26 October 27. EMA/PRAC/782491/2017. 2017.
54. Eick-Cost AA, Hu Z, Rohrbeck P, Clark LL. Neuropsychiatric outcomes after mefloquine exposure among U.S. Military Service Members. Am J Trop Med hyg. 2017;96(1):159–66.
55. Wells TS, Smith TC, Smith B, Wang LZ, Hansen CJ, Reed RJ, et al. Mefloquine use and hospitalizations among US service members, 2002-2004. Am J Trop Med Hyg. 2006;74(5):744–9.
56. Nevin RL. Misclassification and bias in military studies of Mefloquine. Am J Trop Med Hyg. 2017;97(1):305.

57. Tickell-Painter M, Maayan N, Saunders R, Pace C, Sinclair D. Mefloquine for preventing malaria during travel to endemic areas. Cochrane Database Syst Rev 2017;10(10):CD006491.
58. Forrester A. Malaria and insanity. Lancet. 1920;195(5027):16–7.
59. Masters J. The Road Past Mandalay. New York: Bantam; 1979. p. 160–7.
60. Rooney D. Military Mavericks: extraordinary men of battle. London: Cassell Military Paperbacks; 1999. p. 190–1.
61. Stafford J. Unique in medical history – "Guadalcanal Neurosis" plagues invalids returning from fighting in South Pacific. Pittsburgh: The Pittsburgh Press; 1943. p. 1.
62. Greiber MF. Psychoses associated with the administration of atabrine. Am J Psychiatry. 1947;104(5):306–14.
63. Towne AN. Sicily. In: Doctor danger forward: a World War II Memoir of a Combat Medical Aidman, First Infantry Division. Jefferson: McFarland & Company, Inc; 2000. p. 61–78.
64. Couch J. The Day Gen. Patton Slapped a Soldier. The Washington Post. 1979; p. D5.
65. Dekever P. Patton's costly slap; Mishawaka soldier's claim to fame result of battle fatigue — and a general's temper. Sound Bend (Indiana) Tribune. 2002; p. F8.
66. The Science News-Letter. Better antimalarial drug. Sci News Lett. 1946;49(2):30–1.
67. Garrison PL, Hankey DD, Coker WG, Donovan WN, Jastremski B, Coatney GR, et al. Cure of Korean vivax malaria with pamaquine and primaquine. J Am Med Assoc. 1952;149(17):1562–3.
68. Archibald HC, Tuddenham RD. Persistent stress reaction after combat: a 20-year follow-up. Arch Gen Psychiatry. 1965;12:475–81.
69. Hall W, MacPhee D. Do Vietnam veterans suffer from toxic neurasthenia? Aust N Z J Psychiatry. 1985;19(1):19–29.
70. Baskett SJ, Henager J. Differentiating between post-Vietnam syndrome and preexisting psychiatric disorders. South Med J. 1983;76(8):988–90.
71. Van Putten T, Emory WH. Traumatic neuroses in Vietnam returnees. A forgotten diagnosis? Arch Gen Psychiatry. 1973;29(5):695–8.
72. Pettera RL, Johnson BM, Zimmer R. Psychiatric management of combat reactions with emphasis on a reaction unique to Vietnam. Mil Med. 1969;134(9):673–8.
73. Silver SM, Iacono CU. Factor-analytic support for DSM-III's post-traumatic stress disorder for Vietnam veterans. J Clin Psychol. 1984;40(1):5–14.
74. Varney NR, Roberts RJ, Springer JA, Connell SK, Wood PS. Neuropsychiatric sequelae of cerebral malaria in Vietnam veterans. J Nerv Ment Dis. 1997;185(11):695–703.
75. Gunderson CH, Daroff RB. Neurology in the Vietnam War. In: Tatu L, Bogousslavsky J, editors. Frontiers in neurology and neuroscience. Basel, Switzerland: Karger; 2016. p. 201–13. https://doi.org/10.1159/000442657.
76. UNDP-World Bank-WHO. Development of mefloquine as an antimalarial drug UNDP-World Bank-WHO update. Bull World Health Org. 1983;61(2):169–78.
77. Nevin RL. Rational risk-benefit decision-making in the setting of military mefloquine policy. J Parasitol Res. 2015;2015:260106.
78. McCarthy S. Malaria prevention, mefloquine neurotoxicity, neuropsychiatric illness, and risk-benefit analysis in the Australian Defence Force. J Parasitol Res. 2015;2015:287651.
79. Nevin RL. Mefloquine and posttraumatic stress disorder. In: Ritchie EC, editor. Textbook of military medicine forensic and ethical issues in military behavioral health. Washington, DC: Borden Institute; 2015. p. 277–96.
80. Magill A, Cersovsky S, DeFraites R. Special considerations for US Military Deployments. In: Brunette GW, editor. CDC health information for international travel: the Yellow Book 2012. New York: Oxford University Press; 2012. p. 561–5.
81. Nevin RL. Screening for symptomatic mefloquine exposure among veterans with chronic psychiatric symptoms. Fed Pract. 2017;34(3):12–4.
82. Grupp D, Rauber A, Fröscher W. Neuropsychiatric disturbances after malaria prophylaxis with mefloquine. Aktuelle Neurologie. 1994;21:134–6.
83. Stürchler D, Handschin J, Kaiser D, Kerr L, Mittelholzer ML, Reber R, et al. Neuropsychiatric side effects of mefloquine. New Engl J Med. 1990;322(24):1752–3.

84. Jacob RG, Furman JM, Durrant JD, Turner SM. Panic, agoraphobia, and vestibular dysfunction. Am J Psychiatry. 1996;153(4):503–12.
85. Yardley L, Britton J, Lear S, Bird J, Luxon LM. Relationship between balance system function and agoraphobic avoidance. Behav Res Ther. 1995;33(4):435–9.
86. Maxwell NM, Nevin RL, Stahl S, Block J, Shugarts S, Wu AHB, et al. Prolonged neuropsychiatric effects following management of chloroquine intoxication with psychotropic polypharmacy. Clin Case Rep. 2015;3(6):379–87.
87. Summers MR, Nevin RL. Stellate Ganglion Block in the treatment of post-traumatic stress disorder: a review of historical and recent literature. Pain Pract. 2017;17(4):546–53.
88. Gray SN. An overview of the use of neurofeedback biofeedback for the treatment of symptoms of traumatic brain injury in military and civilian populations. Med Acupunct. 2017;29(4):215–9.
89. Nevin RL, Ritchie EC. FDA Black Box, VA Red Ink? A successful service-connected disability claim for chronic neuropsychiatric adverse effects from mefloquine. Fed Pract. 2016;33(10):20–4.
90. Australian Department of Veterans' Affairs. Mefloquine Information. 2016. Available from: http://www.dva.gov.au/health-and-wellbeing/medical-conditions/mefloquine-information
91. Hookham M. MoD cash for soldier hit by malaria drug seizures MoD cash for soldier hit by Lariam drug seizures. The Sunday Times 2018 Jan 14; p. 8.
92. Tigue M. Settlement in malaria drug case. The Irish Times 2017. Available from: https://www.thetimes.co.uk/article/settlement-in-malaria-drug-case-hpknzwf0p
93. Nevin RL. Mefloquine exposure may confound associations and limit inference in military studies of posttraumatic stress disorder. Mil Med. 2017;182(11/12):1757.
94. Nevin RL. Confounding by symptomatic mefloquine exposure in military studies of post-traumatic stress disorder. Behav Med. 2018;44(2):171–2. https://doi.org/10.1080/08964289.2017.1330248.
95. Nevin RL. Re: McGuire JM. The incidence of and risk factors for emergence delirium in U.S. military combat veterans. J Perianesthesia Nurs. American Society of PeriAnesthesia Nurses. 2013;28(6):334–5.

Listening to Trauma, and Caring for the Caregiver: A Psychodynamic Reflection in the Age of Burnout

21

Joseph E. Wise

Introduction

I recently left the Army, where I had served as a psychiatrist for the past 12 years. Upon leaving, I had taken a vacation (as is necessary to care for a mind dedicated to being there for other minds); when I got home, my mailbox was full. There were multiple mailings and flyers from the American Psychiatric Association (APA) on burnout in psychiatrists. In my field, and healthcare as a whole, there has been increasing emphasis on the well-being of providers and acknowledging burnout among physicians. Though it has not been systematically studied, risk for burnout maybe especially important for healthcare systems caring for traumatized patients, such as in the Veterans Affairs (VA) or Department of Defense (DoD) medical systems.

The APA newspaper is providing a year-long column on burnout and wellness through 2017 and 2018, with additional panels at the annual meetings and online resources. Currently, it is estimated that two out of five psychiatrists currently have "burnout" [1]. These numbers have increased among physicians since an earlier 2011 assessment. Burnout in physicians also increased compared with the general US population, and related physician work–life satisfaction has decreased in the same period [17]. Burnout is simply defined as "mental exhaustion and emotional depletion" [2]. Physician burnout is a syndrome characterized by emotional exhaustion, cynicism, and decreased effectiveness at work.

APA publications list some possible causes of burnout: cumbersome electronic health records, excessive productivity quotas, limits on the time physicians can spend with each patient, loss of professional autonomy, and excessive documentation requirements. Specifically, in the current era, psychiatrists have overly

J. E. Wise (✉)
US Army, Walter Reed National Military Medical Center, Brooklyn, NY, USA

Private Practice, Brooklyn, NY, USA

demanding jobs with a high degree of responsibility but little autonomy. Additionally, psychiatrists may be at increased risk due to limited resources (for mental health services), high work demands, and patient violence.

In big healthcare systems like the VA and DoD, doctors often have limited say about workload. A leading psychiatrist, Carol Bernstein, identified lack of autonomy and relocation (from support systems) as key ingredients [1]. Military mental health providers are at increased exposure to these elements, as they are asked to move frequently and often encouraged to sacrifice their own needs for the needs of the military mission.

As a way to assess for burnout, the APA supplies the Oldenburg Burnout Inventory, which measures exhaustion and disengagement from work. It is an easily administered self-report questionnaire with 16 questions on a Likert scale. Scores above 35 are generally associated with burnout [9].

A recent meta-analysis on physician burnout describes multiple levels of intervention. The review defined two main categories of intervention: physician-directed versus organization-directed. Physician-directed interventions are often mindfulness and similar skills that focus on self-care. Organizational interventions seek to reduce stressors by adjusting workloads or schedules to improve work–life balance, or otherwise address elements of organizational culture, such as teamwork. The most effective interventions were at the organizational level, which is consistent with burnout as a workplace phenomenon [17].

Like the APA, many professional organizations have updated their mission to reduce burnout and enhance provider well-being. Unfortunately, the advice is often in the form of stress management, which can be experienced as adding insult to injury by piling more on top of the clinician and making them feel guilty for not doing something. As in the meta-analysis, what is needed is systemic organizational change.

The National Academy of Medicine has developed a graphic to display individual physician factors and systemic organization factors [16]. External (organizational/systemic) factors include sociocultural factors, regulatory and business environment, organizational factors, and learning environment. Internal physician factors include healthcare role, personal factors, and skills and abilities (Fig. 21.1).

In tension with burnout are wellness, resilience, and "grit," which is the ability to continue going despite adversity. I am not suggesting that professional life become leisurely, but we know how difficult being a provider can be, and it is hard and demanding work. (This is not just the oft-cited military aphorism that what does not kill you makes you stronger.) At the same time, burnout is a risk factor for depression, which is a key risk factor for suicide. An optimal work–life balance is what is needed. This prevents compassion fatigue and burnout, which in turn, optimizes patient outcomes. In caring for the caregiver, especially in healthcare systems dealing with trauma such as the VA and DoD, we are also helping patients get better care.

In this chapter reflection, I first establish the personal psychological work providers perform internally to deliver excellent mental healthcare. I next describe organizational dynamics that support the provider–patient pair. Lastly, I make recommendations to organizations, including VA and military healthcare, about how to establish a system, culture, and norms that facilitate such a process.

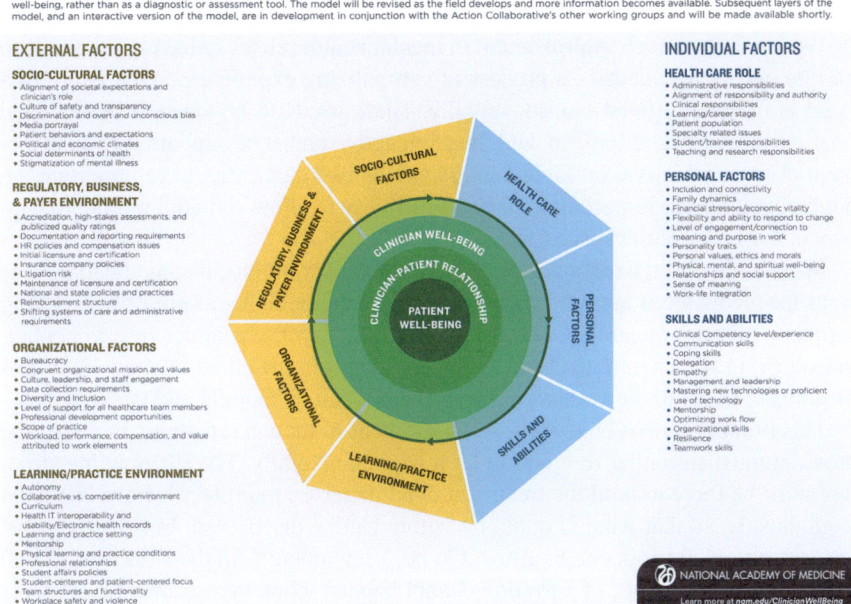

Fig. 21.1 Factors affecting clinician well-being and resilience. (Reprinted with permission from: National Academy of Medicine [16])

Individual Patient-Care: A Relational Home for a Relational Home [7]

The provider must be supported to give him- or herself over to the mind of the patients and acknowledge his or her own complicity in the process [18]. In this way, the provider is the instrument in the change process. As is said, in mental health, the doctor himself is the scalpel. Let us be honest about what we are doing: mental health! We are not lancing boils. This is not a production line!

Moreover, we are in an unusually uncontrolled situation. In the best of circumstances, we do not understand the human mind, brain, and behavior; so how can we treat mental health work as if it is like a controlled process of making widgets? It is not. It is an irreducibly unique human endeavor.

Additionally, patients, despite the best recommendations, make their own decisions, out of the provider's control. In the current era, what is emphasized is simplistic quantification of symptoms only. This has led to a quantification of all care.

Providers are scrutinized by their throughput, their "productivity," rather than quality of caring for the patient. (This is not to say that amount of resources should not be considered, but, in the current era, quality patient-care is often lost.) We cannot forget the complexities of the human situation in mental healthcare, especially in the VA and military systems, which are governmental programs and often publicly scrutinized.

We know that much improvement in mental health relates to having the space to narrate one's experiences—a process of symbolizing experience. What is not narrated is frequently lived out nonverbally. There needs to be space in the clinical relationship for this to happen, and the clinical dyad must be supported by management. As a psychiatrist, biological interventions like medications are important, no doubt, but it is also important to have a sensibility to allow something more to happen, at least a potential space for it.

Specifically, even with concrete and tangible interventions, like medications, the ways the medications are used, as in taking them or not taking as prescribed, calling for them, all have meaning (sometimes called the psychodynamics of psychopharmacology, [15]). There must be a setup—a frame—in the clinic to allow all of this meaning to come to the surface, a place where it can be thought and talked about.

This process cannot be rushed. It is a moment of mutual creativity, in which the provider must surrender to it and to let it happen naturally. The surrounding structure must be there to hold the treatment dyad. It serves to protect it from incursion from outside, so that what is going on within can be discovered. In Freud's terms, the "repetition" must occur, to allow it to be "remembered" in the working through process [10]. This work of narration cannot happen when the treatment dyad fears assault or is not otherwise supported by the organization.

In terms of theorizing, the late British psychoanalytic psychiatrist and Veteran, Wilfred Bion [5], suggests providers must supply the "container" for "thinking" and knowledge to occur. The organization "contains," so that the provider can "contain" what is coming from the patient (beta elements/emotions), and subsequently be transformed by the listening power (alpha function and reverie) of the provider [6].

A contemporary attachment-based modification of Bion's concept of containment is Peter Fonagy's ideas about mentalization. In this model, another mind is necessary to help formulate and find the mind of another. Developmentally, this would be mind of the mother (or primary attachment figure) taking in and relaying the mental state of the infant to the infant, which in turn allows the infant to get a sense of his or her own mental state [3].

Important for the mentalization model is the "marked" (meaning slightly different) quality of the attachment figure's re-presentation of the mental state of infant, such that it is not a perfect mirroring, so the infant implicitly learns interpersonal boundaries. Clinically, similar interpersonal dynamics are recreated in adult therapeutic interactions, indicating once again the implicit psychological work required for the therapist. Fonagy and colleagues have demonstrated the effectiveness of this approach in several empiric studies, especially for Borderline Personality [3]. Like Bion's ideas, the bedrock to allow mentalization to happen is the provider opening up his mind to receive the projections from the patient, which requires a very supportive organization.

As it relates to a Veterans/military population [20], the process of narration, via mentalization, is key to the treatment of PTSD [12]. The telling of the trauma narrative is not just an individual event. The telling in the dyad allows the provider to provide a "witnessing" function that is often needed for healing, especially in cases of moral injury [19]. Witnessing in many ways is narration done in the presence of another.

As it relates to PTSD treatment (the prototypic psychological illness of military and Veterans), current meta-analyses generally demonstrate narration is a key ingredient in psychotherapy. Other common factors include relaxation training, exposure (gradual contact with anxiety stimuli from the trauma, to combat avoidance), and cognitive restructuring (such as reconsidering thoughts of self-blame, guilt) [12].

The unique function of the military and Veterans in our society calls forth even more the need for witnessing. Soldiers are called to provide security for the Nation, even with the possibility of their own death. The self-sacrificial function is borne out in other ways too, such as giving up certain Constitutional rights (such as Freedom of Speech or to Assemble), which would be counter to good military order and discipline.

In the United States, those willing to make these sacrifices are very few, with current estimates at less than 1% of citizens having served in the military. The rest of the citizenry, via their government program, such as the VA, must be willing to bear witness for these Warriors. This witnessing, at the organizational and societal levels, sends the message that those who acted on behalf of society are welcomed back, including hearing what was done on behalf of society.

We know from neuroscientific work on "mirror neurons" (the brain cells and anatomical region that permit humans to get a sense of the mental state of another) that deep empathy usually entails a corresponding state in the therapist [8]. Hence, the need, even more, to account for the impact of difficult material on providers, especially those listening to trauma and combat experiences. Psychiatry is the main field of medicine in which doctor–patient relationship is not only a vehicle to assist medical interventions, but a stand-alone intervention itself, including how therapeutic alliance is the most important factor in any treatment. Once again, in our systems-of-care there needs to be deference to this fact: the therapy relationship is the lynch pin and the relationship needs to be supported as such.

Unfortunately, the thrust of psychiatric treatment has become medications only, which, as above, is a misguided attempted to medicalize and turn psychiatric activities to symptom reduction only, rather than appreciating psychotropic medication in the context of the doctor–patient relationship [13]. Unfortunately, there has also been quantification and monetarization of otherwise fundamentally human activities. Instead, it is the therapy relationship that is internalized, as the mental health provider being the "scalpel" of the treatment. All the more reason that specific efforts must be made to care for the caregiver.

Organizational Factors: Containing Projection

One of the variables in a healthcare system is clinical leadership. In military healthcare, there might be a leadership culture of acquiescing to upper managers and trying to "accomplish the mission" without questioning and without compromise. Though this style might be important on the battlefield, in healthcare it just leads to providers being used up by a system. Leaders need to be able to "manage from the middle" [11] and appropriately push back to make room for the delicate work done by mental health providers, as described above.

The possibility of leaders who might have clinical credentials but do not consider themselves clinicians first, serves to compound this problem. These leaders run the risk of being clinicians in title only, as they do not identify with the clinicians working in the clinics. These leaders are more likely to heap work upon them without attending to the intensity of the work. Sometimes worse, this type of leader might unconsciously counter-identify with the providers, which blocks authentic empathizing with the staff, and they instead become prone to pushing too much work like an assembly-line.

This can become an organizational dynamics scenario of "doer, done to" dynamics [4] rather than mutual and joint creation. Moreover, in a high-anxiety system, as is often the case in VA/DoD, the management may disavow their vulnerable parts (as a worker) and over-identify with those perceived to hold the power (the higher managers in charge). This keeps everything safe in the mind of the managers, but becomes distorted. Adding insult to injury, the disavowed vulnerable parts get projected onto the workers; this gets lived out in the organization, as there can be claims that the workers are not working enough and need to increase their productivity.

Instead, what would allow the organization to grow would be to allow the existence of a Third position (Benjamin) in which there is a mutually and co-constructed place of meeting. This space would be one of recognition of what each brings to the table and a recognition of the shared humanity of each—a place of respectful compromise between the employer and employee.

To get to such recognition of shared humanity, one needs to move from a place of anxiety and fear, which facilitates "doer and done to" dynamics, to a place of containment of anxiety. It is the metabolization of the anxiety that allows feelings of security and safety. The function of leadership is to provide for the basic frame of containment and initial metabolizing of anxiety.

With clinical leaders' attempt to improve resilience, often their intentions are in the right place, but the execution fails. Providers are accustomed to hearing lectures on "take care of yourself" from managers. Once again, the intention is in the right, but telling busy clinicians who are already overwhelmed with caring for others "to take care of yourself" can miss the mark. Instead, managers should make efforts to manage from the middle and push back on efforts to have a throughput productivity-based system. Clinical leaders need to emphasize quality and make space for providers to naturally attend to themselves, not just heaping on more, which they might rationalize with a class on self-care.

In a sense, a Third position is needed. We know from family and child development that a Third is needed to support a dyad. Prototypically, this would be the father (or second parent) supporting the dyad of mother (or primary caregiver) and child. The dyad needs its own space in order to do its own work—a good father takes up this Third position and unlike the Freudian Oedipal, this triad is supportive rather than rivalrous.

Another way to think of it would be concentric circles of support, including a circle around the dyad, another around the triadic, another around the family as a whole, another around the extended family, another around the community, another around the country, and so on. Leaders and managers working with providers need to offer support at their level.

In a perverse form of pseudo-mentalization, similar to gas-lighting, an organization presents itself as if it is interested in attending to the employee and supporting, but says so only in words, but the behavior is only to the contrary. In un-mentalized and uncontained organizational states, conditions are rife for system level scapegoating and mobbing.

Scapegoating occurs when a group locates unwanted qualities in an individual. This is often an unintentional and unconscious group process in the organization (or only partially conscious). Mobbing is similar but happens on a larger organizational scale. In our current era of digital communication, especially email, we have lost some of the face-to-face interpersonal communication feedback, which can naturally attenuate scapegoating; hence, the need for even closer attention to this process.

Recommendations: Toward Patient-Centered Care and Provider-Centered Management

Leaders and managers of clinicians should support flexibility and work choice whenever possible, as long as it does not conflict with overall mission and goals. This allows providers to have maximal professional freedom to feel invested in their work, rather than being dictated to. This facilitates self as agency and a "doer doing" [14]. This is a movement away from "doer, done to" dynamics, and recognition of the individual professional as a contributor.

The professional experience becomes co-constructed and codesigned. It becomes a dialogue rather than a set of orders. Example of professional freedom could be as simple as office setup, collaboration on work times, picking treatment team members, some control over types of clients seen, and most importantly personal control over scheduling of patients.

This allows for the organization to be supportive and not perceived, even unconsciously, as persecutory. Similar to individual dynamics, the organization must provide a secure base upon which the individual provider can do their work. It has been said that you can catch more flies with honey than vinegar, and, in the same way, organizational leaders and managers should reward clinical expertise. This includes academic presentations and publications, which should be facilitated with funding, as part of professional growth. This allows for sustaining and changing behavior through reward.

It is paramount to provide a way to care for the caregiver and psychological space to process what being a provider means. Work even in the best of circumstances is anxiety provoking. Just the mere fact of working is not easy [11], independent of any workplace dynamics.

To facilitate empathy with providers, clinic leaders should make a point of staying in clinical care. This helps them keep a perspective as a provider. It cannot just be a way of maintaining credentials. It has to be full identification as a provider. This will lead to fewer projections onto the "workers" because the leader is also a worker.

The use of ancillary staff, often under the control of the clinic leader and not the providers, must be inculcated with the maxim that they are there to facilitate care. They are not there to exist as a bureaucracy unto itself, but to assist, extend, and facilitate providers doing direct care.

This should be emphasized in all administrative meetings, in a way that respects ancillary staff. "How are we facilitating the patient care?" Hear me, this does not mean the administrative staff are there to be taken advantage of as servants, but the focus on facilitating care by the caregiver should be prominent. Part of this would be to look at evaluations and ratings from the provider staff of their administrator: "How much did X help providers caring for patients?"

With provider-centered management, providers can provide patient-centered care, and organizations can achieve better outcomes with less burned out staff. This would be consistent with leaders at military and Veterans treatment organizations exemplifying the best of military leadership in a "Follow Me" style. This would be leaders taking back their own projections and partnering with their professional employees for better outcomes. In this way, management and provider staff are working together to cocreate a relational home for the relational home.

This is very important since we know military and Veterans organizations are often resource-poor and high-need. In the position of scarcity, organizational dynamics become even more strained. Hence, the need for leaders to be ever more mindful of their own containing role in the organization.

This is about the organization taking care of providers with an openness to organizational process (often implicit or unconscious) rather than just telling providers to take care of themselves, even if the organization provides a tool kit to help the provider. Such resources are not enough and are often felt to be akin to victim-blaming.

Conclusion

Military and Veterans organizations can have difficulty conveying their needs to society at large and asking for help. This might be an artifact of the value of self-sacrifice, or, as Army people might say to themselves "suck it up and drive on". This is a leading edge of growth for these military organizations to ask for what is needed, and it is a tall order to do so because it opens up the organization to vulnerability. These organizations would have to give up their idealized invulnerability, which is so important for the Warrior culture. All the more reason for support structures for those listening to patients, many with trauma, to care for the caregiver. As outlined above, this support comes rooted in a realization of the uniqueness of the provider-patient dyad in mental health and establishing organization dynamics to support that work.

References

1. American Psychiatric Association (APA). Well being and burnout. Retrieved from https://www.psychiatry.org/psychiatrists/practice/well-being-and-burnout 11 Mar 2018.
2. APA, Psych News. Professional News. Active engagement in apa called remedy to burnout. Mark Moran. Published online: July 28, 2017.
3. Bateman A, Fonagy P. Mentalization-based treatment. Psychoanal Inq. 2013;33(6):595–613.
4. Benjamin J. Beyond doer and done to: an intersubjective view of thirdness. Psychoanal Q. 2004;73(1):5–46.
5. Bion WR. Experiences in groups and other papers. London: Tavistock; 1961.
6. Bion WR. Elements of psycho-analysis. London: Heinemann; 1963. p. 1–104.
7. Carr RB. Two war-torn soldiers: combat-related trauma through an intersubjective lens. Am J Psychother. 2013;67(2):109–33.
8. Delgado SV, Strawn JR, Pedapati EV. Contemporary psychodynamic psychotherapy for children and adolescents: integrating intersubjectivity and neuroscience. Berlin/Heidelberg: Springer; 2015.
9. Demerouti E, Bakker AB. Version September 25, 2007. The Oldenburg Burnout Inventory: A good alternative to measure burnout (and engagement). Retrieved from https://www.researchgate.net/publication/46704152_The_Oldenburg_Burnout_Inventory_A_good_alternative_to_measure_burnout_and_engagement 23 Mar 2018.
10. Freud S. Remembering, repeating and working-through (Further recommendations on the technique of psycho-analysis II). In: The Standard Edition of the Complete Psychological Works of Sigmund Freud, Volume XII (1911–1913): The Case of Schreber, Papers on Technique and Other Works. London: The Hogarth Press and the Institute of Psycho-Analysis; 1914. p. 145–56.
11. Hirshhorn L. The workplace within: psychodynamics of organizational life. Cambridge, MA: MIT Press; 1988.
12. Hoge CW. Intervention for war-related posttraumatic stress disorder: meeting veterans where they are. JAMA. 2011;306(5):549.
13. Joseph R. Doctors, revolt! New York Times. 2018:SR12.
14. Lictenberg J, Lachmann F, Fosshage J, editors. Narrative and meaning: the foundation of mind, creativity, and the psychoanalytic dialogue. London/New York: Routledge; 2017.
15. Mintz D, Belnap B. A view from Riggs: treatment resistance and patient authority—III. what is psychodynamic psychopharmacology? An approach to pharmacologic treatment resistance. J Am Acad Psychoanal Dyn Psychiatry. 2006;34(4):581–601.
16. National Academy of Medicine. Clinician well being: factors affecting clinician well-being and resilience. Retrieved from http://nam.edu/clinicianwellbeing/about/ 23 Mar 2018.
17. Shanafelt TD, Hasan O, Dyrbye LN, Sinsky C, Satele D, Sloan J, West CP. Changes in burnout and satisfaction with work-life balance in physicians and the general US working population between 2011 and 2014. Mayo Clin Proc. 2015. https://doi.org/10.1016/j.mayocp.2015.08.023.
18. Slavin MO, Kriegman D. Why the analyst needs to change: toward a theory of conflict, negotiation, and mutual influence in the therapeutic process. Psychoanal Dialogues. 1998;8(2):247–84.
19. Ullman C. Bearing witness: across the barriers in society and in the clinic. Psychoanal Dialogues. 2006;16(2):181–98.
20. Wise JE. Psychoanalytic approaches to treatment-resistant combat PTSD. In: Ritchie EC, editor. Soldiers and veterans case book. Switzerland: Springer; 2015.

Index

A

Acamprosate, AUD, 157, 158, 160, 161
   dosing and precautions, 161, 162
   side effects and monitoring
      parameters, 162
Accelerated Resolution Therapy (ART), 84
Acetaminophen, 173, 203, 219, 224
Active duty service members, 13, 52, 56, 66,
      98, 99, 104, 106, 141, 142, 144,
      146, 152, 285, 288, 289, 291
Activities of daily living (ADLs), 115, 172
Acupuncture, 80–82, 172, 192, 195, 196,
      198–200, 202
Acute alcoholic hepatitis, 146, 150
Adderall, 179, 186
ADDRESSING model, 254
Adherence, TRD, 97
Adult ADHD Self-Report Scale (ASRS-V1.1),
      187
Adzenys XR-ODT, 179
Agency of Healthcare Research and Quality
      (AHRQ), 196
Agent Orange herbicides, 306
Alcohol use, 137, 151
Alcohol use disorder (AUD)
   acamprosate, 157, 161
      dosing and precautions, 161, 162
      side effects and monitoring
         parameters, 162
   comorbidities, 139–141
   disulfiram, 157, 162
      acetaldehyde, accumulation of, 162
      dosing and precautions, 162, 163
      side effects and monitoring
         parameters, 163
   epidemiology, 137–139
   history, 136–137
   medical aspects, 145–147, 149, 150
      alcohol-related hyperglycemia, 147
      alcohol-related neurological
         symptoms, 146
      combat-related traumatic brain injury
         (TBI), 146
      FASD, 147
      hepatitis C, 146
      Korsakoff's syndrome, 146
      liver disease, 146
      liver transplants for alcoholic liver
         disease, 150
      MELD and Child-Pugh scores, 150
      Wernicke's syndrome, 146
   naltrexone, 157
      COMBINE trial, 157
      dosing and precautions, 160
      side effects and monitoring parameters,
         161
   off-label medications
      baclofen, 165
      gabapentin, 164–165
      ondansetron, 165, 166
      topiramate, 163–164
   psychosocial treatments, 141, 145
      Alcoholics Anonymous (AA), 142, 143
      CBT, 143
      community reinforcement approach
         (CRA), 144
      contingency management, 144
      education, 142
      motivational interviewing, 143
      programs, 141
      target behaviors, 144
      Twelve-Step Facilitation Therapy, 142
Alcohol Use Disorders Identification Tests
      (AUDIT) scores, 138
Alcoholics Anonymous (AA), 141–143
Alzheimer's disease, 185, 272, 275, 276
American Professional Society of ADHD and
      Related Disorders (APSARD), 187

American Psychiatric Association (APA), 23, 24, 333, 334
American psychiatry, 21–24
   American Psychiatric Association (APA), 23, 24
   Mental Hygiene, 21, 22
   public/population health interventions, 21
American Society of Addiction Medicine (ASAM) criteria, 142
Americans with Disabilities Act (ADA), 79
Amitriptyline, 202, 224
Amphetamine, 177, 179, 182, 186, 225
Animal-assisted activities, 79, 80
Animal-assisted therapy (AAT), 74, 79, 80
Anticonvulsants, 105
Anti-depressants, 181, 219
Anti-epileptics, 164, 173, 219
Anti-relapse therapy, 323
Anxiety, 77, 135, 181, 287, 318
Apathy, 184, 185
Aripiprazole, 102, 103, 118
Atomoxetine, 181, 186
Attention deficit and hyperactivity disorder (ADHD), 147
   DSM 5 criteria, 178–180
   stimulants, 178, 181–183
      amphetamine compounds, 182
      anti-depressants or anti-anxiolytics, 181
      ASRS-V1.1, 187
      atomoxetine, 181
      bupropion, 181
      CADDRA, 187
      lisdexamfetamine, 182
      long-acting formulations, 182
      long-acting stimulants, 182
      methylphenidate-based compounds, 182
      mood stabilizer, 181
      recommended work up, 186
      risk of, 185
      short-acting formulations, 182
Attention deficit disorder (ADD), 178
AUD, *see* Alcohol use disorder (AUD)
Auditory disturbances, 317
Automated Neuropsychological Assessment Metric (ANAM), 214

B
Baclofen AUD, 159
   dopaminergic neurons, inhibition of, 165
   dosing, 165
   GABA activity, modulation of, 165
Bacterial vaginosis (BV), 287

Balneotherapy, 199
Behavioral Health Interdisciplinary Program (BHIP), 37
Benzedrine, 177, 178
Benzedrine Inhaler, 177, 178
Benzodiazepines, 150, 172–174, 275, 286
Beta-blockers, 219
Biofeedback, 193, 194, 199, 202
Bipolar depression, 184
Bipolar disorder (BPD), 99, 116, 119, 120, 122, 123, 181, 266
Brief Cognitive Behavioral Therapy (BCBT), 63, 64
Buprenorphine, 173, 174
Bupropion-SR, 95, 103, 181, 225
Burnout
   definition of, 333
   depression, 334
   external physician factors, 334
   individual patient-care, 335–337
   internal physician factors, 334
   Oldenburg Burnout Inventory, 334
   organizational factors, 337–339
   organizational interventions, 334
   patient-centered care, 339, 340
   physician-directed intervention, 334
   provider-centered management, 339, 340
   resilience, 334, 335
Butalbital, 203

C
Caffeine, 203, 219, 220
Canadian ADHD Resource Alliance (CADDRA), 187
Cannabis, 85
Cannabis use disorder, 98, 260
Carbamazepine, 105, 150
Cardiovascular disease, 100, 117, 118, 269
Care management, 36, 37, 171
Carfentanil, 173, 174
Cerebral malaria, 315, 321
Chemicals of interest (COIs), 306
Child-Pugh scores, 150
Chlordiazepoxide, 150
Chloroquine, 316, 321, 323
Chronic encephalopathy, 322
Chronic heavy alcohol use, 145, 149
Chronic low back pain (cLBP), 194, 196
Chronic migraine, 202
Chronic pain, complementary and integrative health approach
   acupuncture, 195, 196
   biofeedback, 193, 194

Index

FM (see Fibromyalgia (FM))
massage therapy, 196, 197
migraines
   acupuncture, 202
   CBT, 202
   diet, 201
   feverfew, 203
   HIT, 201
   magnesium, 203
   mindfulness based approach, 202
   nutrition, 201
   riboflavin, 203
   sleep hygiene, 202
   stress management, 202
mindfulness-based interventions, 192, 193
mindfulness meditation, 192, 193
for specific pain conditions, 197
tai chi, 195
yoga, 194
Chronic stimulant, 187
Chronic traumatic encephalopathy (CTE), 222, 223, 273
Cinchonism, 315, 316
Cirrhosis, 146
Citalopram, 101, 184
Classic fetal alcohol syndrome, 146
Clinical illusion, 126
Clinical practice guidelines (CPG), 31, 38, 94, 101, 171, 174
Clinical Video Technology (CVT), 45
Clozapine, 118
Cocaine, 147, 260
Cognitive behavioral therapy (CBT), 33, 64, 76, 81, 103, 143, 183, 202
Cognitive behavioral therapy for insomnia (CBT-I), 45, 220
Cognitive changes in dementia, 184, 185
Cognitive dysfunction, 220, 319
Cognitive impairment, 274
Cognitive processing therapy (CPT), 33, 38, 76, 84, 152, 222
Cognitive Therapy for Suicide Prevention (CT-SP), 63
Collaborative Assessment and Management of Suicidality (CAMS), 65
Co-located collaborative care, 36
Combat environmental exposures, 300
Combat veteran, 10
Combined Pharmacotherapies and Behavioral Interventions (COMBINE) trial, 157
Commission on Accreditation of Rehabilitation Facilities (CARF), 215, 216

Community-based care, 30
Community reinforcement approach (CRA), 144
Comorbid bipolar disorder, 181
Comorbid substance use disorders, 182
Compassion meditation, 79
Compensated Work Therapy (CWT) programs, 129, 237
Compensated Work Therapy-Transitional Residence (CWT-TR), 41
Complementary and alternative medicine (CAM), 75, 77, 78, 82
Complementary and integrative health (CIH), 192
   acupuncture, 195, 196
   biofeedback, 193, 194
   FM (see Fibromyalgia (FM))
   massage therapy, 196, 197
   migraines
      acupuncture, 202
      CBT, 202
      diet, 201
      feverfew, 203
      HIT, 201
      magnesium, 203
      mindfulness based approach, 202
      nutrition, 201
      riboflavin, 203
      sleep hygiene, 202
      stress management, 202
   mindfulness-based interventions, 192, 193
   mindfulness meditation, 192, 193
   for specific pain conditions, 197
   tai chi, 195
   yoga, 194
Comprehensive Addiction and Recovery Act (CARA), 192
Comprehensive care, 294
Comprehensive continuum of homeless programs, 41, 42
   biopsychosocial support, 43
   Housing First programs, 42
   outreach, 43
Comprehensive suicide prevention programs, 33, 34
   Reach Vet, 34
   suicide prevention team, 35
   Suicide Risk Management Consultation Program, 35
   VCL, 34, 35
Concerta, 179
Contingency management (CM), 144
Co-occurring disorder, 97–99
Copy number variant (CNV), 122

Coup-contrecoup injury, 214
Crisis Response Plan (CRP), 61
Cyclobenzaprine, 200

D
Daytrana, 179
Dementia, 272
  Alzheimer's disease, 272
  cognitive impairment, assessment of, 274
  CTE, 273
  decision-making capacity, 274
  DLB, 272
  FTD, 272
  neurocognitive disorders, treatment of, 275, 276
  PDD, 272
  PTSD, 273, 274
  TBI, 273
Dementia with Lewy bodies (DLB), 272
Department of Defense's (DoD's), 10, 51, 52, 56, 141, 170–172, 174, 289, 333
Department of Veterans Affairs healthcare (VHA) system, 29, 30, 301
  American psychiatry, 21–24
  history, 17–21
  military culture and military, 13, 14
  WWI history for, present state and future, 24–26
Department of Veterans Affairs healthcare (VHA) system, 29, 30
Depression, 4, 100, 135, 235
  burnout, 334
  stimulants, 178, 181, 183, 184, 187
  symptoms of, 318
  TBI, 221, 222
Dexedrine, 179
Dextroamphetamine, 184, 225
Diagnostic and Statistical Manual of Mental Disorders (DSM), 178
Dialectical Behavior Therapy (DBT), 64, 65
Diazepam, 150
Diffuse axonal injury (DAI), 214
Distal stressors, 246
Disulfiram, AUD, 157, 162
  accumulation of acetaldehyde, 162
  dosing and precautions, 162, 163
  side effects and monitoring parameters, 163
Dizziness/vestibular, 220, 221
Domiciliary Care for Homeless Veterans (DCHV), 41
Domiciliary posttraumatic stress disorder (Dom PTSD), 41

Domiciliary SA (Dom SA), 41
Donepezil, 225, 275
Duloxetine, 200
Dysautonomia, 318

E
Electroconvulsive therapy (ECT), 82, 104
Electroencenphalographic biofeedback, 199
Electromyography (EMG) biofeedback, 193, 199
Emotional Freedom Technique (EFT), 84
Environmental medicine, 302
Epworth Sleepiness Scale (ESS), 187
Ethanol, 145
Evidence-based psychotherapy (EBP), 32, 33, 222
Exome sequencing (ES), 123, 124

F
Fentanyl, 169, 173
Fetal alcohol spectrum disorders (FASD), 147
Feverfew, 203
Fibromyalgia (FM), 200
  aerobic exercise, 200
  CIH evidence synthesis and clinical guidelines, 198
  acupuncture, 198, 199
  balneotherapy, 199
  biofeedback, 199
  MMT, 198
  tai chi, 198
  water-based therapies, 199
  yoga, 198
  management of, 198
  prevalence of, 197
  symptoms, 197
Focal dysfunction, 306
Frontotemporal dementia (FTD), 272

G
Gabapentin, 159, 164, 165, 260
Galantamine, 275
Garrison occupational exposures, 300
Gender-based violence, 292
Gender difference, 290, 291, 294
Gender identity, 242, 243, 245, 247–249, 252, 253, 255
Gender minority stress, 246
General Domiciliary (General Dom), 41
Generalized Anxiety Disorder scale (GAD-7), 172

Genome-wide association studies (GWAS), 121, 122, 124
Geriatric Depression Scale (GDS), 96
Geriatrics and Extended Care (GEC) services, 276
Glutamate and inhibitory γ-aminobutyric acid (GABA), 161, 164, 165
Glutamate receptor modulators, 105
Group therapy, 270
Guided imagery (GI), 198, 200
Gulf War Illness (GWI), 307

H
Hamilton Depression Scale (HAM-D), 96
Healthcare for Homeless Veterans (HCHV), 43
Health Care for Re-Entry Veterans (HCRV), 236
Health-related quality of life (HRQOL), 198, 199
Heavy alcohol use, 145, 147–149
Hepatic steatosis, 146
Hepatitis serology, 149
Hepatotoxicity, 160, 161, 163
High-intensity interval training (HIT), 201
Homeless Patient Aligned Care Teams (HPACTs), 43
Homeless veterans
  background and historical perspective, 233
  demographics of, 234
  mental illness
    female, 235
    metal health treatment challenges, 235–237
    PTSD, 234, 235
    suicidal ideation, 235
  veteran administration initiatives to end, 237, 238
Homelessness, 250, 292
Hormone therapy, 255, 259
Hospital Anxiety and Depression Scales (HADS), 96
Housing First programs, 42, 238
Hydrotherapy, 199
Hyperglycemia, 118, 119, 147
Hyperkinetic impulse disorder, 178
Hypnosis, 84, 192, 198, 199

I
Identity-related factors, 246
Implicit cognition, 59
Improvised explosive device (IED), 287
Incentive Therapy (IT), 129

Infertility, 290
Inflammation, 105
Insomnia, 33, 45, 165, 183, 187, 219, 220, 316, 319, 322
Instrumental activities of daily living (IADLs), 115
Integrated Disability Evaluation System (IDES), 14
Integrative medicine, 77
International Classification of Diseases (ICD), 24
Intimate partner violence (IPV), 285
Irritable heart syndrome, 21

J
Joint Pain Education Program (JPEP), 171, 172

K
Ketamine infusion therapies, 84, 85
Korsakoff's syndromes, 146

L
Lamotrigine, 105
Late-Onset Stress Symptomatology (LOSS), 268
Lesbian, gay, bisexual, transgender, queer or questioning (LGBTQ), 243, 251, 261
Limbic encephalopathy, symptoms of, 316
Lisdexamfetamine, 182, 184
Lithium augmentation, 103
Long-term opiate therapy (LOT), 170
Lorazepam, 150
Low-dose aspirin, 119

M
Machine learning, 58, 59
MagVenture (MagVita system), 82
Major depressive disorder (MDD), 94
  definition of, 93
  military veterans, 93
  optimizing depression treatment outcomes
    clinical practice guidelines and seminal research studies, 94
    STAR * D, 95
  treatment-resistant depression (TRD) (*see* Treatment-resistant depression (TRD))
  women veterans, 284

Major neurocognitive disorder, 271
Malaria, 319–321, 323
Mandate military treatment facilities (MTFs), 170
Mania, 177, 181, 184, 185, 188, 315, 316, 318
Mantram meditation, 79
Marijuana, 85
Massage therapy, 192, 196, 197
Medical board, 14
Medical comorbidities, 99, 100
Medication-assisted therapy (MAT), 39, 173
Meditation
　compassion meditation, 79
　mantram meditation, 79
　mental training, 78
　mindfulness meditation, 78
　self-management approach, 78
Meditative movement therapies (MMT), 198, 200
Mefloquine, 4, 300, 308, 316, 321, 323
Melatonin, 220, 225
Memantine, 275
Mental health care
　alcohol misuse, 39, 40
　BMHI, 37
　comprehensive continuum of homeless programs, 41, 42
　　biopsychosocial support, 43
　　Housing First programs, 42
　　outreach, 43
　comprehensive suicide prevention programs, 33, 34
　　Reach Vet, 34
　　suicide prevention team, 35
　　Suicide Risk Management Consultation Program, 35
　　VCL, 34, 35
　evidence-based psychotherapies, 32, 33
　mental health practices, 31–32
　mental health services, use of technology, 44, 45
　mission driven, 29
　MST, 38
　opioid use disorders, 40
　PC-MHI, 36, 37
　PTSD, 37, 38
　RRTP, 40, 41
　SUD, 39
　telemedicine, 45, 46
　tobacco use, 39
　Vet Center Program, 43, 44
Mental health disorders, 266, 282, 287
Mental health practices, 31, 32

Mental health providers, 9, 37, 51, 300, 334, 337, 338
Mental Health Residential Rehabilitation Treatment Programs (MH RRTP), 41
Mental Health Treatment Coordinator (MHTC), 32
Mental Hygiene, 21, 22
Mental illness, in homeless veterans
　female, 235
　mental health treatment challenges, 235–237
　PTSD, 234, 235
　suicidal ideation, 235
Metabolic syndrome
　medication treatment, 117, 118
　patient with SMI, 119
Metadate ER, 179
Methadone, 173, 174
Methylphenidate, 184–186, 220, 225, 276
Metoprolol, 203
Migraines
　characterization, 200
　CIH evidence synthesis and clinical guidelines
　　acupuncture, 202
　　CBT, 202
　　diet, 201
　　feverfew, 203
　　HIT, 201
　　magnesium, 203
　　mindfulness based approach, 202
　　nutrition, 201
　　riboflavin, 203
　　sleep hygiene, 202
　　stress management, 202
　integrative approach, 201
Mild to moderate depression, 101
Military Acute Concussion Evaluation (MACE) test, 214
Military competence for provider, 12
Military culture and military, 23
　administrative discharges and retirement, 12, 13
　administrative separations, 9
　disability evaluations, 14
　importance of time periods, 11–12
　military competence for provider, 12
　military health-care system, 13, 14
　time periods, importance of, 11–12
　transition issues, 14, 15
　VA health care system, 13, 14
Military environmental exposures
　challenges and pitfalls, 303, 304

clinical exposure evaluation, 305
combat environmental exposures, 300
exposure routes, 303
garrison exposures, 300
historical military exposures, 300–301
neuropsychiatric conditions, 307, 308
neuropsychiatric symptoms
    Agent Orange herbicides, 306
    Gulf War Illness, 307
occupational and environmental hazards, 302
occupational and environmental medicine, 302
potential neuropsychiatric and behavioral symptoms, 305, 306
prevalence, 301
protective mechanisms, 302
risk communication, 308, 309
significance, 301, 302
Military health-care system (MHS), 13, 14
Military sexual trauma (MST), 38, 41, 237, 284, 285
Military suicide, 53–55, 98
Mindfulness-based intervention (MBIs), 192, 193
Mindfulness-based stress reduction (MBSR), 192, 193, 202
Mindfulness meditation (MM), 78, 192, 193
Mindfulness-Oriented Recovery Enhancement (MORE) program, 192, 193
Mini-Mental State Exam (MMSE), 274
Minority stress, 256
Minority stress theory, 246
Mirtazapine, 95, 103
Mixed Vascular-Alzheimer's disease, 272
Model for End-stage Liver Disease (MELD) scores, 150
Monotherapy, 102, 196
Montreal Cognitive Assessment (MOCA), 274
Mood disorders, 172
Moral injury, 5, 6
Morphine milligram equivalents (MME), 173
Motivational interviewing (MI), 143
Moxibustion, 81, 195

N

Naltrexone, 164
    AUD, 157, 160
        COMBINE trial, 157
        dosing and precautions, 160
        side effects and monitoring parameters, 161

opiates use in military context, 173
Naproxen, 224
Narcan®, 174
Narcolepsy, 177, 178, 180, 183, 187
Narrative medicine, 270, 271
National Defense Authorization Act, 52
Neurobehavioral Symptom Inventory (NSI), 215
Neurocognitive disorders, 100
Neurodegeneration, 222, 223
Neuromodulation, 103, 104
Neuronetics (Neurostar system), 82
Neuropsychiatric quinism
    clinical features of, 317–319
    diagnosis of, 322–324
    epidemiology, 319–320
    implications, 326, 327
    management of, 325, 326
    PTSD, 322
    in recent military history, 320–321
    TBI, 322
Non-combat missions, 10
Non-steroidal anti-inflammatory drugs, 173
Nonveteran women, 282, 283
Nutrition, 105, 106, 201

O

Obstructive sleep apnea, 99, 219, 318
Occupational exposures, 300, 303, 305
Occupational medicine, 302
Occupational Safety and Health Administration (OSHA), 302
Olanzapine, 102, 118
Older veterans
    dementia (*see* Dementia)
    demographics of, 265–266
    geriatrics care in VHA, 276
    mental health disorders, 266
    military cohesion, 269, 270
        group therapy, 270
        narrative medicine and film, 270, 271
        training, 269
    military/combat-related PTSD, 267
        assessment of, 267
        course of, 267, 268
        treatment of, 268
    serious mental illness, 266
    social connectedness and health, 269
    substance use disorder, 266
Ondansetron, AUD, 165, 166
Ontario Neurotrauma Foundation guidelines, 183
Operations other than war (OOTW), 10

Opiates use in military context
   clinical practice guidelines (CPGs), 171, 174
   epidemiology, 170–171
   overdose reversal, 174
   pain management
      benzodiazepines, 173
      buprenorphine, 173
      dosage and duration of opiate prescription, 172
      ER use, 172
      evidence-based therapies, 173
      functional activity, 172
      methadone, 173
      MME, 173
      mood disorders, 172
      naltrexone, 173
      non-pharmacologic therapies, 173
      pain severity, 171
      primary care physician (PCP), 172
      referrals and visits, 172
      refractory pain, 171
      self-care, 172
      sleep, 172
      stepped care model, 171
      substance use disorder, 172
Opioid treatment program (OTP), 40
Opioid use disorders, 40, 170
Opioids, 147, 191
Oral contraceptives (OCPs), 287
Oxazepam, 150

P

Parkinson's disease (PD), 272, 275
Parkinson's disease dementia (PDD), 272
Paroxetine (Paxil), 76, 101
Patient Aligned Care Teams (PACT), 36
Persistent posttraumatic headaches, 218
Persistent stress reaction, 321
Personality disorders, 98
Pharmacotherapy, 157
Phenytoin, 105
Pneumothorax, 196
Polygenic risk scores (PRSs), 120
Polytrauma, 211, 215, 216, 221
Polytrauma Network Sites (PNSs), 215, 216
Polytrauma Point of Contacts (PPOCs), 215, 216
Polytrauma Rehabilitation Centers (PRCs), 215
Polytrauma Support Clinic Teams (PSCTs), 215, 216
Polytrauma System of Care Assessment, 215
Polytrauma Transitional Rehabilitation Programs, 215
Postconcussive syndrome, 218
Posttraumatic headaches (PTH), 218, 219
Posttraumatic stress disorder (PTSD), 3, 25, 53, 94, 97, 99, 106, 139, 152, 183, 185, 201, 234, 321
   arousal, 74
   avoidance, 74
   burnout, 337
   comorbidity, 75
   DSM-5 criteria, 74
   Gulf War Illness (GWI), 307
   heterogeneous group, 73
   negative cognitions and mood, 74
   neuropsychiatric quinism, 322
   older veterans, dementia, 273, 274
   older veterans, military/combat-related, 267
      assessment of, 267
      course of, 267, 268
      treatment of, 268
   re-experiencing, 74
   SGM veterans, 246, 249, 250
   symptoms, 116
   TBI, 222
   three buckets concept (*see* Three buckets models)
   VA mental health care, 37, 38
   women veterans, 284–286, 288, 289, 291, 292
Posttraumatic Stress Disorder Residential Rehabilitation Treatment Program (PTSD-RRTP), 41
Post-Vietnam syndrome, 321
Prazosin (Minipress), 76, 268
Pregabalin, 200
Pregnant servicewomen, 288
Prescription drug monitoring programs (PDMPs), 170
Primaquine, 321, 323
Primary Care-Mental-Health Integration (PC-MHI), 36, 37
Primary care physician (PCP), 172
Procentra, 179
Prolonged Exposure (PE), 38
Propranolol, 77, 224
Proximal stressors, 246
Pseudo-mentalization, 339
Psychodynamics of psychopharmacology, 336
Psychoeducation, 128, 221
Psychosis, 236
   genetics and boundaries of, 119, 120

Index 351

in military, 114
symptoms of, 319
Psychosocial Rehabilitation and Recovery Centers (PRRC), 127, 128
Psychosocial Residential Rehabilitation Treatment Programs (PRRTP), 41
Psychostimulants
  in pregnancy, risk of, 185, 186
  recommended medical work up, 186
Psychotherapy, 37, 64, 75–77, 103, 200, 221, 250, 261, 284, 337
Psychotic disorders, 325
  active duty military epidemiology and prevalence, 114, 115
  antipsychotic medication, monitoring, 118, 119
  differential diagnosis, 124, 125
  improving transition of care, 127
  innovations in treatments, 127, 128
  metabolic syndrome
    medication treatment, 117, 118
    patient with SMI, 119
  mortaliy of, 117
  prevalence, 115, 116
  psychosis
    genetics and boundaries of, 119, 120
    in military, 114
  psychotic illness, heritability of, 121
  schizophrenia
    CNV, 122
    genetics and clinical heterogeneity of, 120, 121
    GWAS, 121, 122
    minimization of symptoms, 117
    public health impact and disability, 116
    rare SNV, 122, 123
    symptoms, 116
    WGS, 123, 124
  serious mental illness (SMI), stigma of, 125–127
  SMITREC data, 115
  TSES, 129
    sheltered workshops, 129
    Supported Employment (SE), 129
    TWE, 129
    VCT, 129
Psychotic illness, heritability of, 121
Psychotropic Drug Safety Initiative (PDSI), 32
PTSD, *see* Posttraumatic stress disorder (PTSD)
Pyridostigmide bromide, 300
Pyridostigmine bromide, 307

Q
Quetiapine (Seroquel), 76, 102
Quick Inventory of Depressive Symptomatology-Self-Report (QIDS SR), 96
Quillichew ER (chewable), 179
Quinine, 315, 320
Quinolines, 318, 320, 322, 323, 326, 327
  encephalopathy, 318
  limbic encephalopathy, symptoms of, 316
  pathophysiology, 316–317
  signs and symptoms, 316

R
Readjustment Counseling Services (Vet Center Program), 43, 44
Recovery Engagement and Coordination for Health (Reach Vet), 34
Refractory pain, 171
Reproductive mental health issues, 287
Residential Rehabilitation Treatment Programs (RRTP), 40, 41, 43
Resilience, 246, 251, 252, 334, 335
Riboflavin, 203, 204
Risk communication
  characterization of, 308
  definition, 308
  principles of, 309
Risperidone (Risperdal), 76, 102
Ritalin, 178, 179, 186
Rivastigmine, 275

S
Safety Planning Intervention (SPI), 60
Schizophrenia (SCZ), 113–115, 266
  CNV, 122
  genetics and clinical heterogeneity of, 120, 121
  GWAS, 120–122
  minimization of symptoms, 117
  polygenic score of, 120
  public health impact and disability, 116
  rare SNV, 122, 123
  symptoms, 116
  WGS, 123, 124
Second-generation antipsychotics, 102
Selective serotonin reuptake inhibitors (SSRI), 76, 81, 100, 101, 183, 184, 222, 268, 275, 276
Self-Rating Depression Scale (SDS), 96
Sequenced Treatment Alternatives to Relieve Depression study (STAR * D), 95, 96, 101, 102

Serious mental illness (SMI), 117, 266
  definition of, 115
  metabolic syndrome in patient, 119
  stigma of, 125
    provider stigma, 125
    public stigma, 125–127
    self-stigma, 125, 126
Serious Mental Illness Treatment Resource and Evaluation Center (SMITREC), 115
Serotonin and norepinephrine reuptake inhibitors (SNRIs), 76, 276
Sertraline (Zoloft), 76, 101, 184, 224
Severe depression, 102
Sexual and gender minority (SGM) veterans, 241, 245
  affirming clinical practice with, 255, 256
  barriers to healthcare, 248, 249
  culturally responsive assessment and treatment, 253–255
  definition, 243
  diverse population among
    aging, 249
    of color, 250
    homeless, 250
    in rural areas, 250
  gender identity, 243
  health disparities and social determinants of health, 246, 247
  identity, pronouns and sexual risk, 252, 253
  integrated psychosocial assessments, 256, 257
  lesbian, gay and bisexual, 243
  policy and legislation, impact of, 247, 248
  provider-patient interactions, 244
  resilience factors, 251, 252
  sexual identity, 243, 245
  sexual minority men, 242
  sexual minority women, 242
  transgender care and resources, 257–261
  transgender individuals, 242
  VHA, 242, 243
Sexual identity, 242, 243, 245, 247, 248, 253
Sexual orientation identity, 243
Sexually transmitted infections (STIs), 287
Sildenafil (Viagra), 76
Single nucleotide variants (SNV's), 122, 123
Sleep disturbances, 219, 220
Sleep issues, 99
SMI, *see* Serious mental illness (SMI)
Stellate ganglion block (SGB), 84, 85
Stepped care model, 171
Stimulants
  in ADHD, 181–183
  in apathy, 184, 185
  chronic stimulant use, ongoing monitoring for, 187
  clinical indication for, 180, 181
  cognitive changes in dementia, 184, 185
  definition, 177
  in depression, 184
  history, 177–180
  mechanism of action, 185
  psychostimulants
    in pregnancy, risk of, 185, 186
    recommended medical work up, 186, 187
  risk of, 185
  in TBI, 183, 184
Strategic Analytics for Improvement and Learning (SAIL), 31
Stress management, 202
Substance Abuse Residential Rehabilitation Treatment Program (SARRTP), 41
Substance use disorder (SUD), 39, 139–141, 143, 145, 146, 149, 150, 152, 172, 173, 181, 236, 286
  CBT, 143
  CM, 144
  older veterans, 266
  treatment, 141
  women veterans, 285, 286
Suicidal ideation, 53, 61–66, 101, 136, 139, 150, 161, 162, 219, 235, 261, 267, 273, 276, 318
Suicide Assessment and Follow-up Engagement–Veteran Emergency Treatment (SAFE VET), 61, 62
Suicide prevention, 4, 5, 51, 52, 286
  annual suicide rates, 53
  combat, 53
  DoD Task Force, 52
  identified military prevention initiatives, 55
  RAND corporation, 54
  Task Force, 56
  US Air Force, 54
  veteran-specific, 56, 57
    evidence-based suicide-prevention, 57
    identification, 57–59
Suicide Prevention Application Network (SPAN), 35
Suicide Prevention Coordinators (SPC), 35
Suicide prevention team, 35
Suicide Risk Management Consultation Program, 35
Suicide Status Form (SSF), 65
Sumatriptan, 224
Supermarket syndrome, 325
Supported Employment (SE), 129

Supportive Services for Veteran Families
    (SSVF) program, 238

T
Tafenoquine, 316, 321, 323
Tai chi, 192, 195, 198
Team-based care, 30
Telemental Health technology, 45
Temporal lobe seizure disorder, 325
Theoretical maximum heart rate (TMHR), 215
Therapeutic and supported employment
    services (TSES) program, 129
  sheltered workshops, 129
  Supported Employment (SE), 129
  TWE, 129
  VCT, 129
Three buckets models
  acupuncture, 80–82
  animal-assisted activities, 79, 80
  animal-assisted therapy, 80
  ART, 84
  complementary and aternative medicine/
      integrative medicine, 77
  EFT, 84
  everything else, 75
  evidence-based therapies, 75
  ketamine infusion therapies, 84, 85
  medications, 76
  meditation
    compassion meditation, 79
    mantram meditation, 79
    mental training, 78
    mindfulness meditation, 78
    self-management approach, 78
  psychotherapies, 76, 77
  stellate ganglion block, 84, 85
  TMS, 82
  yoga and exercise therapy, 82, 83
Tobacco use, 39
Tobacco use disorder, 39, 98, 247
Tobacco-related disorders, 39
Topiramate, AUD, 105, 224
  dising and side effects, 164
  GABAergic transmission, enhancing, 163
  inhibiting gluametergic transmission, 163
  mechanism of action, 163
Toxic neurasthenia syndrome, 321
Toxic shock syndrome (TSS), 287
Transcranial magnetic stimulation (TMS), 82, 104
Transgender care and resources, 257–261
Transgender veterans, 241, 243, 247, 248, 250, 251, 257–259, 261
Transition Assistance Program (TAP), 14

Transitional Work Experience (TWE), 129
Transmagnetic cranial stimulation (TMS), 75
Tranylcypromine, 95, 103
Trauma, 334, 336, 337, 340
Traumatic brain injuries (TBI), 25, 180, 273
  assessment of, VA, 217
  definitions of, 212
  epidemiology with causes, blast wave
      physics, 213, 214
  evaluation and management of common
      symptoms
    cognitive impairments, 220
    depression, 221, 222
    dizziness/vestibular, 220, 221
    PTH, 218, 219
    sleep disturbances, 219, 220
  mild
    initial in-theater evaluation and
        management, 214–216
    pharmacology, 223–225
  in military veterans, 211
  neurodegeneration/CTE in veterans, 222, 223
  neuropsychiatric quinism, 322
  postconcussive syndrome, 218
  PTSD, 222
  severity grading, 212
  stimulants, 183, 184
Trazodone, 225
Treatment-refractory depression (TRD), 184
Treatment-resistant depression (TRD)
  adherence, 97
  clinical vignette, 101
  co-occurring disorder, 97–99
  factors, 96
  management of, 102
    anticonvulsants, 105
    exercise and nutrition, 105, 106
    glutamate receptor modulators, 105
    inflammation, 105
    integrated care, 102
    medication, 102, 103
    neuromodulation, 103, 104
    prevention, 101
    psychotherapy, 103
    TMS, 104
  measurement based care, 96–97
  medical comorbidities, 99, 100
  neurocognitive disorders, 100
  nonpharmacologic options, 104
  personalized level of care, 106
  sleep issues, 99
  treatment dose and duration, 100, 101
TRICARE, 13, 14, 25, 288
Triiodothyronine (T3), 95, 103

U

Unhealthy alcohol use, 137, 139–141
United States Armed Forces, 10
United States Coast Guard (USCG), 10
Urinary tract infections (UTIs), 287

V

Venlafaxine, 224
Venlafaxine-XR, 95, 102, 222, 224
Vet Center Program, 43, 44
Veteran Benefits Administration (VBA), 14
Veteran Health Administration (VHA), 56–58, 66
Veteran population
  clinical issues, 4
  cultural competence, 4
  Department of Veterans Affairs (VA), 4
  mefloquine, 4
  military culture, 4
  moral injury, 5, 6
  service member, 3, 4
  stigma vs fitness for duty, 6
  themes, 5
Veterans Benefit Administration (VBA), 14
Veterans Construction Team (VCT), 129
Veterans Crisis Line (VCL), 34, 35, 59, 60
Veterans Health Administration (VHA), 12, 13, 115, 170–172, 174, 192, 242, 243, 247–249, 258, 276, 282
Veterans Health Information System and Technology Architecture (VISTA) system, 44
Veterans Integrated Service Networks (VISNs), 29, 40, 216
Veterans Justice Outreach Program (VJO), 43
Veteran-specific suicide prevention, 56, 57
  barriers to treatment, 66
  Brief Cognitive Behavioral Therapy (BCBT), 63, 64
  CAMS, 65
  clinical treatment, 62, 63
  crisis intervention
    Crisis Hotline and On-Line Chat, 59, 60
    Crisis Response Plan (CRP), 61
    SAFE VET, 61, 62
    safety planning, 60
  CT-SP, 63
  DBT, 64, 65
  evidence-based, 57
  identification, 57
  implicit cognition, 59
  machine learning, 58, 59
Vitamin B2, 203
Vyvanse, 179

W

Water-based therapies, 199, 200
Wernicke's syndrome, 146
Whole-genome sequencing (WGS), 123, 124
Women veterans, 247
  amputation, 290, 291
  biological considerations, 286, 287
  biological function in deployment, 287
  breastfeeding, 289
  demographics of, 282–283
  gender-sensitive mental healthcare, 292, 293
    childcare, 294
    effect of driving distance on access to care, 293
    eligibility requirements and scope of services, 293
    integrated care, acceptability of, 294
    mental health stigma, 294
    outreach, effectiveness of, 293
  infertility, 290
  mental healthcare needs, 283
  MST, 284, 285
  pregnancy, 287–289
  prosthetic devices, 290, 291
  PTSD and MDD, 284
  reproductive health, 295
  social and cultural factors
    homelessness, 292
    marriage, 291, 292
  SUD, 285, 286
  suicide, 286
World Professional Association for Transgender Health's (WPATH's) Standards of Care, 258, 259

Y

Yoga, 82, 83, 192, 194, 198, 202

Z

Z-drugs, 220
Zero tolerance policy for illicit drug use, 137
Ziprasidone, 118
Zolpidem, 225

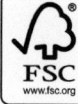

MIX
Papier aus verantwortungsvollen Quellen
Paper from responsible sources
FSC® C105338

If you have any concerns about our products,
you can contact us on
ProductSafety@springernature.com

In case Publisher is established outside the EU,
the EU authorized representative is:
**Springer Nature Customer Service Center GmbH
Europaplatz 3, 69115 Heidelberg, Germany**

Printed by Libri Plureos GmbH
in Hamburg, Germany